Imaging of Alimentary Tract Perforation

Luigia Romano • Antonio Pinto
Editors

Imaging of Alimentary Tract Perforation

Springer

Editors
Luigia Romano
Department of Radiology
"A. Cardarelli" Hospital
Naples
Italy

Antonio Pinto
Department of Radiology
"A. Cardarelli" Hospital
Naples
Italy

ISBN 978-3-319-08191-5 ISBN 978-3-319-08192-2 (eBook)
DOI 10.1007/978-3-319-08192-2
Springer Cham Heidelberg New York Dordrecht London

Library of Congress Control Number: 2014951824

Printed on acid-free paper

Springer is part of Springer Science+Business Media (www.springer.com)

Preface

Alimentary tract perforations represent an emergency and life-threatening condition requiring prompt diagnosis and surgical treatment in most cases. Diagnosis depends on clinical suspicion: The clinical symptoms of free perforation are associated with the underlying cause of the perforation, and the clinical presentations of patients with a perforated viscus are quite variable. Imaging examinations play an important role in order to determine the correct diagnosis and ensure an appropriate treatment to the patient.

The purpose of this book is to illustrate and discuss causes and imaging features related to cases of alimentary tract perforation from the esophagus to the rectum, occurring in radiology practice. Signs of a pneumoperitoneum on plain abdominal film, on abdominal ultrasonography, and on Multi-detector row Computed Tomography are extensively illustrated; moreover, the role of plain abdominal film, abdominal ultrasonography, and Multi-detector row Computed Tomography are addressed. In addition, imaging of gastrointestinal tract perforation in the pediatric patient, in the elderly patient, and in the oncological patient are presented.

We hope that this book will provide important information to Residents in Radiology, Radiologists, and Physicians daily involved in the Emergency Department in the management of patients with suspected alimentary tract perforation.

Naples, Italy — Luigia Romano
Naples, Italy — Antonio Pinto
September 2014

Contents

Diagnostic Approach to Alimentary Tract Perforations

1

Francesca Iacobellis, Daniela Berritto, and Roberto Grassi

1.1 Introduction

Alimentary tract perforations represent an emergency and life-threatening condition requiring prompt diagnosis and surgical treatment [1].

Diagnosis depends on clinical suspicion and especially on imaging examinations that allow us to define the presence, the level, and cause of perforation [2].

These details are essential to define an appropriate management and the surgical approach.

Bowel perforation can be spontaneous, traumatic, or iatrogenic in etiology and can occur both in the upper and lower intestines [1–4].

The clinical diagnosis, particularly in the early stage, is difficult as the symptoms may be variable and nonspecific [5].

The standard treatment is prompt surgery, and if the diagnosis and treatment are delayed, the patient morbidity (sepsis and multiorgan failure) results in 75 % and mortality in 30 % [1, 6]. The imaging plays an important role to determine the diagnosis and ensure an appropriate treatment to these patients.

Plain abdominal X-ray still remains the most frequently requested imaging examination in the emergency department even if its role is currently debated; ultrasound (US) and computed tomography (CT) traditionally have been the dominant cross-sectional imaging modalities for evaluating acute thoracic, abdominal, and pelvic conditions; magnetic resonance (MR) is not yet widely used in diagnostic work-up of patients with acute abdominal pain, but can be useful in the differential diagnosis of acute abdomen in specific patients (pregnancy, pediatric patients) [7].

1.2 Clinical Symptoms and Etiology

The *clinical symptoms* are related to the cause and the site of the perforation, so the clinical presentation is variable. Nevertheless, an "acute abdomen" is usually present [7].

Other clinical manifestations include nausea, vomiting, fever, localized abscess formation, inflammatory mass, fistulas, and gastrointestinal hemorrhage. Rare complications secondary to perforation are septicemia, portal pyemia or pyogenic abscess, enterovascular fistulas, and even endocarditis.

Usually the pain is initially localized in the suggested site of origin but may move to a different site by the time the patient is examined to culminate – if not promptly treated – in diffuse, poorly localized abdominal pain [8].

The *etiology* spontaneous, traumatic, or iatrogenic is suggested by the clinical history.

F. Iacobellis, MD (✉) • D. Berritto • R. Grassi
Department of Radiology, Second University of Naples, Piazza Miraglia 2, Naples, 80138, Italy
e-mail: francesca.iacobellis@libero.it; berritto.daniela@gmail.com; roberto.grassi@unina2.it

L. Romano, A. Pinto (eds.), *Imaging of Alimentary Tract Perforation*,
DOI 10.1007/978-3-319-08192-2_1,

The esophageal perforation is more commonly iatrogenic, caused by endoscopic procedures – dilatation for strictures and achalasia [9] – or by surgical complications [10].

The traumatic etiology, which is less common, can result from penetrating sharp injuries or from gunshot [11].

A spontaneous rupture – 15 % of cases – can be due to intensive vomiting or Boerhaave syndrome [12, 13].

Other causes are represented by foreign body ingestion and esophageal tumors [1, 14, 15].

Peptic ulcers are the main cause of gastroduodenal perforation, followed by necrotic or ulcerated malignancies, blunt or penetrating trauma, and iatrogenic causes [1, 2, 8].

The main etiologies for small bowel perforation are inflammatory, infectious, and ischemic conditions, small bowel diverticulitis, mechanical obstruction, trauma, malignancy, iatrogenic causes, and foreign bodies [1, 16].

Colon and rectum perforations are related to tumors, inflammatory pathologies, iatrogenic causes, and foreign bodies [1, 15, 17].

1.3 Imaging

1.3.1 Plain Abdominal X-Ray

Even if in the American College of Radiology (ACR) appropriateness criteria [18] the enhanced CT of the abdomen and pelvis is considered the most appropriate examination for patients with fever, non-localized abdominal pain, and no recent surgery, plain radiography remains the most frequently requested examination performed as initial imaging in the assessment of patients who present with acute abdominal pain to the emergency department [7, 19, 20, 21, 22]. Plain abdominal radiograph is widely available and can be easily performed. It can exclude major illness such as bowel obstruction and perforated viscus [7]. However, it should be considered that plain abdominal film exposes the patient to 35 times the radiation dose of a chest X-ray (0.7 mSv) and then its use must be carefully assessed anyway [7].

In the available literature, it is emphasized that plain abdominal X-ray should not be used as a routine investigation in patients with undifferentiated abdominal pain, unless there is clinical suspicion of bowel obstruction [20].

The detection of free intraperitoneal gas on the plain X-ray usually indicates bowel perforation. The reported specificity of plain X-ray for pneumoperitoneum ranges from 50 to 70 % according to some AA [8] and from 53 to 89.2 % according to other AA [23], but the site of perforation is almost never elucidated. It is also reported that pneumoperitoneum or retroperitoneum may be not be detected in up to 49 % of patients [24].

Experimental studies [25] have shown that as little as 1 ml of gas can be detected below the right hemidiaphragm on properly exposed erect chest radiographs [5].

Signs of esophageal perforation can be seen on posteroanterior and lateral plain chest radiographs. Such signs are indirect findings and include pleural effusion, pneumomediastinum, subcutaneous emphysema, hydrothorax, pneumothorax, and collapse of the lung. If a water-soluble contrast medium is administered, it will reveal a contrast leak in most cases of esophageal perforation [13]; water-soluble contrast should be used instead of barium contrast to avoid barium-related inflammation of mediastinum if there is perforation. If the initial contrast swallowing study is negative, imaging should be repeated after 4–6 h if the clinical suspicion remains [12].

Plain abdominal radiograph is usually performed in upright and supine decubitus; in addition, upright chest films and/or left lateral decubitus abdominal films can also be used (in the detection of small amounts of free air that may be interposed between the free edge of the liver and the lateral wall of the peritoneal cavity). In critically ill patients, the supine decubitus is preferred, with anteroposterior and lateral views of the abdomen and anteroposterior view of the thorax [19].

Supine abdominal radiograph allows detection of moderate or large amounts of free intraperitoneal air, but is insensitive in detecting small amounts of free intraperitoneal air; upright abdominal radiographs are better than supine in showing pneumoperitoneum; however, because the X-ray beam is centered on the mid-abdomen, and the exposure is high, small amounts of free air can be obscured. Left lateral decubitus radiograph of the abdomen can show small amounts of free air if the heavy exposure does not compromise the detection. On upright posteroanterior chest radiograph, the central X-ray beam penetrates air in the superior portion of the subdiaphragmatic recess along its long axis and usually does not burn out small amount of free air. The upright lateral chest radiograph is more sensitive than the posteroanterior chest radiograph in detecting small amounts of pneumoperitoneum as the long axis of X-ray beam can show small air collection that may remain trapped anterior to the liver [5, 8, 19, 26, 27].

Several signs of intraperitoneal free air, direct finding of perforation, were described: in the upright thoracic film, the air in the subdiaphragmatic regions and, on the supine abdominal films, the outlining of various peritoneal reflections between the mesenteric folds.

In other cases, indirect sign of perforation could be visible such as translucent triangle, lucent liver, perihepatic gas collections, Rigler's sign, and cupola sign, and football and cap of Doge signs can be detected [19, 28–30].

Some AA retain that in the presence of clinical signs of acute abdominal pathology, pneumoperitoneum identified on plain X-ray obviates the need for further imaging and constitutes an indication for laparotomy [31, 32] even if in the majority of cases, further imaging is useful to clarify the site and the etiology of perforation.

1.3.2 US

Abdominal US examination is particularly indicated in patients in whom radiation should be avoided, as well as children and pregnant woman, being a noninvasive, rapid diagnostic, wide available and low-cost method [33]. It represents an optimal first-line imaging method in emergency department [7, 34].

Some AA reports that US could provide useful information in 56 % of patients with acute abdominal pain, and in another study it is reported that US allows diagnosing or confirming one of the possible differential diagnosis or provides information in 65 % of patients [7].

Diagnostic value of plain X-ray (erect chest film) compared versus US in the detection of pneumoperitoneum in patients with suspected bowel perforation showed US sensitivity of 92 % (versus 78 % of plain abdominal film), a negative predictive value of 39 % (versus 20 %), and specificity of 53 % (versus 53 %) concluding that ultrasound is more sensitive than plain radiography in the diagnosis of pneumoperitoneum [23], even if establishing the cause and location of the perforation is difficult with US [7].

Other AA detected a lower sensitivity for the US if compared with radiography (76 % versus 92 %, respectively), suggesting the use of US only in selected cases [35].

The US examination is conducted with patient in supine position, preferably with the thorax slightly elevated (10–20°) [36]; the linear array transducers (10–12 MHz) are more sensitive than convex transducers(2–5 MHz) in the detection of intraperitoneal free air for their size and shape and for their resolution [36].

US signs of free intraperitoneal air are represented by echogenic lines or spots with comet-tail reverberation artifacts adjacent to the abdominal wall. These signs are best detected in the prehepatic space using linear probes.

If a pneumoretroperitoneum is present, the detection of the air around the duodenum and the head of the pancreas and especially ventral to the great abdominal vessel lead to the picture of "vanishing" vessels [37].

Indirect signs of bowel wall perforation detectable at US are represented by intraperitoneal free fluid and/or reduced intestinal peristalsis [36].

US main limits are represented by the operator dependence and by the poor cooperation of some patients due to the abdominal pain; obese patients and patients with subcutaneous emphysema are difficult to scan too [36]. Furthermore, US has low sensitivity in the detection of retropneumoperitoneum; so, it should not be considered definitive in excluding a pneumoperitoneum [7, 35].

1.3.3 Multidetector CT (MDCT)

MDCT is considered most valuable imaging technique for identifying the presence, site, and cause of alimentary tract perforations [2, 3, 38, 41, 42] and some AA consider CT as the primary technique for the diagnosis of acute abdominal pain, except in patients clinically suspected for acute cholecystitis – in which US represents the technique of choice [7].

MDCT is superior to single helical CT allowing a rapid execution of the diagnostic exam also in patients with difficulties to perform prolonged breath holds; the thinner collimation may improve the visualization of CT findings suggestive of colonic perforation too [8].

The CT examination in emergency setting is performed with the administration of intravenous (iv) contrast medium and includes the thorax if an esophageal perforation is suspected and/or the entire abdomen, from the dome of the diaphragm to the pelvic floor; the administration of iv contrast medium facilitates a good accuracy and a high level of diagnostic confidence [7].

The range of sensitivity and specificity of MDCT for gastrointestinal perforation is between 80 and 100 % [43]. The CT diagnosis of alimentary tract perforation is based on direct CT findings, such as discontinuity of the bowel wall and the presence of extraluminal air and on indirect CT findings, such as bowel wall thickening, abnormal bowel wall enhancement, abscess, and inflammatory mass adjacent to the bowel [40].

Bowel wall discontinuity is a pathognomonic image finding for bowel perforation and can predict the perforation site before surgery, the CT detection rate of bowel wall discontinuity was low. A previous study with single spiral CT reported 0–8 % detection rate of bowel wall discontinuity on initial CT scans [44, 45]. The relatively infrequent detection of this finding is partly due to the small size of the lesion [39].

Free air was detected using CT in only approximately 50 % of the cases of small bowel perforation [29, 40, 42].

The detection of *extraluminal air* bubbles, focal defects of bowel wall, and segmental bowel wall thickening allows us to correctly identify the site of perforation [38] even if CT detection of pathognomonic image findings of bowel perforation is uncommon [39, 44, 47]; CT multiplanar reconstruction is very helpful in the identification of alimentary tract perforations, and the lung window setting could be used to assist in detection of free gas [7, 42].

In patients with esophageal perforation, a collection of air or fluid in the mediastinum, pleural effusions, pneumocardium, and pneumoperitoneum are important diagnostic findings. The site and the degree of perforation may be easier to judge by CT than by plain chest X-ray [12].

Free air located around the liver and stomach is suggestive for a gastroduodenal perforation. If free air is detected predominantly in the pelvis and supramesocolic and inframesocolic regions, a perforation of the colon or appendix is more likely [38].

Extraluminal intra- or retroperitoneal air can occur without GI tract perforation too. Various causes were described, such as mechanical ventilation and pulmonary barotraumas, peritoneal lavage performed prior to CT, pneumothorax, chest injury, and entry of air via the female genital tract [39].

MDCT accuracy in predicting the site of perforation may rise to 86 % [5, 38], and the additional information gained may be useful in either directing or avoiding surgery in patients with pneumoperitoneum on plain X-ray.

In the last years, with the increased use of CT, the diagnosis of contained perforations is more common, and it is possible to consider a conservative treatment [7]. The monitoring of selected patients with alimentary tract perforations with repeated CT studies helps in nonoperative management. However, in patients with peritonitis, the CT does not significantly alter the management or the surgical approach [31].

A further specific finding of alimentary tract perforations is the *extraluminal leakage* of oral contrast medium that is also considered diagnostic for bowel perforation, so it could be useful to opacify the entire alimentary tract with a sufficient quantity of contrast agent especially when an upper intestinal tract perforation is suspected [8] even if the overall detection rate of extraluminal oral contrast material reported is lower than 31 % [39, 44, 46]. However, it should be considered that patients may not be able to cooperate if they complain for pain, nausea, or vomiting and if there is a paralytic ileus, the peristalsis is impaired, and oral contrast medium cannot go through the entire bowel; in these cases, the use of oral contrast medium is questionable [3].

Free peritoneal fluid can be detected in alimentary tract perforation, but there was no consensus regarding the diagnostic value of free peritoneal fluid. It has been considered a sign of bowel or mesenteric injury and a useful indication for exploratory laparotomy [48].

The disadvantage of CT is represented by the exposure to ionizing radiation. The effective radiation dose for abdominal CT is approximately 10 mSv, and the radiation exposure-related risks should be weighed against the direct diagnostic benefit and related to the lifetime cancer risk, especially in young patients [21].

1.3.4 Magnetic Resonance

MR can be used in the diagnostic work-up of patients with acute abdominal pain, especially in pediatric patients and in pregnant woman. It has demonstrated promising accuracy for the assessment and diagnosis of appendicitis, diverticulitis, and intestinal infarctions [49] and is more accurate than CT for the diagnosis of acute cholecystitis and the detection of common bile duct stones [50]. Therefore, MR has a role in the differential diagnosis of acute abdomen only in special conditions.

The major advantage of MR imaging is the lack of ionizing radiation and the possibility to avoid the use of intravenous contrast medium associated with the high intrinsic contrast resolution. With high-speed techniques, MR imaging protocols for patients with acute abdominal pain shorter than 15 minutes were introduced [7, 50].

The limitations are represented by its high cost, the lack of full-time availability at many hospitals, claustrophobia, or the incompatibility of MR imaging systems and pacemakers or the equipment used for intensive care and monitoring of patient status [7, 50].

References

1. Del Gaizo AJ, Lall C, Allen BC, Leyendecker JR (2014) From esophagus to rectum: a comprehensive review of alimentary tract perforations at computed tomography. Abdom Imaging
2. Furukawa A, Sakoda M, Yamasaki M, Kono N, Tanaka T, Nitta N, Kanasaki S, Imoto K, Takahashi M, Murata K, Sakamoto T, Tani T (2005) Gastrointestinal tract perforation: CT diagnosis of presence, site, and cause. Abdom Imaging 30(5):524–534
3. Maniatis V, Chryssikopoulos H, Roussakis A, Kalamara C, Papadopoulos A, Andreou J, Stringaris K (2000) Perforation of the alimentary tract: evaluation with computed tomography. Abdom Imaging 25:373–379
4. Sherck J, Shatney C, Sensaki K, Selivanov V (1994) The accuracy of computed tomography in the diagnosis of blunt small-bowel perforation. Am J Surg 168:670–675
5. Singh JP, Steward MJ, Booth TC, Mukhtar H, Murray D (2010) Evolution of imaging for abdominal perforation. Ann R Coll Surg Engl 92:182–188
6. Espinoza R, Rodriguez A (1997) Traumatic and non traumatic perforation of hollow viscera. Surg Clin North Am 77(6):1291–13042
7. Stoker J, van Randen A, Laméris W, Boermeester MA (2009) Imaging patients with acute abdominal pain. Radiology 253(1):31–46
8. Scaglione M, Linsenmaier U, Schueller G (2012) Emergency radiology of the abdomen imaging features and differential diagnosis for a timely management approach. Springer, Milan/New York
9. Merchea A, Cullinane DC, Sawyer MD, Iqbal CW, Baron TH, Wigle D, Sarr MG, Zielinski MD (2010) Esophagogastroduodenoscopy-associated gastrointestinal perforations: a single-center experience. Surgery 148:876–880, discussion 881–872
10. Sanchez-Pernaute A, Aguirre EP, Talavera P, Valladares LD, de la Serna JP, Mantilla CS, de Leon AR, Torres A (2009) Laparoscopic approach to esophageal perforation secondary to pneumatic dilation for achalasia. Surg Endosc 23:1106–1109
11. Enguidanos L, Pfleiderer A, Smith W, Ramkumar S (2005) Pneumomediastinum secondary to an apparently trivial stab wound to the neck: the value of the Hamman's sign and thorough radiological investigation. Emerg Med J 22:230–231
12. Søreide JA, Viste A (2011) Esophageal perforation: diagnostic work-up and clinical decision-making in the first 24 hours. Scand J Trauma Resusc Emerg Med 19:66
13. De Lutio di Castelguidone E, Pinto A, Merola S, Stavolo C, Romano L (2005) Role of Spiral and Multislice Computed Tomography in the evaluation of traumatic and spontaneous oesophageal perforation. Our experience. Radiol Med 109(3):252–259
14. Pinto A, Muzj C, Gagliardi N, Pinto F, Setola FR, Scaglione M, Romano L (2012) Role of imaging in the assessment of impacted foreign bodies in the hypopharynx and cervical esophagus. Semin Ultrasound CT MR 33(5):463–470

15. Pinto A, Muzj C, Stavolo C, Pepe M, Cinque T, Romano L (2004) Pictorial essay: foreign body of the gastrointestinal tract in emergency radiology. Radiol Med 107(3):145–152
16. Pinto A, Grassi R, Rossi G, Romano L, Scaglione M, Pinto F (1998) Computerized tomography in the study of jejuno-ileal perforations. Personal case load. Radiol Med 96(6):602–606
17. Pinto A, Reginelli A, Pinto F, Sica G, Scaglione M, Berger FH, Romano L, Brunese L (2014) Radiological and practical aspects of body packing. Br J Radiol 87(1036):20130500
18. ACR appropriateness criteria, 2006. American College of Radiology Web site. http://www.acr.org/SecondaryMainMenuCategories/quality_safety/app_criteria/pdf/ExpertPanelonGastrointestinal Imaging Acute AbdominalPainandFeverorSuspected AbdominalAbscessDoc1.aspx. Accessed 15 Oct 2008
19. Grassi R, Romano S, Pinto A, Romano L (2004) Gastro-duodenal perforations: conventional plain film, US and CT findings in 166 consecutive patients. Eur J Radiol 50(1):30–36
20. Smith JE, Hall EJ (2009) The use of plain abdominal x rays in the emergency department. Emerg Med J 26(3):160–163
21. Reginelli A, Mandato Y, Solazzo A, Berritto D, Iacobellis F, Grassi R (2012) Errors in the radiological evaluation of the alimentary tract: part II. Semin Ultrasound CT MR 33(4):308–317
22. Grassi R, Di Mizio R, Pinto A, Romano L, Rotondo A (2004) Serial plain abdominal film findings in the assessment of acute abdomen: spastic ileus, hypotonic ileus, mechanical ileus and paralytic ileus. Radiol Med 108(1–2):56–70
23. Chen SC, Yen ZS, Wang HP, Lin FY, Hsu CY, Chen WJ (2002) Ultrasonography is superior to plain radiography in the diagnosis of pneumoperitoneum. Br J Surg 89:351–354
24. Hefny AF, Abu-Zidan FM (2011) Sonographic diagnosis of intraperitoneal free air. J Emerg Trauma Shock 4(4):511–513
25. Miller RE, Nelson SW (1971) The roentgenologic demonstration of tiny amounts of free intraperitoneal gas: experimental and clinical studies. AJR Am J Roentgenol 112:574–585
26. Pendergrass EP, Kirk E (1995) Significance of gas under right dome of diaphragm with discussion of hepatoptosis. Am J Roentgenol 22:238–246
27. Woodring JH, Heiser MJ (1995) Detection of pneumoperitoneum on chest radiographs: comparison of upright lateral and posteroanterior projections. AJR Am J Roentgenol 165(1):45–47
28. Grassi R, Pinto A, Rotondo A, Smaltino F (1996) Pneumoperitoneo. Idelson-Gnocchi
29. Grassi R, Pinto A, Rossi G, Rotondo A (1998) Conventional plain-film radiology, ultrasonography and CT in jejuno-ileal perforation. Acta Radiol 39(1):52–56
30. Grassi R, Catalano O, Pinto A, Fanucci A, Rotondo A, Di Mizio R (1996) Case report: identification of the transverse mesocolon and root of small bowel mesentery; a new sign of pneumoperitoneum. Br J Radiol 69(824):774–776
31. Solis CV, Chang Y, De Moya MA, Velmahos GC, Fagenholz PJ (2014) Free air on plainfilm: do we need a computed tomography too? J Emerg Trauma Shock 7(1):3–8
32. Grassi R, Di Mizio R, Pinto A, Cioffi A, Romano L, Rotondo A (1996) Sixty-one consecutive patients with gastrointestinal perforation: comparison of conventional radiology, ultrasonography, and computerized tomography, in terms of the timing of the study. Radiol Med 91(6):747–755
33. Catalano O, Grassi R, Rotondo A (1994) Diagnosis of free air in the abdomen. Role of echography. Radiol Med 87(5):632–635
34. Pinto F, Scaglione M, Pinto A, Lassandro F, Romano L, Grassi R (2000) Gastrointestinal perforations: ultrasound diagnosis. Emerg Radiol 7:263–267
35. Chen SC, Wang HP, Chen WJ, Lin FY, Hsu CY, Chang KJ, Chen WJ (2002) Selective use ultrasonography for the detection of pneumoperitoneum. Acad Emerg Med 9(6):643–645
36. Coppolino F, Gatta G, Di Grezia G, Reginelli A, Iacobellis F, Vallone G, Giganti M, Genovese E (2013) Gastrointestinal perforation: ultrasonographic diagnosis. Crit Ultrasound J 5(Suppl 1):S4
37. Nurberg D, Mauch M, Spengler J, Holle A, Pannwitz H, Seitz K (2007) Sonographical diagnosis of pneumoretroperitoneum as a result of retroperitoneal perforation. Ultraschall Med 28(6):612–621
38. Hainaux B, Agneessens E, Bertinotti R, De Maertelaer V, Rubesova E, Capelluto E, Moschopoulos C (2006) Accuracy of MDCT in predicting site of gastrointestinal tract perforation. AJR Am J Roentgenol 187:1179–1183
39. Brofman N, Atri M, Hanson JM, Grinblat L, Chughtai T, Brenneman F (2006) Evaluation of bowel and mesenteric blunt trauma with multidetector CT. Radiographics 26:1119–1131
40. Kim SH, Shin SS, Jeong YY, Heo SH, Kim JW, Kang HK (2009) Gastrointestinal tract perforation: MDCT findings according to the perforation sites. Korean J Radiol 10(1):63–70
41. Rossi G, Grassi R, Pinto A, Ragozzino A, Romano L (1998) New computerized tomography sign of intestinal infarction: isolated pneumoretroperitoneum or associated with pneumoperitoneum or late findings of intestinal infarction. Radiol Med 95(5):474–480
42. Pinto A, Scaglione M, Giovine S, Romano S, Lassandro F, Grassi R, Romano L (2004) Comparison between the site of multi slice CT signs of gastrointestinal perforation and the site of perforation detected at surgery in forty perforated patients. Radiol Med 108(3):208–217
43. Cadenas Rodríguez L, Martí de Gracia M, Saturio Galán N, Pérez Dueñas V, Salvatierra Arrieta L, Garzón Moll G (2013) Use of multidetector computed

tomography for locating the site of gastrointestinal tract perforations. Cir Esp 91:316–323
44. Scaglione M, de Lutio di Castelguidone E, Scialpi M, Merola S, Diettrich AI, Lombardo P, Romano L, Grassi R (2004) Blunt trauma to the gastrointestinal tract and mesentery: is there a role for helical CT in the decision-making process? Eur J Radiol 50:67–73
45. Brody JM, Leighton DB, Murphy BL, Abbott GF, Vaccaro JP, Jagminas L, Cioffi WG (2000) CT of blunt trauma bowel and mesenteric injury: typical findings and pitfalls in diagnosis. Radiographics 20:1525–1536
46. Romano S, Scaglione M, Tortora G, Martino A, Di Pietto F, Romano L, Grassi R (2006) MDCT in blunt intestinal trauma. Eur J Radiol 59:359–366
47. Hawkins AE, Mirvis SE (2003) Evaluation of bowel and mesenteric injury: role of multidetector CT. Abdom Imaging 28:505–514
48. Elton C, Riaz AA, Young N, Schamschula R, Papadopoulos B, Malka V (2005) Accuracy of computed tomography in the detection of blunt bowel and mesenteric injuries. Br J Surg 92:1024–1028
49. Saba L, Berritto D, Iacobellis F, Scaglione M, Castaldo S, Cozzolino S, Mazzei MA, Di Mizio V, Grassi R (2013) Acute arterial mesenteric ischemia and reperfusion: macroscopic and MRI findings, preliminary report. World J Gastroenterol 19(40):6825–6833
50. Singh A, Danrad R, Hahn PF, Blake MA, Mueller PR, Novelline RA (2007) MR imaging of the acute abdomen and pelvis: acute appendicitis and beyond. Radiographics 27(5):1419–1431

2 Plain Film Signs of Pneumoperitoneum

Antonio Pinto, Roberta Grassi, and Carlo Liguori

2.1 Introduction

Pneumoperitoneum is caused by rupture of a hollow viscus which includes the stomach, small bowel, and large bowel, with the exception of those portions that are retroperitoneal in the duodenum and colon. The most frequent cause of spontaneous pneumoperitoneum is perforation of a gastric or duodenal ulcer. The magnitude of free air is variable, being related to the size and site of the ulcer. A large perforation allows more rapid passage of air. Pneumoperitoneum may also be observed with a variety of other conditions including recent abdominal surgery, trauma, infection, paracentesis, and pneumatosis intestinalis [1]. After laparotomy, air will usually be present for 3–7 days, gradually decreasing in volume daily [2].

Upright posteroanterior chest radiography traditionally has been used for the initial examination of patients suspected of having pneumoperitoneum. Pneumoperitoneum is visualized as a translucent crescent or area below the diaphragm [3]. The upright chest radiograph can enable detection of as little as 1 mL of free air located beneath the right or left hemidiaphragm [4]. In the emergency setting, in critically ill patients, radiographic examination is performed in the supine decubitus, with anteroposterior and lateral view of the abdomen and anteroposterior view of the thorax [5].

It is crucial that the radiologist become familiar with the signs of pneumoperitoneum that can be discerned on the supine film of the abdomen because that may be the only radiograph available for interpretation [2].

2.2 Etiology and Clinical Presentation

There are four etiologic categories of pneumoperitoneum: iatrogenic, spontaneous, traumatic, and miscellaneous [6]. Iatrogenic causes include surgery, recent endoscopy, peritoneal dialysis, feeding tube placement, use of gynecologic instruments, and vigorous respiratory resuscitation. Spontaneous causes comprise peptic ulcer perforation, intestinal ischemia, bowel obstruction, toxic megacolon, and inflammatory conditions such as acute appendicitis, tuberculosis, and necrotizing enterocolitis. Traumatic causes can be blunt or penetrating, either of which can determine intestinal perforation. Miscellaneous causes include drugs (steroidal drugs, nonsteroidal anti-inflammatory drugs) and pneumatosis coli or

A. Pinto (✉) • C. Liguori
Department of Radiology,
"A. Cardarelli" Hospital,
Via Cardarelli 9, Naples I-80131, Italy
e-mail: antopin1968@libero.it;
carlo.liguori@gmail.com

R. Grassi (✉)
Department of Internal and Experimental Medicine
Magrassi-Lanzara, Institute of Radiology,
Second University of Naples, Naples I-80131, Italy
e-mail: email_roberta@libero.it

L. Romano, A. Pinto (eds.), *Imaging of Alimentary Tract Perforation*,
DOI 10.1007/978-3-319-08192-2_2, © Springer International Publishing Switzerland 2015

intestinalis. Miscellaneous causes may also be female genital tract related (after coitus, orogenital sex, and even sometimes following exercise in the postpartum period) [6, 7].

Because the clinical symptoms of free perforation are associated with the underlying cause of the perforation, the clinical presentations of patients with perforated viscus are quite variable. Patients will typically present with the acute onset of abdominal pain that is persistent, progressive, and unremitting. Severity of the pain will depend on the type and amount of intestinal contents released into the peritoneal cavity. Patients may have associated symptoms including fever, nausea, and vomiting. On physical examination, a patient with intestinal perforation will typically manifest diffuse tenderness to palpation and peritonitis [8]. Recognizing a perforation and establishing the cause and site of the perforation can yield crucial information for the surgeon [3].

2.3 Plain Abdominal Radiographs

Conventional radiography is commonly the initial imaging examination performed in the diagnostic workup of patients who present with acute abdominal pain to the emergency department. Plain radiography can demonstrate 55–85 % of patients with pneumoperitoneum [9]. This examination is widely available, can be easily performed in admitted patients, and is used to exclude major illness such as perforated viscus, bowel obstruction, and foreign body ingestion [10]. Moreover, plain abdominal film is useful in the evaluation of the different types of ileus (spastic ileus, hypotonic ileus, mechanical ileus, and paralytic ileus) [10].

Conventional radiography includes supine and upright conventional abdominal radiography and upright chest radiography [3]. On upright posteroanterior chest radiography, pneumoperitoneum is visualized as a translucent crescent or area below the diaphragm. As reported in literature [11] the upright lateral chest radiograph is more sensitive than the upright posteroanterior chest radiograph in detecting small amounts of pneumoperitoneum. However, many patients with an acute abdomen are too sick or debilitated to stand erect for the time necessary to permit air to migrate to the least dependent portion of the peritoneal cavity. Miller and Nelson [12] showed that as little as 1–2 mL of free air could be detected if a strict protocol of positioning the patient in the left lateral decubitus position for 10–20 min and then in the upright position for an additional 10 min was followed. This protocol is of limited use for patients with clinical symptoms that preclude a wait of this duration and in those patients unable to cooperate by maintaining the optimal position described.

The left lateral decubitus position is also uncomfortable, raising further questions about patient compliance. In the emergency setting, in critically ill patients, radiographic examination is generally performed in the supine decubitus, with anteroposterior and lateral view of the abdomen and anteroposterior view of the thorax [5].

2.4 Signs of Pneumoperitoneum on Plain Radiographs

There are many possible radiographic appearances of pneumoperitoneum.

On upright posteroanterior chest radiography, pneumoperitoneum is visualized as a translucent crescent or area below the diaphragm (Fig. 2.1). Pneumoperitoneum can also be detected on left lateral decubitus radiograph of the abdomen (Fig. 2.2) and on cross-table lateral abdominal radiograph (Fig. 2.3).

On supine abdominal radiograph, free peritoneal air may become visible and, in various shapes and sizes, may be located in different positions. These free air signs can be categorized into four groups: bowel-related signs, right upper quadrant signs, peritoneal ligament-related signs, and other signs [13].

Bowel-related signs include the following:

- Rigler sign. The Rigler sign (Fig. 2.4), also known as the bas-relief sign or the double-wall sign, is the visualization of both sides of the bowel wall, on a radiograph of the

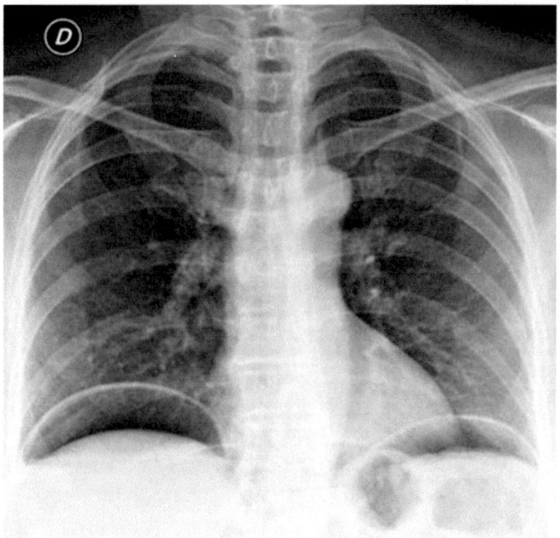

Fig. 2.1 Upright posteroanterior chest radiograph: evidence of free air beneath the right and left hemidiaphragms

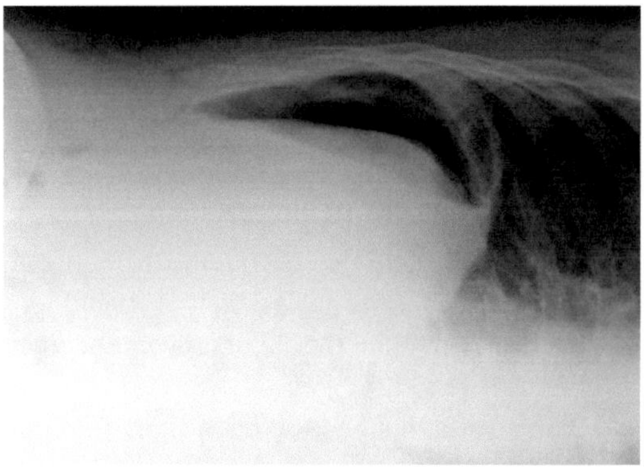

Fig. 2.2 Left lateral decubitus film of the abdomen in a patient with free peritoneal air resulting from gastric perforation

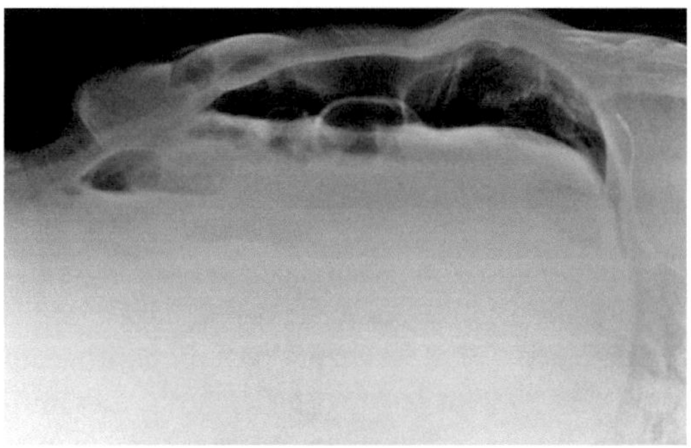

Fig. 2.3 Cross-table lateral abdominal radiograph demonstrating the presence of pneumoperitoneum

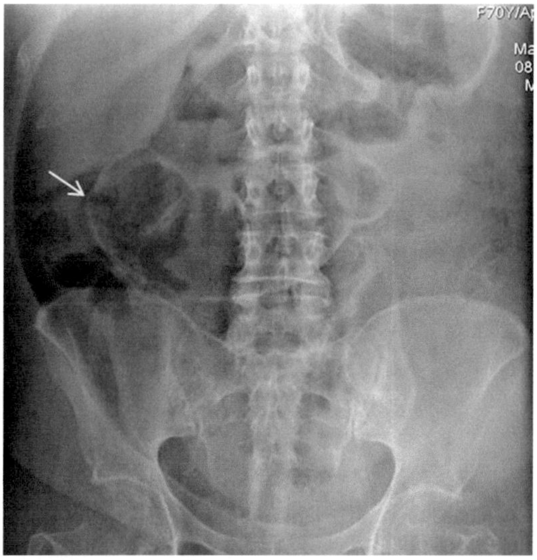

Fig. 2.4 Anteroposterior supine abdominal radiograph shows the Rigler sign (*arrow*)

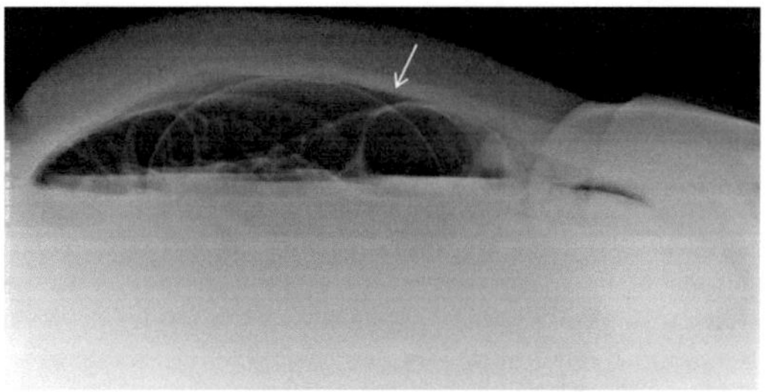

Fig. 2.5 Cross-table lateral radiograph of the abdomen showing the triangle sign (*arrow*)

abdomen obtained with the patient in the supine position, in the presence of a large volume of free air so that the bowel loops can be separated from each other [14].

- Triangle sign. Free intraperitoneal air accumulating among three adjoining bowel loops or two bowel loops and the parietal peritoneum (Fig. 2.5) appearing as a triangular radiolucency is called the triangle sign [15].

Right upper quadrant signs include the following:

- Hyperlucent liver sign. On the supine radiographs, the blacker density of the large intraperitoneal free gas anterior to the ventral hepatic surface replacing the brightness of the hepatic shadow is called the hyperlucent liver sign (Figs. 2.6 and 2.7) [15].

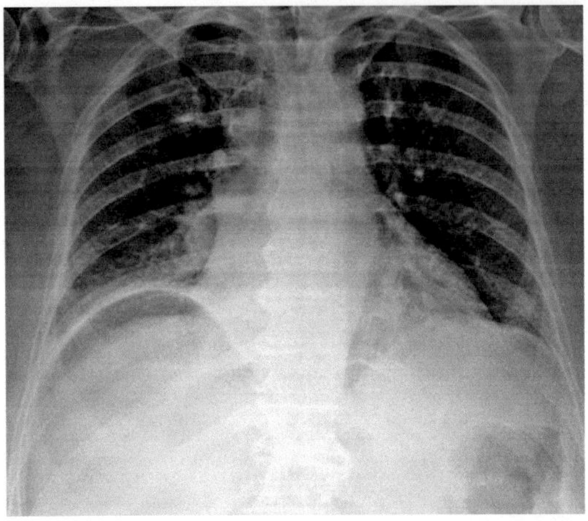

Fig. 2.6 Anteroposterior supine chest radiograph shows the hyperlucent liver sign

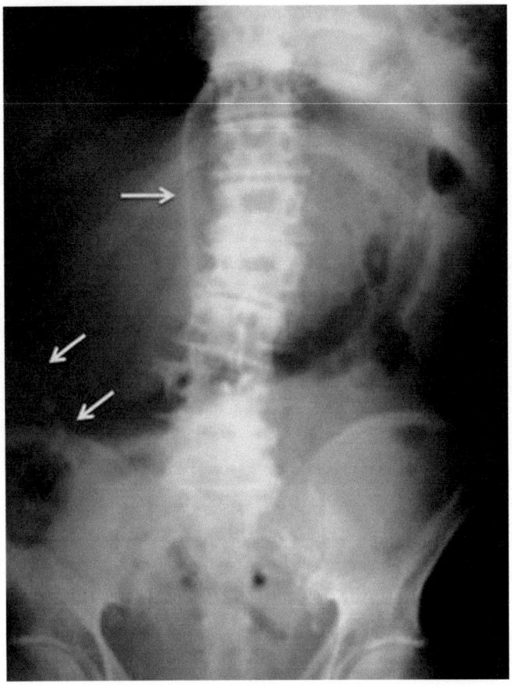

Fig. 2.7 A supine radiograph of the abdomen showing the hyperlucent liver sign, the falciform ligament sign (*arrow*), and the mesoappendix sign (*arrows*) in a perforated patient

- Anterior superior oval sign. This sign refers to a single or multiple oval, round, or pear-shaped gas bubbles projected over the liver shadow [15, 16].
- Fissure for ligamentum teres sign. This sign refers to a characteristic elongated area of hyperlucency that represents intraperitoneal gas trapped within the fissure for the ligamentum teres [17].
- The visible gallbladder. On supine abdominal radiograph, the gallbladder is seen as a homogeneous opacity because of surrounding free intraperitoneal air [18].
- Doge cap sign. This sign refers to triangle-shaped free air accumulated in Morison pouch on supine abdominal films [15, 19].
- Hepatic edge sign. An oblong saucer or cigar-shaped collection of free air may be seen in the subhepatic space with its long axis directed superomedially following the liver contour [15, 20].
- Dolphin sign. The undersurface of the long costal muscle slips of the diaphragm that indented the adjacent air-filled space in the right upper quadrant on supine films is a sign of pneumoperitoneum [21].

Peritoneal ligament-related signs include the following:

- Falciform ligament sign. The intraperitoneal free air may outline the falciform ligament, which is seen as a linear density situated longitudinally within the right upper abdomen (Fig. 2.7) [15, 22].
- Extrahepatic ligamentum teres sign. The ligamentum teres is another anterior peritoneal ligament that can be visualized on plain radiographs. It is a firm fibrous cord representing the remnant of an obliterated left umbilical vein. On supine radiographs, the extrahepatic ligamentum teres may be seen when outlined by free air anywhere along the course of the ligament [23].
- The "inverted V" sign. Free air outlining the lateral umbilical ligaments makes these structures visible in the lower abdomen, forming an "inverted V" as they course inferiorly and laterally from the umbilicus [24, 25].
- Urachus sign. When pneumoperitoneum occurs, the urachus may be seen as a thin midline linear structure in the lower abdomen from the umbilicus to the dome of the urinary bladder [26].

- The transverse mesocolon and root of small bowel mesentery signs. The intraperitoneal free air can determine the identification of the transverse mesocolon and the root of the small bowel mesentery on plain abdominal radiographs obtained in the supine and in the prone position [27].
- The mesoappendix sign. In the presence of a large amount of pneumoperitoneum, the mesoappendix may be observed on the supine radiograph as a radiopaque linear stripe directed from the cecum to the middle of the abdomen (Fig. 2.7).

Other signs of pneumoperitoneum are the following:

- Football sign. It refers to a large oval radiolucency in the shape of an American football producing a sharp interface with the parietal peritoneum on a supine abdominal radiograph. The oval radiolucency seen in the football sign represents massive pneumoperitoneum which distends the peritoneal cavity [28, 29].
- Cupola sign. The cupola sign is seen as an arcuate lucency overlying the lower thoracic spine and projecting caudad to the heart on supine radiograph [30]. The term *cupola* is used to indicate the inverted cup-shaped configuration of the lucency.
- Left-sided anterior superior oval sign. Chiu et al. [13] defined a single or multiple oval, round, or pear-shaped free air projected over the left upper quadrant abdomen as the "left-sided anterior superior oval sign."
- Subphrenic radiolucency. Radiolucency that appeared beneath the diaphragm, either right or left side on the supine chest radiographs, has been defined as "subphrenic radiolucency" [13].
- Focal radiolucency. The abnormal gas pattern presenting on the supine films without fitting any sign mentioned above has been called "focal radiolucency" [13].

Conclusions

The diagnosis of hollow-organ perforation is based on the evidence of pneumoperitoneum. Pneumoperitoneum can be an indicator of potentially serious intraperitoneal disease. Although the upright and left decubitus projections are the most sensitive views for the radiographic recognition of small collections of free intraperitoneal air, the role of the supine projection should not be minimized especially in the critically ill patients. There are many useful signs that may contribute to a diagnosis of free air at supine radiography.

References

1. Pinto A, Scaglione M, Pinto F et al (2000) Helical computed tomography diagnosis of gastrointestinal perforation in the elderly patient. Emerg Radiol 7:259–262
2. Baker SR (1990) Plain film radiology of the peritoneal and retroperitoneal spaces. In: Baker SR (ed) The abdominal plain film. Appleton & Lange, Norwalk/San Mateo, pp 71–125
3. Stoker J, van Randen A, Laméris W et al (2009) Imaging patients with acute abdominal pain. Radiology 253:31–46
4. Miller RE, Becker GJ, Slabaugh RA (1980) Detection of pneumoperitoneum: optimum body position and respiratory phase. AJR Am J Roentgenol 138:487–490
5. Grassi R, Romano S, Pinto A et al (2004) Gastroduodenal perforations: conventional plain film, US and CT findings in 166 consecutive patients. Eur J Radiol 50:30–36
6. Ly JQ (2003) The Rigler sign. Radiology 228:706–707
7. Manchanda R, Refaie A (2005) Acute pneumoperitoneum following coitus. CJEM 7:51–53
8. Brown CVR (2014) Small bowel and colon perforation. Surg Clin North Am 94:471–475
9. Roh JJ, Thompson JS, Harned RK et al (1983) Value of pneumoperitoneum in the diagnosis of visceral perforation. Am J Surg 146:830–833
10. Grassi R, Di Mizio R, Pinto A et al (2004) Serial plain abdominal film findings in the assessment of acute abdomen: spastic ileus, hypotonic ileus, mechanical ileus and paralytic ileus. Radiol Med 108:56–70
11. Woodring JH, Heiser MJ (1995) Detection of pneumoperitoneum on chest radiographs: comparison of upright lateral and posteroanterior projections. AJR Am J Roentgenol 165:45–47
12. Miller RE, Nelson SW (1971) The roentgenological demonstration of tiny amounts of free intraperitoneal gas: experimental and clinical studies. Am J Roentgenol Radium Ther Nucl Med 112:574–585
13. Chiu Y-H, Chen J-D, Tiu J-D et al (2009) Reappraisal of radiographic signs of pneumoperitoneum at emergency department. Am J Emerg Med 27:320–327
14. Rigler LG (1941) Spontaneous pneumoperitoneum: a roentgenologic sign found in the supine position. Radiology 37:604–607

15. Cho KC, Baker SR (1994) Extraluminal air diagnosis and significance. Radiol Clin North Am 32:829–844
16. Cho KC, Baker SR, Thornhill BA et al (1988) Supine film diagnosis of pneumoperitoneum: new observations in the right upper quadrant. Radiology 169:405
17. Cho KC, Baker SR (1991) Air in the fissure for the ligamentum teres: new sign of intraperitoneal air on plain radiographs. Radiology 178:489–492
18. Radin R, Van Allan RJ, Rosen RS (1996) The visible gallbladder: a plain film sign of pneumoperitoneum. AJR Am J Roentgenol 167:69–70
19. Brill PW, Olson SR, Winchester P (1990) Neonatal necrotizing enterocolitis: air in Morison pouch. Radiology 174:469–471
20. Menuck L, Siemers PT (1976) Pneumoperitoneum: importance of right upper quadrant features. AJR Am J Roentgenol 127:753–756
21. Cho KC, Baker SR (1997) Depiction of diaphragmatic muscle slips on supine plain radiographs: a sign of pneumoperitoneum. Radiology 203:431–433
22. Han SY (1980) Variations in falciform ligament with pneumoperitoneum. Can Assoc Radiol J 31:171–173
23. Cho KC, Baker SR (1997) Visualization of the extrahepatic segment of the ligamentum teres: a sign of free air on plain radiographs. Radiology 202:651–654
24. Weiner CI, Diaconis JN, Dennis JM (1973) The inverted V: a new sign of pneumoperitoneum. Radiology 107:47–48
25. Bray JF (1984) The "inverted V" sign of pneumoperitoneum. Radiology 151:45–46
26. Jelaso DV, Schultz EH (1969) The urachus – an aid to the diagnosis of pneumoperitoneum. Radiology 92: 295–296
27. Grassi R, Catalano O, Pinto A et al (1996) Case report: identification of the transverse mesocolon and root of small bowel mesentery; a new sign of pneumoperitoneum. Br J Radiol 69:774–776
28. Miller RE (1960) Perforated viscus in infants: a new roentgen sign. Radiology 74:65–67
29. Rampton JW (2004) The football sign. Radiology 231:81–82
30. Mindelzun RE, McCort JJ (1986) The cupola sign of pneumoperitoneum in the supine patient. Gastrointest Radiol 11:283–285

3 Ultrasonographic Assessment of Gastrointestinal Perforation

Massimo Valentino and Libero Barozzi

3.1 Introduction

Gastrointestinal perforation is diagnosed by demonstrating air or intestinal content in the peritoneum or retroperitoneum. The diagnosis of free air in the abdominal cavity is usually made with x-ray, both chest radiography in the standing position and abdominal radiography in the upright and left lateral position. Miller et al. reported that as little as 1–2 ml of free intraperitoneal air can potentially be imaged [1]. However, in clinical practice, x-ray may not detect small amount of air on radiography, and CT is often requested.

Recently, ultrasonography (US) has emerged as a useful diagnostic technique in patients with acute abdomen also for detecting pneumoperitoneum [2]. US is routinely performed to investigate patients with abdominal pain, including those having gastrointestinal perforation as final diagnosis [3]. During abdominal examination of these patients, US images all the contents of the abdominal cavity, including bowel and mesentery. In case of gastrointestinal perforation, a correct interpretation of the artifact due to free air eventually present can lead to the correct diagnosis.

3.2 Technique

The concept of visualizing abdominal air using US is not new. In fact, one of the most comprehensive and detailed studies on the topic was published nearly 30 years ago [4]. Seitz et al. observed that US examination of patients with recent cholecystectomy was impeded by strong hyperechoic reverberation and shadowing artifacts caused by postoperative free air.

Most authors agree that the best place to look for pneumoperitoneum by US is in the right hypochondrium, superficial to the liver, with the patient in the supine position with the thorax slightly elevated or in a semilateral decubitus position [5]. If the patient is studied in a left semilateral decubitus, free air collects in the ventral hepatoperitoneal space. In his study, Asrani was able to demonstrate that air at US can be observed in all quadrants of the abdomen, with 83 % being observable in the right hypochondrium, 75 % in the umbilical region, and in 8.3 % in the right lumbar region [6]. Another study suggests positioning the patient supine with 10–20° inclination for a better visualization of air [7].

In the clinical practice, patients are studied in the supine position, searching for the same

M. Valentino (✉)
Dipartimento Diagnostico, U.O. di Radiologia, Ospedale S. Antonio Abate, Tolmezzo (UD), Via Morgagni, 18, Tolmezzo (UD) 33028, Italy
e-mail: mvm.valentino@gmail.com

L. Barozzi
Dipartimento Servizi, U.O. Radiologia OM e Area Nord-Ovest, Ospedale Maggiore, Bologna, Largo Nigrisoli 2, Bologna 40100, Italy
e-mail: l.barozzi@ausl.bologna.it

L. Romano, A. Pinto (eds.), *Imaging of Alimentary Tract Perforation*,
DOI 10.1007/978-3-319-08192-2_3, © Springer International Publishing Switzerland 2015

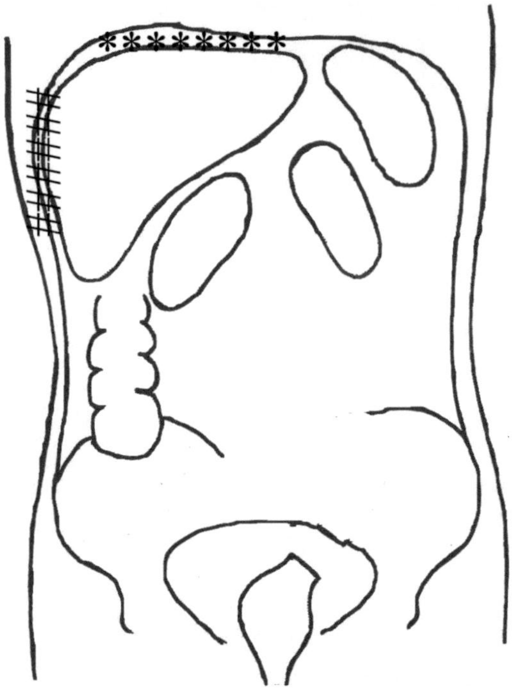

Fig. 3.1 Sites of free intraperitoneal air in the abdomen on US examination (Modified from Beyer and Modder [21])

findings of the trauma (free fluid in the abdominal space), and if a perforation is suspected, the semilateral decubitus position is added (Fig. 3.1).

3.2.1 US of Pneumoperitoneum

Free air in abdominal cavity can give direct or indirect signs. The main US signs of the presence of pneumoperitoneum include strong reverberation anterior to the liver surface, the shifting phenomenon, and the enhancement of the peritoneal stripe. The indirect signs are the presence of intraperitoneal free fluid and the decreased bowel motility.

3.2.1.1 Reverberations

Air is a medium posing high resistance and impermeability to ultrasound waves, making it a strong reflector. Free air can be visualized as horizontal or vertical reverberations originating in the peritoneum and extending to the lower edge of the monitor. The reverberation echo, generated by an air structure, was well described by Linchenstein [8]. It consists in a succession of roughly horizontal (or slightly curved) lines that generate a striped pattern, alternating dark and clear lines at regular intervals. They can be large or very narrow. The reverberation echo hides the information below, as does an acoustic shadow. Larger air collections make bright, highly echogenic lines with distal reverberation and shadowing artifacts (Fig. 3.2). Smaller air bubbles can appear as bright punctuate foci with or without ring-down artifacts (Fig. 3.3).

3.2.1.2 Shifting Phenomenon

Reverberation is not specific for pneumoperitoneum unless it is possible to demonstrate the "shifting" of air in the cavity when the patient was repositioned. It is therefore needed to move the patient on the left semilateral decubitus position observing the shifting of the air in the space between peritoneum and liver or in the hepatorenal space. Excessive gas in an abscess can mimic the shifting phenomenon. For this reason, Karahan and colleagues proposed an original method for the detection of pneumoperitoneum [9]. While the patient is in the supine position, if the reverberation artifact is visible, a slight pressure is applied to the abdominal wall using the probe. During this maneuver, the free intraperitoneal air is expelled from the region anterior to the liver to other parts of the peritoneal cavity, and consequently, the reverberation artifact became much less prominent. Conversely, when the pressure on the probe is released, maintaining the contact with the skin surface, the free gas return to the epigastric region and the artifact echo pattern became more prominent. On real-time US examination, repetition of this maneuver appears like the opening and closing of scissors, leading to the term "scissors maneuver." The diagnostic accuracy values in the diagnosis of pneumoperitoneum obtained by the authors with the adding of this maneuver was very high, and they reported a sensitivity of 94 %, specificity of 100 %, PPV of 100 %, and NPV of 98 %.

3.2.1.3 Peritoneal Stripe

This finding was first described by Muradali et al. [10], and it was termed the "peritoneal stripe."

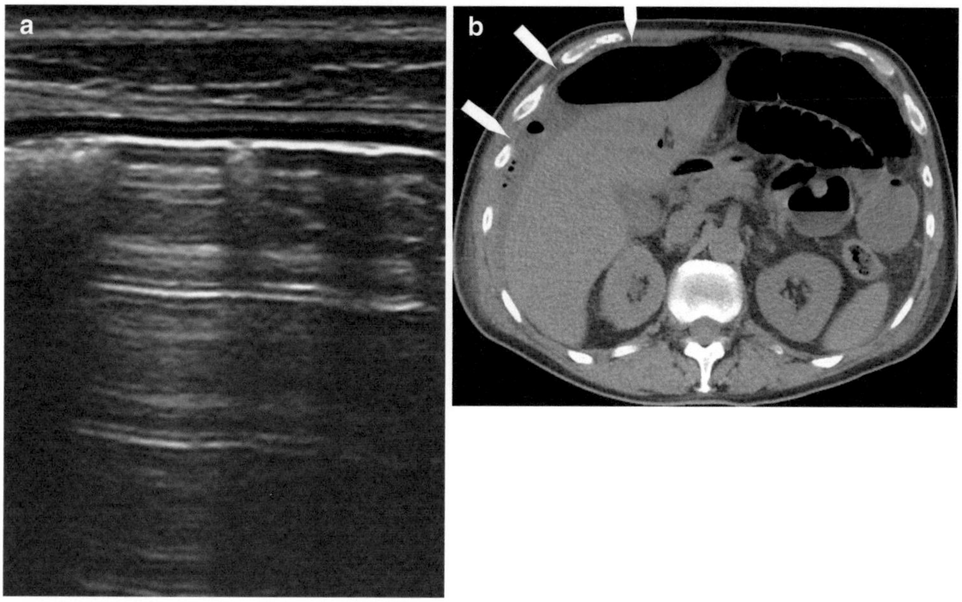

Fig. 3.2 Sagittal sonographic section of the right hypochondrium using a linear probe showing reverberation artifacts which obscure the right lobe of the liver (**a**). Computed tomography confirms the large amount of air superficial to the liver (**b**, *white arrows*). At laparotomy, the patient had perforated peptic ulcer

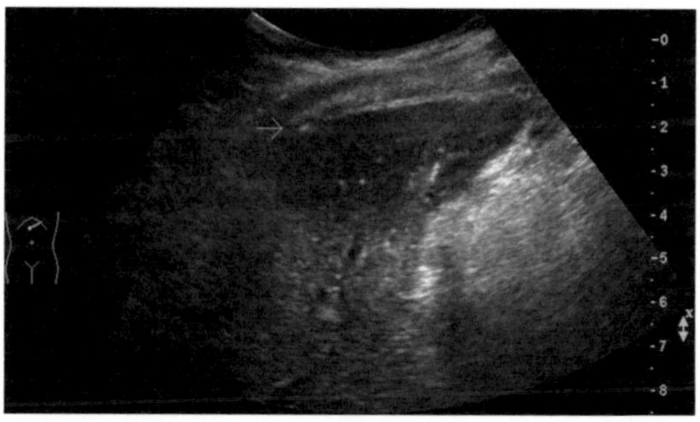

Fig. 3.3 Sagital sonographic section of the right hypochondrium using a curvilinear probe. Small air bubble anterior to the liver causing ring-down artifact (*white arrows*). This patient presented with normal vital signs had moderate abdominal pain due to perforated diverticulitis.

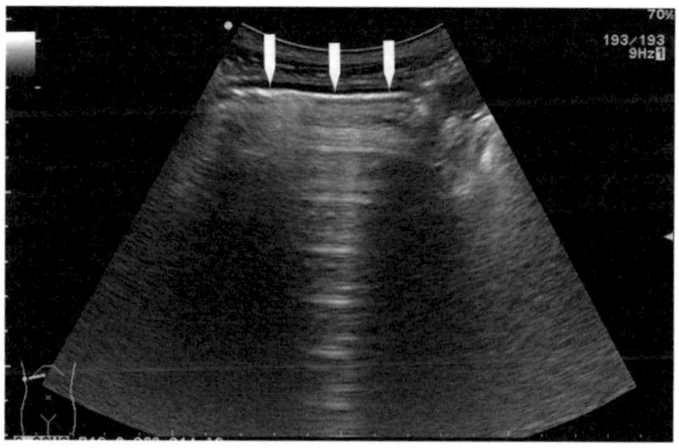

Fig. 3.4 Sagittal sonographic section of the right hypochondrium with curvilinear probe. Enhanced peritoneal stripe (*white arrows*)

Under an animal experimental model, they were able to demonstrate that tiny bubbles of free air produced focal enhancement and apparent thickening of the peritoneal stripe with or without multiple reflection artifacts, depending on the amount of the peritoneal air. In the cases of air within the intestinal bowel, overlying peritoneal stripe was normal, whereas in the cases of extraluminal (intraperitoneal) air, the peritoneal stripe was thickened. The animal model was than demonstrated in nine patients who underwent laparoscopy, and it was documented for all four quadrants of the abdomen. The enhanced peritoneal stripe indicates free intraperitoneal air and permits its differentiation from intraluminal bowel gas (Fig. 3.4). In the US imaging of the abdomen, it is possible to identify a single or a double thin echogenic line between the anterior abdominal wall and the anterior liver surface.

Intraperitoneal free fluid and decreased bowel motility are indirect signs, but in the adequate clinical context can help in the diagnosis [11]. Peritonitis caused by gastrointestinal perforation leads to a paralytic or adynamic ileus, a condition characterized by gas-fluid stasis, with a reduction in intestinal movement [12].

3.3 Causes of Bowel Perforation

The most common causes of gastrointestinal perforation are as follows:

- Peptic ulcer
- Appendicitis
- Sigmoid diverticulitis
- Bowel malignancy
- Crohn's disease
- Sharp foreign body

One of the hallmarks of bowel perforation useful for identification of the site of the perforation is the inflamed fat, like in appendicitis and diverticulitis. "Inflamed fat" represents the defense mechanism of omentum and mesentery to stop the bowel perforation. Sometimes this mechanism is effective; sometimes it is less effective, and an open perforation can lead to the surgery treatment. Whether this process is going to be successful (and a nonoperative management can be indicated) cannot be judged from the imaging findings alone, and a combination of clinical and imaging findings needs to be considered.

- Peptic ulcer. Uncomplicated duodenal ulcer is becoming quite rare, since most symptomatic patients have already been treated with proton pump inhibitors before any test is done. Pneumoperitoneum can sometimes be visualized by US: small amount of air with fluid can be visualized in the falciform ligament or medially to the gallbladder wall (Fig. 3.5).
- Appendicitis. Appendiceal perforation is a common complication of acute appendicitis. The criteria for the diagnosis of acute appendicitis by sonography are well established: identification of a noncompressible blind-ending structure in the right lower quadrant with an outer diameter of greater than 6 mm. A small quantity of periappendiceal fluid is often present and aspecific. It may be present in both nonperforated and perforated appendicitis and in many other conditions, both surgical and nonsurgical. A large quantity of fluid in the presence of an inflamed appendix may represent pus from perforated appendicitis and then is usually accompanied by paralytic ileus [13]. In case of perforation, an appendiceal abscess can be visible as a circumscribed collection, walled off by omentum, mesentery, and bowel (Fig. 3.6).
- Sigmoid diverticulitis. Diverticulitis is inflammation of a diverticulum. It can be uncomplicated, or it can result in complications such as perforation. Uncomplicated diverticulitis consists in inflammation of colonic diverticulitis and/or microperforation of the wall of the diverticulum, which results in peridiverticulitis or phlegmon. In complicated diverticulitis that ensues, the process is associated with an abscess, a free perforation, or a fistula. In the past decade, US has been largely proposed in this diagnosis because of its ability to identify the disease and to detect its complications [14].

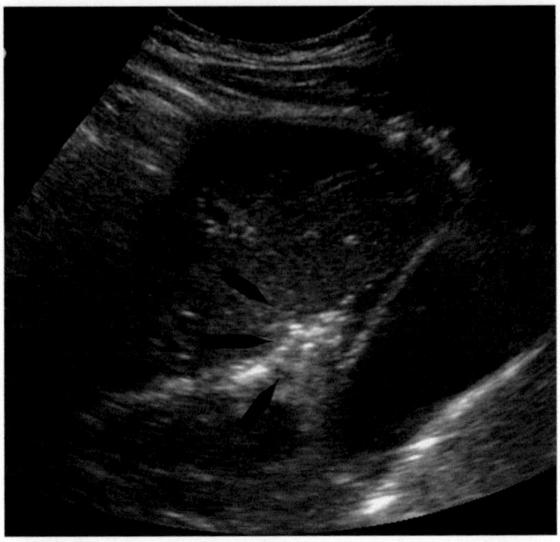

Fig. 3.5 Pneumoperitoneum due to peptic ulcer perforation: small amount of air visualized in the falciform ligament medially to the gallbladder wall (*black arrows*)

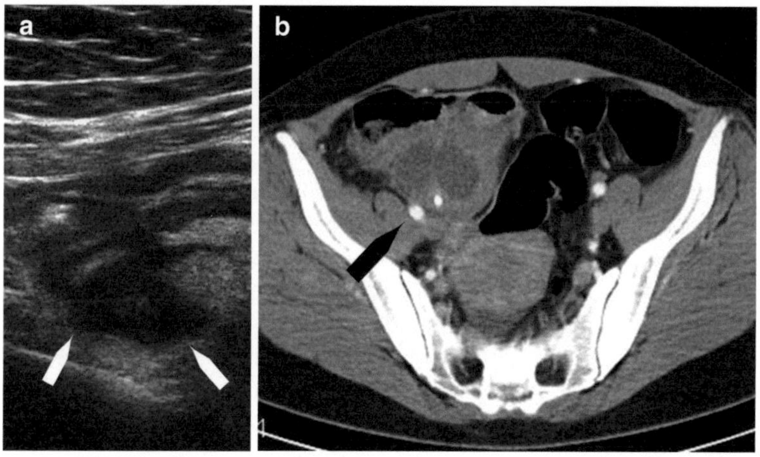

Fig. 3.6 Acute appendicitis with appendiceal abscess visible as a circumscribed collection at US (**a** *white arrows*) and confirmed at contrast-enhanced CT (**b**). Note the appendicoliths within the collection (*black arrow*)

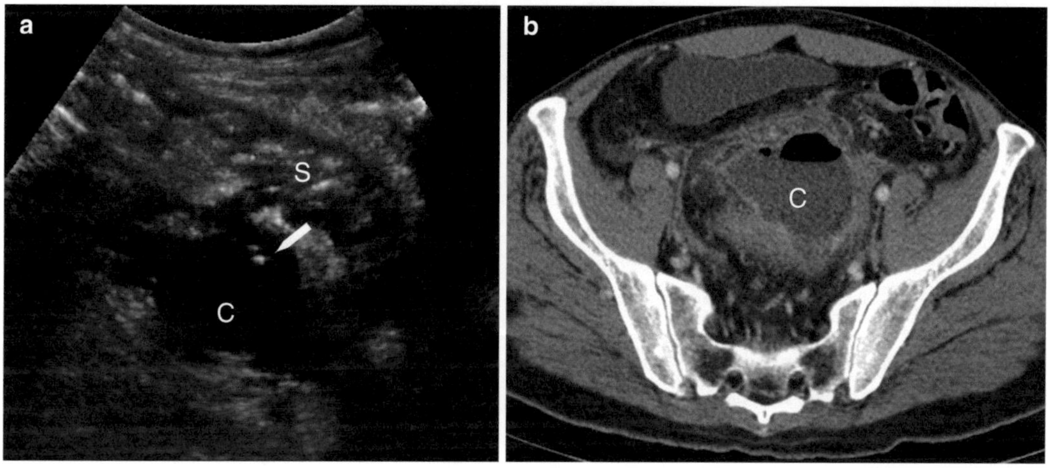

Fig. 3.7 Abscess from perforated acute sigmoid diverticulitis (*S*). At US (**a**) it appears as a fluid collection containing (*C*) echoes and producing dirty shadowing from air (*white arrow*). Contrast-enhanced CT confirmed the diagnosis (**b**)

The complications of diverticulitis depend on the location of the diverticulum, whereas an intraperitoneal diverticulum can result in a free perforation into the peritoneal cavity, or an intraperitoneal abscess, or sometimes in a fistula formation with the neighbor organs. The free air in the peritoneal cavity can be depicted as a hyperechoic line along the hepatic surface or the peritoneal line. An abscess appears as a fluid collection usually containing echoes and producing dirty shadowing from contained air (Fig. 3.7). A fistula is identified as a linear hypoechoic tract extending from the tip of the diverticulum into the inflamed fat. It can involve an adjacent bowel loop, the bladder, or the uterus [15].

- Crohn's disease. Inflammatory bowel diseases, such as Crohn's disease, may produce inflammation of various intensities, including perforation with abscesses formation. Intra-abdominal abscesses occur up to 30 % of Crohn's disease, as a consequence of fistulas or as a postsurgical complication [16]. At US, abscesses appear as hypoechoic mass containing internal ring-down artifacts due to the presence of air. US sensitivity for detection of intra-abdominal abscesses in Crohn's disease is quite high [17].

- Bowel malignancy. The most common presenting symptoms of bowel carcinoma are related to changes in bowel habits, bleeding, abdominal pain, abdominal mass, weight loss, anorexia, and other characteristics related to metastasis. It is not uncommon for patients having such diseases to present with perforation, which might be free or contained or result in a fistula formation. Free perforation leads to secondary peritonitis, while contained or fistulous perforation has a variable outcome. Cecal and sigmoid carcinomas are the most common malignant diseases that may present with abscess or free perforation. The US appearances in these cases are the same as the previous reported for Crohn's disease and sigmoid diverticulitis. It can be helpful to identify a segmental, eccentric mass of the intestinal wall eventually with liver metastasis [18].
- Sharp foreign body. Gastrointestinal perforation is most often secondary to extrinsic or intrinsic obstruction, but occasionally it may be due to other factors such as foreign bodies. A lot of cases of bowel perforation caused by foreign bodies have been reported in the literature, with fish bones and chicken bones being the most common objects, followed by toothpicks and cocktail sticks [19]. Foreign body-associated perforation commonly occurs at the point of acute angulation and narrowing, and the most common sites of perforation are the terminal ileum and colon, the appendix, and the right side or left side diverticulum. The case of colon perforation by foreign body due to previously undiagnosed colon cancer is also not uncommon [20]. Ultrasonography may a useful modality for the identification of foreign bodies that may appear as a linear echogenic structure usually accompanied by a posterior acoustic shadow, embedded in a large reactive inflammatory mass. In such cases, computed tomography may easily confirm the diagnosis.

Conclusions

US plays an important role in patients with acute abdominal pain as a first-line imaging method able to provide the correct diagnoses in a high percentage of cases. In gastrointestinal diseases, it can identify specific signs of perforation, such as reverberation, the shifting phenomenon, and the enhancement of the peritoneal stripe. Emphasis on air artifacts may establish the final diagnosis and guiding the correct workup.

References

1. Miller RE, Nelson SW (1971) The roentgenologic demonstration of tiny amounts of free intraperitoneal gas: experimental and clinical studies. Am J Roentgenol Radium Ther Nucl Med 12:574–585
2. Lee DH, Lim JH, Ko YT, Yoon Y (1990) Sonographic detection of pneumoperitoneum in patients with acute abdomen. AJR Am J Roentgenol 154:107–109
3. Puylaert J, van der Zant F, Rijke A (1997) Sonography and the acute abdomen: practical considerations. AJR Am J Roentgenol 168:179–186
4. Seitz K, Reising KD (1982) Ultrasound detection of free air in the abdominal cavity. Ultraschall Med 3:4–6
5. Ghaffar A, Siddiqui TS, Haider H, Khatri H (2008) Postsurgical pneumoperitoneum – comparison of abdominal ultrasound findings with plain radiography. J Coll Physicians Surg Pak 18:477–480
6. Asrani A (2007) Sonographic diagnosis of pneumoperitoneum using the 'enhancement of the peritoneal stripe sign'. A prospective study. Emerg Radiol 14: 29–39
7. Grechenig W, Peicha G, Clement HG, Grechenig M (1999) Detection of pneumoperitoneum by ultrasound examination: an experimental and clinical study. Injury 30:173–178
8. Linchenstein D (2005) US in the critically ill. Springer, Berlin/Heidelberg
9. Karahan O, Kurt A, Yikilmaz A, Kahriman G (2004) New method for the detection of Intraperitoneal free air by sonography: scissors maneuver. J Clin Ultrasound 32:381–385
10. Muradali D, Wilson S, Burns PN, Shapiro H, Hope-Simpson D (1999) A specific sign of pneumoperitoneum on sonography: enhancement of the peritoneal stripe. AJR Am J Roentgenol 173:1257–1262
11. Grassi R, Romano S, D'Amario F et al (2004) The relevance of free fluid between intestinal loops detected

by sonography in the clinical assessment of small bowel obstruction in adults. Eur J Radiol 50(1):5–14
12. Grassi R, Di Mizio R, Pinto A, Romano L, Rotondo A (2004) Serial plain abdominal film findings in the assessment of acute abdomen: spastic ileus, hypotonic ileus, mechanical ileus and paralytic ileus. Radiol Med 108:56–70
13. Puylaert J (2003) Ultrasonography of the acute abdomen: gastrointestinal conditions. Radiol Clin North Am 41:1227–1242
14. Liljegren G, Chabok A, Wickbom M, Smedh K, Nilsson K (2007) Acute colonic diverticulitis: a systematic review of diagnostic accuracy. Colorectal Dis 9:480–488
15. Valentino M, Serra C, Ansaloni L, Mantovani G, Pavlica P, Barozzi L (2009) Sonographic features of acute colonic diverticulitis. J Clin Ultrasound 37:457–463
16. Nagler SM, Poticha SM (1979) Intra-abdominal abscesses in regional enteritis. Am J Surg 173:350–354
17. Maconi G, Bollani S, Bianchi Porro G (1996) Ultrasonographic detection of intestinal complications in Crohn's disease. Dig Dis Sci 41:1643–1648
18. Lim JH (1996) Colorectal cancer: sonographic findings. Am J Roentgenol 167:45–47
19. McGregor DH, Liu X, Ulusarac O, Ponnuru KD, Schnepp SL et al (2011) Colonic perforation resulting from ingested chicken bone revealing previously undiagnosed colonic adenocarcinoma: report of a case and review of literature. World J Surg Oncol 9:24
20. Rathaus V, Erez I, Zissin R (2006) Ileal perforation due to an ingested fragment of a skewer. J Ultrasound Med 25:389–391
21. Beyer D, Modder U (1988) Diagnostic imaging of the abdomen. Springer, Berlin

Esophageal Perforation: Assessment with Multidetector Row Computed Tomography

4

Nicola Gagliardi, Ciro Stavolo, and Angela De Gennaro

4.1 Introduction

Esophageal perforation is still associated with a high mortality rate, even after surgical repair. A variety of stresses can result in an esophageal perforation as a dramatic increase in intraluminal pressure caused by retching as in Boerhaave's syndrome, blunt chest injury or abdominal trauma, and iatrogenic manipulation by instrumentation. These events can result in an increased wall tension followed by perforation [1]. We must consider also perforations due to ingestion of foreign bodies that can directly penetrate the esophageal wall, perforations due to caustic ingestion (Fig. 4.1), and neoplastic perforations. Perforations caused by gunshots or penetrating chest trauma are extremely rare [2, 3]. The majority of injuries (>80 %) are iatrogenic, and the increasing use of endoscopic procedures such as esophagogastroscopy (EGS), transesophageal echocardiography (TEE), and endosonography (EUS) resulted in an increased incidence of EP. Patients who have a history of similar events and present with Mackler's classic triad of vomiting followed by lower thoracic pain and subcutaneous emphysema may quickly be suspected of having an EP [4]. Many patients, however, present with less specific symptoms such as severe respiratory distress, thoracic pain, hypotension, or shock suggestive of myocardial infarction or acute aortic dissection. Because EP is a life-threatening condition that may rapidly progress to acute mediastinitis and septic shock, clinical suspicion of EP must follow a quick and accurate diagnosis with the aim to improve prognosis for these patients. An accurate diagnosis indeed provides therapeutic indications for conservative or surgical treatment [5]. In most cases the site of perforation is the thoracic esophagus (50–55 %), and distal esophagus is perforated with a lower frequency (25–30 %). Cervical esophagus is seldom perforated (15–18 %) [1, 6].

4.2 Iatrogenic Injuries

Iatrogenic injuries are the most common causes of EP. Many endoscopic procedures such as EGS, TEE, and EUS can result in an abnormal wall tension from instrumentation and subsequent transmural perforation (Fig. 4.2a, b). CT appearances of iatrogenic EP are variable depending on the site and size of perforation and the time elapsed since the onset of symptoms [7]. Beyond these frequent causes, we must remember palliative treatment of esophageal ste-

N. Gagliardi (✉) • C. Stavolo
Department of Radiology, "A. Cardarelli" Hospital, Via Antonio Cardarelli, 9, Naples 80131, Italy
e-mail: n.gagliardi@katamail.com; cirostavolo@alice.it

A. De Gennaro
Department of Diagnostic Imaging and Radiotherapy, Federico II University, Via S. Pansini, 5, Naples 80131, Italy
e-mail: angela.degennaro@hotmail.it

L. Romano, A. Pinto (eds.), *Imaging of Alimentary Tract Perforation*,
DOI 10.1007/978-3-319-08192-2_4,

nosis using laser therapy, electrothermal therapy, and stent placement (Fig. 4.3a, b). EP can also be a complication of sclerotherapy of esophageal varices and surgery of hiatal hernias and rarely occur during placement of Sengstaken-Blakemore tube or insertion of nasogastric tube [8]. A large number of most patients present the

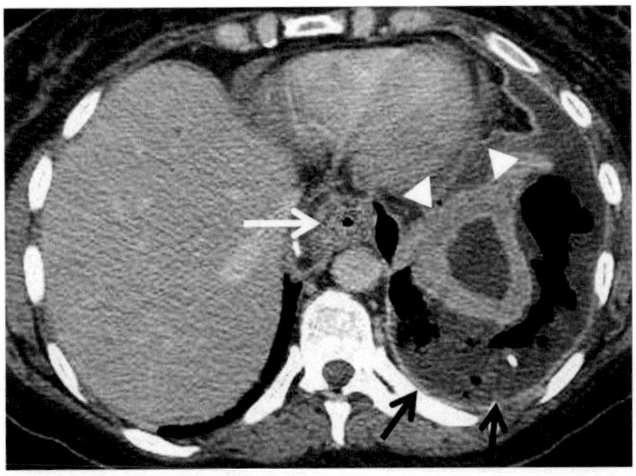

Fig. 4.1 Esophageal-pleural fistula after caustic ingestion: thickened esophageal (*white arrow*) and gastric (*white arrowheads*) walls; left pleural effusion (*black arrows*)

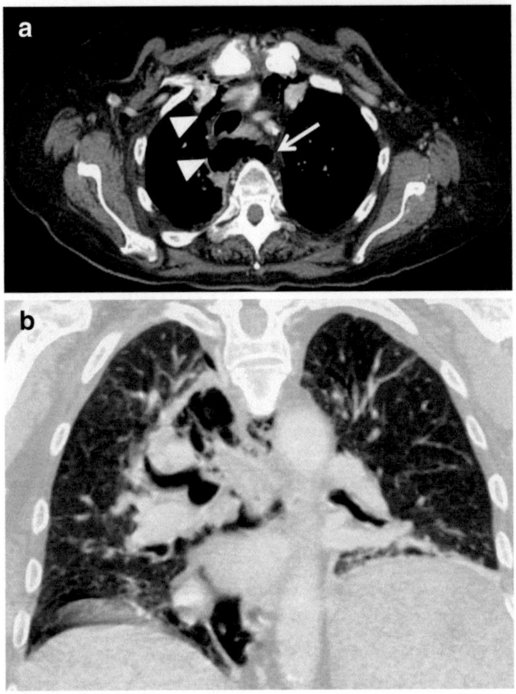

Fig. 4.2 (**a**, **b**) Iatrogenic perforations during endoscopy: esophagus (*arrow*) and extensive pneumomediastinum (*arrowheads*) with early subcutaneous emphysema on the right axilla

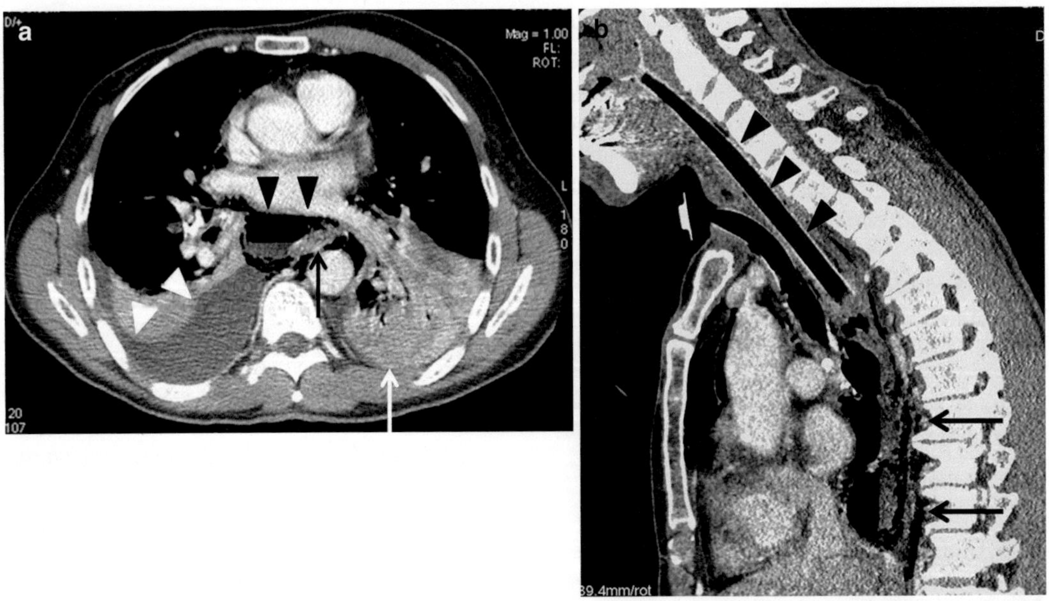

Fig. 4.3 (**a**, **b**) Esophageal perforation after stent placement: (**a**) pneumomediastinum (*black arrowheads*); Rigth pleural effusion (*white arrowheads*) left pleural effusion (*white arrow*); thickened esophageal wall (*black arrow*); (**b**) intraluminal esophageal stent (*black arrowheads*); pneumomediastinum (*black arrows*)

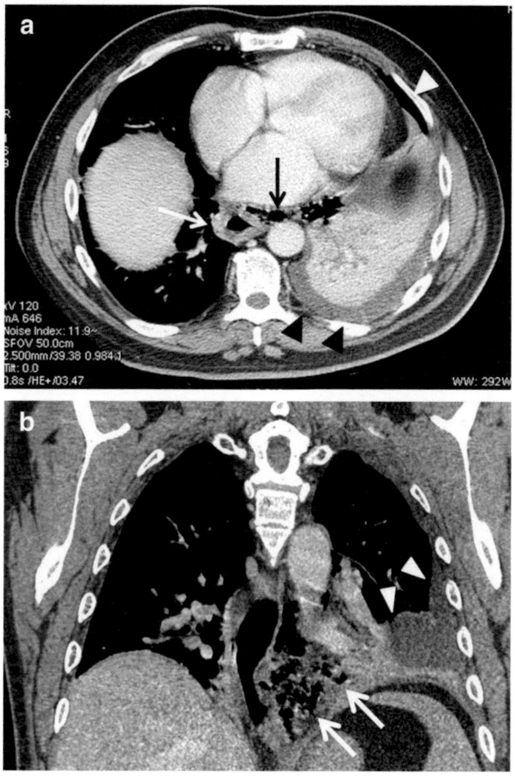

Fig. 4.4 (**a**, **b**) Esophageal perforation after stricture dilatation in achalasia: (**a**) thickened esophageal wall (*white arrow*); pneumomediastinum (*black arrow*); left pleural effusion (*black arrowheads*); pneumothorax (*white arrowhead*); (**b**) pneumomediastinum (*white arrows*); pleural effusion (*white arrowheads*)

classic Mackler's triad but someone have atypical symptoms and the diagnosis of EP is not initially suspected. Other patients have only one or two of the Mackler's triad symptoms. In these cases, a history of a recent endoscopic procedure should recommend the execution of a CT scan because an early diagnosis improves the prognosis of these patients [2, 9].

4.3 Intraluminal Pressure Increase

Intraluminal pressure increase is a frequent cause of EP. This increase may occur for iatrogenic causes, such as during stricture dilation as in achalasia (Fig. 4.4a, b) or, spontaneously, as in Boerhaave's syndrome, in which an incomplete cricopharyngeal relaxation during vomiting results in abruptly intraluminal pressure increase, sufficient to breach esophageal wall [10]. In these cases the distal left posterior wall is the most common site of rupture, which results in a pneumomediastinum and left pleural effusion.

4.4 Foreign Bodies and Other Causes

The esophagus is a common site of impaction of swallowed foreign bodies. EP can occur directly, by full-thickness wall lesion, or indirectly by snap intraluminal pressure increase due to vomiting with an esophageal obstruction [11]. Direct wall perforation may be caused by sharp objects such as bones, dental work with hooks, pins and screws, or nails. In these cases, it can realize a periesophageal abscess formation [11, 12]. Improper foreign body removal by endoscopy can also cause determinate EP. In more difficult cases with a transfixed foreign body, you would prefer to shatter and then pull it out. Sometimes foreign bodies can cause only a mucosal lesion which can cause parietal pneumatosis (Fig. 4.5a, b). Neoplasm can also cause determinate EP. This happens in advanced lesions that cause a progressive wall erosion. Such events are often associated with bleeding [3]. EP due to gunshot or penetrating chest trauma are extremely rare. In most cases it comes to autopsy. However, in patients who have a thoracic gunshot or knife lesion that are submitted to CT scanning, EP must be considered [13].

4.5 CT Findings

The most frequent useful CT findings of EP are manifested by extraluminal variable amounts of air, in relationship with elapsed time, secondly periesophageal fluid collection. CT allows the visualization of very small air or fluid collections, otherwise undetectable, in cases of small tears [5, 14]. Pleural effusions, combined or not with pneumothorax, are most frequently present. Distal perforations are usually asso-

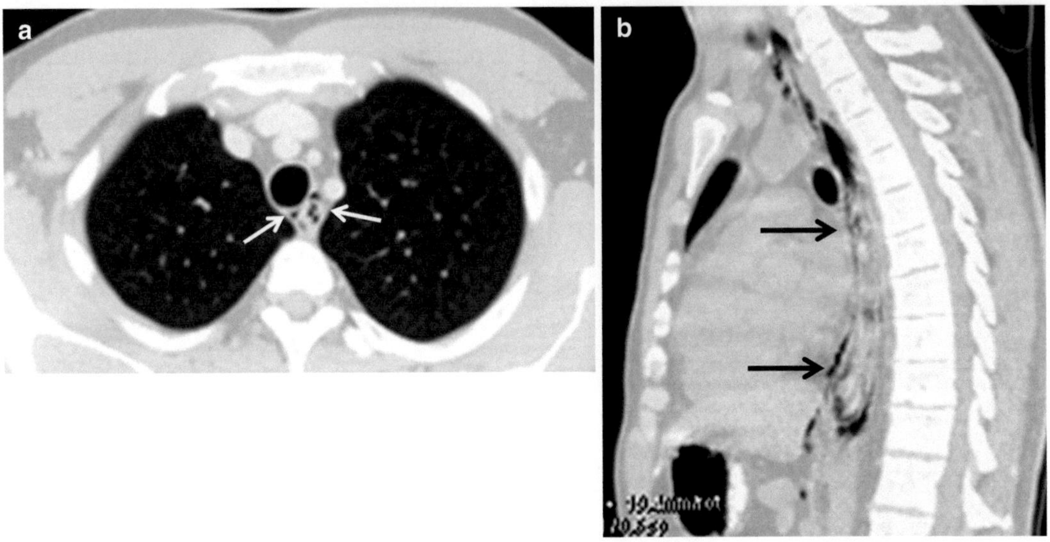

Fig. 4.5 (**a**, **b**) Esophageal parietal pneumatosis after foreign body ingestion: (**a**) *white arrows*; (**b**) *black arrows*

ciated with a left-side pleural effusion or a hydropneumothorax, while a middle perforation is often associated with a right-side pleural effusion. This allows to detect makes it possible to assume the location of the EP [15]. Another CT sign such as esophageal thickening may allow further characterization of the process. In patients with foreign body ingestion, CT allows you to identify the size and the exact spatial position of the foreign body, very useful data for removing.

4.6 Complications

Whatever its cause and the site of perforation, EP is a common point of origin for potentially life-threatening complications which may involve different intrathoracic organs. Mediastinitis at first and then pneumonia, lung abscess, and empyema are among the most commonly seen complications [16]. Tissue destruction due to mediastinitis may result in development of a fistula between the esophagus and adjacent structures including pleural cavity, tracheobronchial tree, and stomach and very rarely aorta (Fig. 4.6a, b) [17]. Due to these reasons, you must use CT because contrast esophagograms allow identification of EP but not all its complications. CT helps to delineate complications and provides valuable information for early initiation of an appropriate management strategy [17, 18].

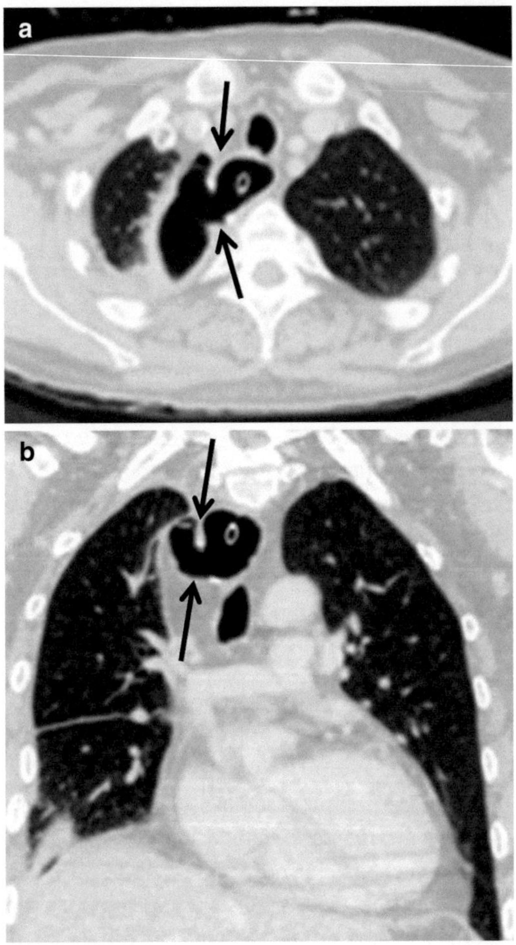

Fig. 4.6 (**a**, **b**) Esophageal-pleural fistula after iatrogenic injury: (**a**, **b**) *black arrows*

Conclusions

Contrast-enhanced CT evaluation of EP requires a high index of suspicion in relation to anamnesis of the patient and attention to findings that may be subtle yet significant. Due to particular anatomic orientation of the esophagus, multiplanar reformatted images are ideally suited to this purpose. They allow a better appreciation of the extent of perforation and their complications and also the possible involvement of adjacent structures. Multidetector CT promotes the radiologist's ability to diagnose accurately EP, reducing delays in diagnosis and improving outcomes in these patients [19].

References

1. Hhuber-Lang M, Henne-Bruns D, Schmitz B, Wurel P (2006) Esophageal perforation: principles of diagnosis and surgical management. Surg Today 36: 332–340
2. Eisen GM, Baron TH, Dominitz JA et al (2002) Guide-line for the m management of ingested foreign bodies. Gastrointest Endosc 55(7):802–806
3. Ferguson MK (1997) Esophageal perforations and caustic injury: management of perforated esophageal cancer. Dis Esophagus 10(2):90–94
4. Brinster CJ, Singhal S, Lee L, Marshall BM, Kaiser LR, Kucharczuk JC (2004) Evolving options in the management of esophageal perforation. Ann Thorac Surg 77(4):1475–1483
5. With CS, Templeton PA, Attar S (1992) Esophageal perforation: CT findings. AJR Am J Roentgenol 160:767–770
6. Pate JW, Walker WA, Cole FH Jr, Owen EW, Johnson WH (1989) Spontaneous rupture of the esophagus: a 30-years experience. Ann Thorac Surg 47:689–692
7. Younes Z, Johnson DA (1999) The spectrum of spontaneous and iatrogenic esophageal injuries: perforations, Mallory-Weiss tears and hematomas. J Clin Gastroenterol 29(4):306–317
8. Jackson RH, Payne DK, Bacon BR (1990) Esophageal perforation due to Nasogastric intubation. Am J Gastroenterol 85(4):439–442
9. Shcmidt SC, Strauch S, Rosch T et al (2010) Management of esophageal perforations. Surg Endosc 24:2809–2813
10. Pinto A, Romano L (2014) Imaging of foreign bodies. Springer, Milan
11. Li ZS, Sun ZX, Zou DW, Xu GM, Wu RP, Liao Z (2006) Endoscopic management of foreign bodies in the upper-GI tract: experiences with 1088 cases in China. Gastrointest Endosc 64(4):485–492
12. Wu JT, Maxott KL, Wall MJ Jr (2007) Esophageal perforations: new perspectives and treatment paradigms. J Trauma 63(5):1173–1184
13. Cabrera-Hinojosa J, Diaz-Rosales J, Lenin ED, Arambula-Melendez P (2009) Esophageal perforation by gunshot: conservative surgical treatment. Calicut Med J 7(3):4–6
14. Backer CL, Lo Cicero J III, Hartz RS et al (1990) Computed tomography in patients with esophageal perforation. Chest 98:1078–1080
15. Gimenez A, Franquet T, Erasmus JJ, Martinez S, Estrada P (2002) Thoracic complications of esophageal disorders. Radiographics 22:247–258
16. Port JL, Kent MS, Korst RJ, Bacchetta M, Altroki NK (2003) Thoracic esophageal perforations: a decade of experience. Ann Thorac Surg 75(4):1071–1074
17. Eroglu A, Turkyilmaz A, Aydun Y, Yekeler E, Karaoglanoglu N (2009) Current management of esophageal perforations: 20 years experience. Dis Esophagus 22(4):374–380
18. Exaros DN, Malagri K, Tsatalou EG et al (2005) Acute mediastinitis: spectrum of computed tomography findings. Eur Radiol 15:1569–1574
19. Soreide JA, Viste A (2011) Esophageal perforation: diagnostic work-up and clinical decision-making in the first 24 hours. Scand J Trauma Resusc Emerg Med 19:66

5 Role of Multidetector Row Computed Tomography in the Diagnosis of Gastroduodenal Perforation

Daniela Vecchione, Giovanna Russo, and Raffaella Niola

Gastroduodenal perforation is an emergency clinical situation that usually requires early recognition and well-timed surgical treatment. It can arise from different natural, iatrogenic, or traumatic causes, and it can present with various symptoms especially in the early phase.

A precise diagnostic classification is fundamental in order to propose the best therapeutic approach and is usually based on detecting presence, site, cause, and extension of the extraluminal leakage [1].

5.1 Etiology and Mechanism of Perforation

The most common reported cause of gastroduodenal perforation is ulcer disease linked to both infection with *Helicobacter pylori* and frequent use of aspirin (ASA) and other nonsteroidal anti-inflammatory drugs (NSAID) [2].

The presence of a peptic ulcer induces loss of normal mucosal integrity, local inflammation, and focal penetration that leads to local pathologic changes of the normal mural anatomy. Gastroduodenal perforation related with peptic ulcer is usually located at level of the gastric antrum and duodenal bulb (Figs. 5.1 and 5.6) Variable location of the ulcer produces different consequences; a deep anterior ulcer may perforate directly into the peritoneal cavity, whereas posterior stomach or duodenal ulcers often cause a confined perforation.

Other reported causes are traumatic, neoplastic, foreign body ingestion, and iatrogenic.

With regard to iatrogenic causes, blunt trauma usually induces perforation of the descending and horizontal segments of duodenum because of their firm attachment and the compression against the vertebral column.

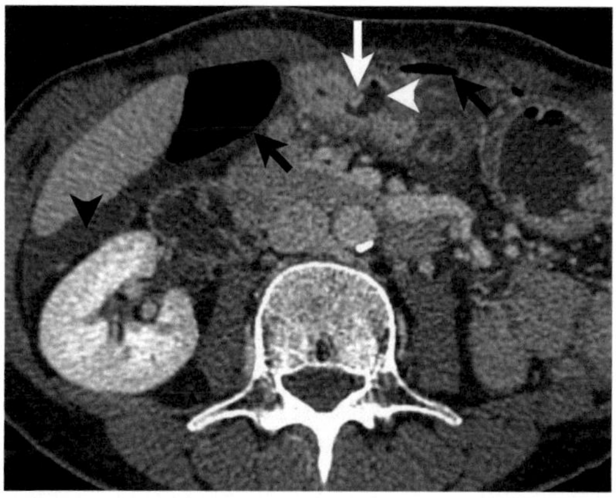

Fig 5.1 Axial MPR CT image. Perforation of the anterior wall of the gastric antrum. Focal defect in the anterior wall of the gastric antrum associated with surrounding mural thickening (*white arrow*). Pneumoperitoneum (*black arrow*). Extraluminal fluid with small free air bubble inside (*white arrowhead*). Intraperitoneal fluid in subhepatic space (*black arrowhead*)

D. Vecchione (✉) • G. Russo • R. Niola
Department of Radiology, "A. Cardarelli" Hospital, A. Cardarelli, Naples 80131, Italy
e-mail: danielavecchione@hotmail.it; giovyrusso1976@gmail.com; raffaellaniola@tiscali.it

L. Romano, A. Pinto (eds.), *Imaging of Alimentary Tract Perforation*,
DOI 10.1007/978-3-319-08192-2_5, © Springer International Publishing Switzerland 2015

Neoplastic causes usually depend on the presence of a tumor that can lead to obstruction or increased endoluminal pressure (Fig. 5.7).

Perforation can also arise from foreign bodies that can be ingested either intentionally or accidentally; this injury can cause perforation either through direct damage or endoluminal obstruction.

In the era of diagnostic and therapeutic use of esophagoduodenoscopy, iatrogenic lesion represents an increasing cause of gastroduodenal perforation. Other iatrogenic causes are related to the placement of inferior vena cava filter, ERCP, and biliary stents [3] (Fig. 5.5).

5.2 Diagnosis

A correct diagnosis of gastroduodenal perforation strictly relies on signs and symptoms referred by the patient and detected during clinical examination. For example, the presence of intermittent abdominal pain, gastroesophageal reflux, ongoing symptoms and sudden exacerbation of pain in known peptic ulcer disease, and recent trauma or diagnostic/therapeutic intervention followed by worsening pain should alert the clinician for the presence of injury [2].

The location of the pain facilitates definitive diagnosis, because with the time a localized peritoneal inflammation develops exactly at level of the injured organ involving a correspondent abdominal wall segment.

Patients with gastroduodenal perforation usually present with signs and symptoms of either local or generalized peritonitis due to the leakage of luminal contents in the peritoneal cavity.

For instance, a lesion of the gastroduodenal wall provokes intra-abdominal contamination with peritonitis or abscesses [4].

The type and the intensity of peritoneal contamination strictly rely on the site, size, and duration of perforation other than other factors such as time from the last meal, coexistent diseases, presence or absence of an ileus or bowel obstruction, etc.

The anatomic site of perforation heavily influences the type and the severity of enteric contamination [5, 6].

Microbiological contamination increases from proximal to distal side of the gastrointestinal tract; the stomach and duodenum show the lowest number of vital microorganisms per gram of luminal contents due to a hostile local environment from acidic, biliary, and pancreatic secretions, and in fact the bacterial load is inversely related to the toxicity of organ fluid composition [7, 8].

Organ-specific fluid composition affects not only bacterial load but also bacterial species composition with consequent different early presenting symptoms from a perforated hollow viscus that can be helpful for the diagnosis. For example, patients suffering from gastric or duodenal perforation usually present with highly acute pain due to a rapid chemical peritonitis usually followed by a systemic inflammatory response. In the untreated patients or in those who have late presentation, the perforation can also proceed to an infected peritonitis and sepsis [9].

Laboratory tests are usually performed to get a correct diagnosis or to facilitate the differential diagnoses. Routinely ordered tests include a complete blood cell count with differential, coagulation panel, electrolyte panel, liver function tests, urinalysis, lipase or amylase, arterial blood gas, and serum lactate level [10, 11].

Laboratory tests are usually nonspecific, but leukocytosis, metabolic acidosis, and hyperamylasemia may be indicative of the presence of perforation.

Plain abdominal films are the initial diagnostic tool in patients with clinically suspected gastroduodenal perforation. In addition to upright and supine abdominal radiographic images, upright chest films and/or left lateral decubitus abdominal films should be included for the accurate evaluation of perforation [1].

The radiologic feature of perforation is the presence of air and/or fluid in the peritoneal cavity, retroperitoneal spaces, mesentery, or ligaments of organs. In some cases, pneumomediastinum or subcutaneous emphysema can also be detected. About one-third of cases of gastroduodenal perforation do not present with pneumoperitoneum on abdominal radiographs. This situation is usually caused by a very small perforation, perforation well contained by adjacent organs, or empty stomach at the time of perforation [12].

The reported sensitivity in the detection of extraluminal air on plain radiography is 50–70 % [13, 14].

US is considered a useful diagnostic tool because even if it is not actually helpful to identify intraperitoneal free gas, it could identify some suggestive findings of gastrointestinal perforation such as the decreased peristalsis and the presence of intraperitoneal free fluid. It is worth to note that usually in the case of gastroduodenal perforation the evidence of free peritoneal fluid is the only finding of injury, but unfortunately US study is not able to define the exact cause for its presence (peritoneal reaction or perforated intestinal loop) [15, 16].

When a perforation of the gut is not proved by plain radiograph and more accurate assessment regarding the site and cause of perforation is needed, a contrast examination may be indicated. Water-soluble iodinated contrast material is administrated orally, if gastroduodenal tract is the suspected site of perforation. It may demonstrate extraluminal contrast material leakage as a direct sign of bowel perforation. However, the reported sensitiveness of extravasation of oral contrast material on plain radiograph varies from 19 to 42 % [17–19].

CT is now estimated the most valuable imaging technique to identify the presence, site, and etiology of gastrointestinal (GI) tract perforation [17].

CT is indicated in two different cases: when clinical suspicion is high, but there is no pneumoperitoneum on the plain abdominal radiograph; the clinical signs are atypical, or, instead, peritonitis is present with no etiological explanation [20].

Several authors have illustrated the direct and indirect CT findings of bowel perforation, and free extraluminal air has been regarded as a major imaging finding to identify the GI tract perforation [17, 21–24].

CT is more sensitive than plain radiography in determining the presence of perforation because it can also display a small amount of free extraluminal, intraperitoneal, or retroperitoneal air. The overall accuracy of CT for predicting the site of bowel perforation has been reported to range between 82 and 90 %. However, the recent introduction of multidetector row CT has improved the accuracy of CT for predicting the site of GI tract perforation [16, 21, 24–26].

According to the perforation site the CT findings may be different. In this chapter, CT findings of gastroduodenal tract perforation will be reported.

5.3 CT Technique

Whole abdomen, from the dome of the diaphragm to the pelvic floor, should be scanned with a multidetector CT (MDCT). The protocol used with a 64-row MDCT included, after the pre-contrast images have been acquired, a helical axial acquisition at 70 s after the intravenous injection of contrast material (400 mgI/mL; 100–150 mL at a rate of 2–3 mL/s), a 1- to 2.5-mm collimation and reconstruction in 0.625 mm contiguous slices.

The analysis was immediate on a workstation, allowing multiplanar reconstructions that were used systematically. In our hospital, we use CT scanning without oral contrast administration for evaluating bowel perforation. In fact, even if the contrast may improve the detection of the lesions site of the posterior gastrointestinal wall, on the other site, it becomes difficult to identify a perforation in the axial scan, when the lesion lies just near the anterior bowel wall.

Although extraluminal leakage of oral contrast material has been reported to be a specific finding for bowel perforation, several authors queried about the extra benefit of oral contrast [13, 17, 22, 27]. Several reports adduce safety issues (i.e., the risk of aspiration and the subsequent complications), the potential delay in the diagnosis, and the lack of substantial extra benefit for detecting bowel perforation.

Further, the slow progression of the oral contrast material in the GI tract in a patient suffering from paralytic ileum, and the quick sealing of the perforation site, may preclude extraluminal leakage of oral contrast material in patients with GI tract perforation [17].

5.4 CT Findings

We classified the CT findings of GI tract perforation as direct and indirect findings. The first one included extraluminal air (free air) and direct visualization of GI tract wall rupture. The second one included focal bowel wall thickening (>8 mm in gastroduodenal wall), abnormal bowel wall enhancement, inflammatory changes (abscess and an inflammatory mass adjacent to the bowel), or a fluid collection in the surrounding soft tissues or organs [1, 21, 23, 28, 29]. Direct visualization of the discontinuity of the bowel wall can specify the presence and site of GI tract perforation, which is marked by a low-attenuating cleft that usually runs perpendicular to the bowel wall on CT [17, 24] (Figs. 5.1 and 5.2). However, this cleft has been reported to be observed less frequently than free air on CT, and a cleft is usually seen in less than 50 % of the patients with GI tract perforation [21, 23, 24, 28]. The relatively infrequent detection of this finding is partly due to the small size of the lesion [23]. MDCT with multiplanar reformation images may help identify discontinuity of the bowel wall, and especially when the axial CT images are indeterminate. Although extraluminal air is highly specific for making the diagnosis of GI tract perforation, it may be absent in gastroduodenal perforation, and especially at the onset of symptom [16]. The sensitivity of plain radiograph to detect free extraluminal air is not high [1, 24]; in contrast, CT is highly sensitive for detecting pneumoperitoneum and very small free air bubbles. To enhance this sensitivity, CT images should also be assessed in the wide window setting that distinguishes air from fat densities [11, 14]. The amount and location of free air could be different according to the perforation site. A large amount of intraperitoneal air usually indicates gastroduodenal perforation, except for bowel perforation, which is caused by obstruction or an endoscopic procedure. Air in the lesser sac is commonly due to posterior perforation of the stomach or duodenum. Free air or an air-fluid level crossing the midline and an accentuating falciform ligament (the "falciform ligament sign") (Fig. 5.6) and free air confined in the intrahepatic fissure for the ligamentum teres (the "ligamentum teres sign") have been considered to be useful findings in patients with perforation of the duodenal bulb or stomach. Air trapped in the mesenteric folds is seldom seen in gastric perforation. Pneumoretroperitoneum is caused by perforation of descending horizontal duodenal tract. Gas in the retroperitoneum does not spread freely as in the peritoneal space; specifically, when the amounts is small, it tends to remain regional with respect to the boundaries of the retroperitoneal compartment in which it arises. Extraluminal free air in the right anterior pararenal space is the reliable CT finding for diagnosing duodenal perforation beyond the bulbar segment [1, 17, 28, 30] (Fig. 5.5).

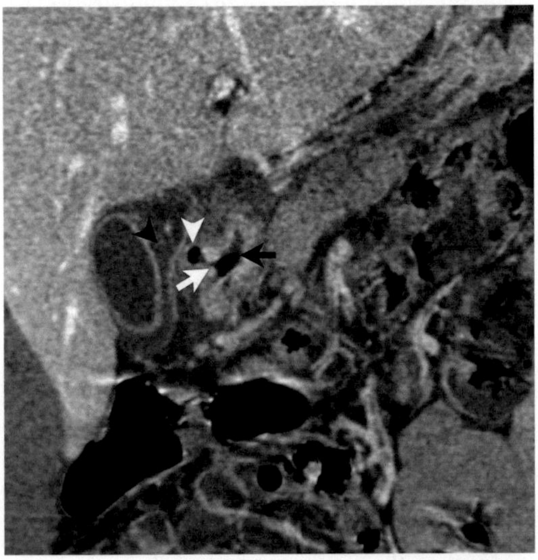

Fig. 5.2 Coronal MIP CT image. Covered perforation of the duodenal bulb. Focal defect in the wall of the duodenal bulb (*white arrow*). Intraluminal air (*black arrow*). Small extraluminal free air bubble (*white arrowhead*). Intraperitoneal fluid (*black arrowhead*)

It should be noted that extraluminal intra- or retroperitoneal air could occur without GI tract perforation. Various causes can produce air, such as mechanical ventilation and pulmonary barotraumas, peritoneal lavage that is performed prior to CT, pneumothorax, chest injury, and entry of air via the female genital tract. Thus, additional CT findings that are indicative of GI tract perforation intensify the significance of extraluminal free air [17, 23].

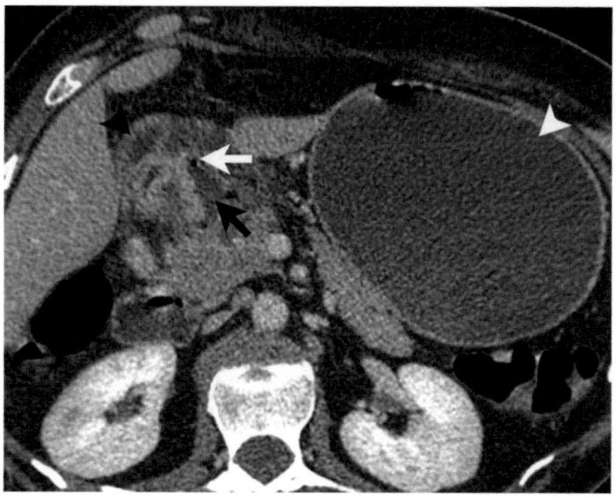

Fig. 5.3 Axial MIP CT image. Covered perforation on the 2nd tract of the duodenum. Very small free air bubble adjacent to the duodenal wall (*white arrow*). Small amount of free fluid in the lesser sac (*black arrow*). Fluid gastric distension (*white arrowhead*). Duodenal wall thickening (*black arrowhead*)

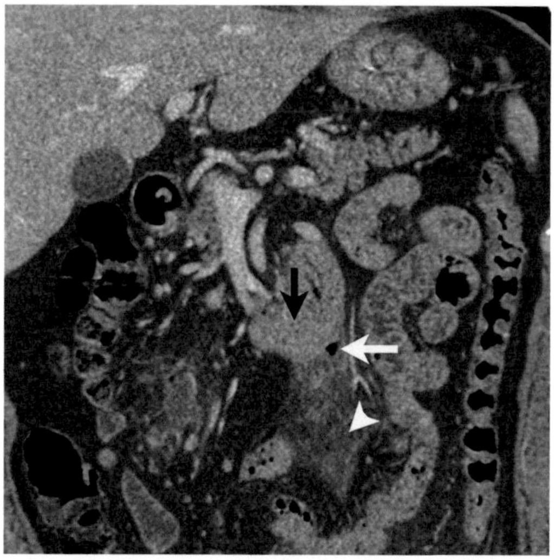

Fig. 5.4 Coronal MIP CT image. Perforation on the 3rd tract of the duodenum. Small free air bubble in close proximity to the duodenal wall (*white arrow*). Wall of the 3rd tract of the duodenum (*black arrow*). Free fluid in left anterior pararenal space associated with local "dirty fat" density (*white arrowhead*)

In addition to the presence of GI tract perforation, concentrated free air bubbles in close proximity to the bowel wall may help determine the site of perforation because free air bubbles tend to be in the vicinity of the bowel wall from which they arise, and especially when the amount of air is small [17, 21].

Among various disease entities, peptic ulcer disease is a major cause of gastroduodenal perforation, followed by necrotic or ulcerated malignancies, iatrogenic injuries, and traumatic injuries [1, 17]. Accuracy of MDCT in predicting site of gastrointestinal tract perforation is 86 %. Three findings were statistically significant predictors of a correct localization of the perforation: ulceration or focal defect of the gastroduodenal wall, air bubbles in close contact with the stomach or the duodenum, segmental bowel wall thickening [1, 21] (Figs. 5.1, 5.2, and 5.3). These findings can be associated with adjacent "dirty fat" density and local fluid between the duodenum and the pancreatic head (Fig. 5.4). Overall, the supramesocolic location of the peritoneal fluid is a persuasive argument for the diagnosis of ulcer perforation [20].

The breach in the gastroduodenal wall is found in 36 % of the cases using conventional, whereas the contribution of the multiplanar reconstructions, provided by MDCT, is huge for the advantages in the search for wall opening when it is not visible on the axial slides [20]. In our experience, multiplanar reconstruction images were routinely performed, which we found to be useful of determining the precise location of bubbles of extraluminal air and defects in the gastroduodenal wall.

However, a large percentage of perforated gastric and duodenal ulcers seal off quickly. Furthermore, ulcers on the posterior wall of the stomach and duodenum may perforate into the pancreas, lesser omentum, transverse mesocolon, liver, spleen, biliary tree, or colon.

Posterior wall peptic ulcers most commonly perforate into the pancreas, resulting in pancreatitis or true abscess formation. Ulcers that perforate into the biliary tree or colon also may lead to fistula. Abscess in the left lobe of the liver or spleen may result from posterior wall penetrating ulcers. As a result, MDCT may be the first modality to suggest the diagnosis of a perforated posterior wall peptic ulcer. Small bubbles of gas or pockets of fluid may be seen trapped near the wall of the stomach or

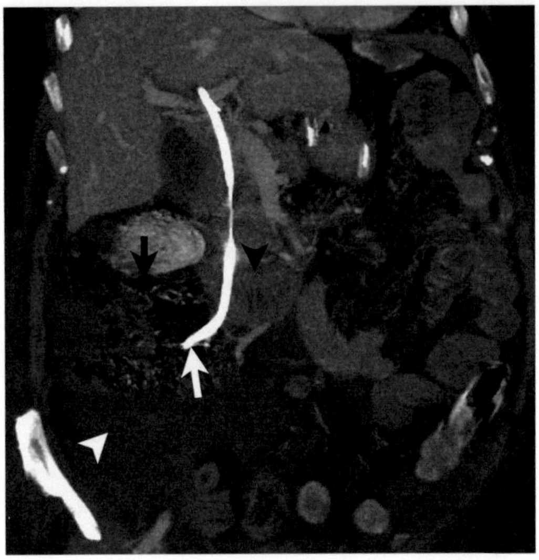

Fig. 5.5 Coronal MIP image: Iatrogenic perforation of the duodenum inferior knee caused by biliary stent. Distal tip of biliary stent located in right pararenal anterior space (*white arrow*). Retroperitoneal free air (*back arrow*). Retroperitoneal free fluid, right pararenal anterior space (*white arrowhead*). The 3rd tract of the duodenum (*black arrowhead*)

duodenum, near the surface of the pancreas, or in the mesenteries near the duodenal bulb and stomach (hepatogastric and hepatoduodenal ligaments). Small bubbles of air also may be detected in the greater or lesser peritoneal sac. MDCT may also reveal evidence of pancreatitis, especially in the pancreatic head, or ascites [31, 32].

Surgeons frequently choose to oversee a perforated ulcer because there is less than a 20 % recurrence rate with therapy. So in patients who have not had surgery, MDCT is an excellent modality for detecting the extraluminal changes associated with a perforation.

A CT-demonstrated postoperative abscess may be caused by the persistence of the inflammatory reaction, continuing or previous perforation at the treated site, or continuing or sealed off anastomotic or staple line leak. Determination of the cause of a postoperative abscess may require a luminal contrast study. Luminal contrast studies are not unfailing in detecting the leaks, because a leak may have sealed off by the time a contrast study is performed (Figs. 5.5, 5.6, and 5.7) [31, 33].

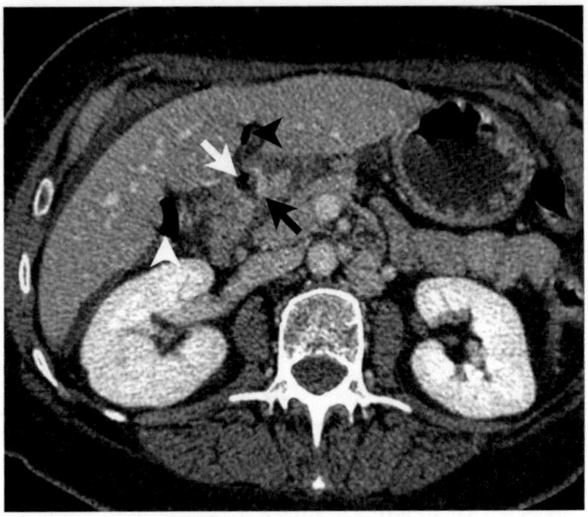

Fig. 5.6 Axial MPR CT image. Perforation of the duodenal bulb. Extraluminal free fluid with a very small air bubble inside (*white arrow*). Focal defect in thickened wall of the duodenal bulb (*black arrow*). Pneumoperitoneum (*white arrowhead*). Falciform ligament sign (*black arrowhead*)

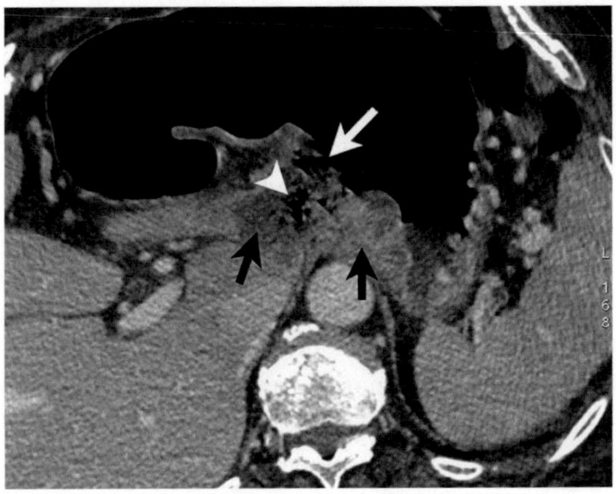

Fig. 5.7 Axial MIP CT image. Neoplastic lesion infiltrating and perforating the posterior wall of the gastric body. Discontinuity in the posterior wall of the gastric body (*white arrow*). Neoplastic lesion infiltrating the posterior wall of the gastric body and the fundus, portal vein, and caudate lobe of liver (*black arrow*). Free air bubbles in the lesser sac (*white arrowhead*)

Anastomotic leaks may be detected at gastroenteric anastomoses. Leaks may also occur at the overseen proximal duodenal stump after Billroth II surgery or after Graham plication of perforated duodenal ulcers. The postoperative contrast examination may show contrast material outside the expected lumen of the bowel filling a collec-

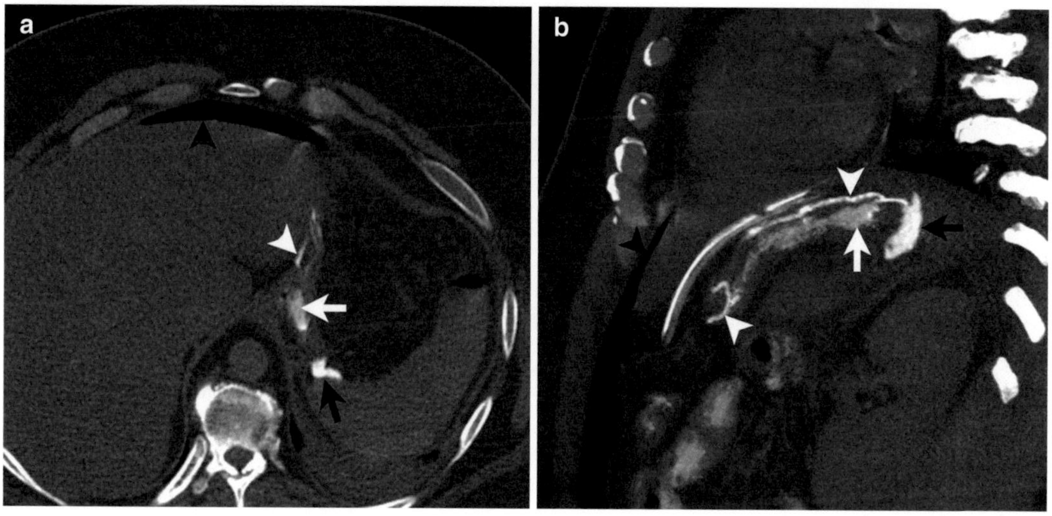

Fig. 5.8 (**a**) Axial MIP CT image (CT performed after oral administration of Gastrografin®). Anastomotic dehiscence in sleeve gastrectomy. Gastrografin® in gastric lumen (*white arrow*). Gastrografin® extraluminal leakage (*black arrow*). Metal stitches (*white arrowhead*). Pneumoperitoneum (*black arrowhead*). (**b**) Sagittal MIP CT image (CT performed after oral administration of Gastrografin®). Anastomotic dehiscence in sleeve gastrectomy. Gastrografin® in gastric lumen (*white arrow*). Gastrografin® extraluminal leakage (*black arrow*). Metal stitches (*white arrowhead*). Pneumoperitoneum (*black arrowhead*)

tion or fistula. MDCT also is useful for demonstrating the size and location of an abscess cavity or guiding percutaneous drainage of an abscess collection. At last, anastomotic or staple line dehiscence also may occur after vertical banded gastroplasty or gastric bypass procedures for morbid obesity [34] (Fig. 5.8).

Conclusion

It is crucial to make a prompt and correct diagnosis of GI tract perforation with respect to the presence, site, and cause of perforation, and this helps the physician choose the optimal therapeutic option. MDCT allows radiologists not only to detect intra-abdominal free air but also to precisely determine the anatomic site of GI tract perforation without the use of oral contrast material. CT findings such as discontinuity of the bowel wall, concentrated bubbles of extraluminal air in close proximity to the bowel wall, and abrupt bowel wall thickening with or without an associated phlegmon or abscess are useful for assessing the site of perforation.

CT examination is considered more sensitive than abdominal plain film in detection of peritoneal free air, but our advice is, it cannot become the first step imaging technique in a busy emergency department and in all patients with clinical suspicion of gastroduodenal tract perforation, because of its costs and availability of the equipment [29].

In our experience, sensitivity of the plain films allowed a correct identification of a huge percentage of patients with direct findings of perforations. When the first plain film is negative, it is useful to repeat it few hours later [13, 29].

MDCT is useful in the diagnosis of gastroduodenal ulcer perforation when the clinical examination combined with the plain abdominal films does not provide a clear diagnosis or when a pneumoperitoneum or atypical signs have not been detected on plain film.

The use of three-dimensional reformatting is mandatory to improve the detection of the wall breach when it has not been showed on the axial slices [20].

References

1. Furukawa A, Sakoda M, Yamasaki M (2005) Gastrointestinal tract perforation: CT diagnosis of presence, site, and cause. Abdom Imaging 30:524–534

2. Luy FY, Davis KA (2010) Gastroduodenal perforation: maximal or minimal intervention? Scand J Surg 99:73–77
3. Langel JT, Mulvihill SJ (2008) Gastrointestinal perforation and the acute abdomen. Med Clin North Am 92:599–625a
4. Ordonez CA, Puyana JC (2006) Management of peritonitis in the critically ill patient. Surg Clin North Am 86:1323–1349
5. Sjostedt S, Kager L, Heimdahal A et al (1998) Microbiological colonization of tumors in relation to the upper gastrointestinal tract in patients with gastric carcinoma. Ann Surg 207:341–346
6. Sjostedt S, Heimdahal A, Kager L et al (1985) Microbiological colonization of oropharynx, esophagus and stomach in patients with gastric disease. Eur J Clin Microbiol 4:49–51
7. Guarner F (2006) Enteric flora in health and disease. Digestion 73(Suppl 1):5–12
8. Guarner F, Malageleda JR (2003) Gut flora in health and disease. Lancet 361:512–519
9. Wittman DH, Shein M, Condon RE (1996) Management of secondary peritonitis. Ann Surg 224(1):10–18
10. Lyon C, Clark DC (2006) Diagnosis of acute abdominal pain in older patients. Am Fam Physician 74(9):1537–1544
11. Gerhardt RT, Nelson BK, Keenan S et al (2005) Derivation of a clinical guideline for the assessment of nonspecific abdominal pain: the guideline for abdominal pain in the ED setting (GAPEDS) phase 1 study. Am J Emerg Med 23:709–717
12. Pinto A, Scaglione M, Pinto F et al (2000) Helical computed tomography diagnosis of gastrointestinal perforation in the elderly patient. Emerg Radiol 7:259–262
13. Maniatis V, Chryssikopoulos H, Roussakis A et al (2000) Perforation of the alimentary tract: evaluation with computed tomography. Abdom Imaging 25:373–379
14. Cho KC, Baker SR (1994) Extraluminal air. Diagnosis and significance. Radiol Clin North Am 32:829–844
15. Grassi R, Romano S, Pinto A, Romano L (2004) Gastro-duodenal perforations: conventional plain film, US and CT findings in 166 consecutive patients. Eur J Radiol 50:30–36
16. Grassi R, Pinto A, Rossi G, Rotondo A (1998) Conventional plain film radiology, ultrasonography and CT in jejuno-ileal perforation. Acta Radiol 39:52–56
17. Kim SH, Shin SS, Jeong YY et al (2009) Gastrointestinal tract perforation: MDCT findings according to perforations sites. Korean J Radiol 10:63–70
18. Jacobsen G, Berne CJ, Meyers HI et al (1961) The examination of patients with suspected perforated ulcer using water-soluble contrast medium. Am J Roentgenol Radium Ther Nucl Med 86:37–49
19. Buecker A, Wein BB, Neuerburg JM et al (1997) Esophageal perforation: comparison of use of aqueous and barium-containing contrast media. Radiology 202:683–686
20. Cazejust J, Castaglioli B, Bessoud B et al (2007) Gastroduodenal perforation: the role of MDCT. J Radiol 88:53–57
21. Hainaux B, Agneessens E, Bertinotti R et al (2006) Accuracy of MDCT in predicting site of gastrointestinal tract perforation. AJR Am J Roentgenol 187:1179–1183
22. Ghekiere O, Lesnik A, Hoa D et al (2007) Value of computed tomography in the diagnosis of the cause of nontraumatic gastrointestinal tract perforation. J Comput Assist Tomogr 31:169–176
23. Brofman N, Atri M, Hanson JM et al (2006) Evaluation of bowel and mesenteric blunt trauma with multidetector CT. Radiographics 26:1119–1131
24. Imuta M, Awai K, Nakayama Y et al (2007) Multidetector CT findings suggesting a perforation site in the gastrointestinal tract: analysis in surgically confirmed 155 patients. Radiat Med 25:113–118
25. Kim HC, Shin HC, Park SJ et al (2004) Traumatic bowel perforation: analysis of CT findings according to the perforation site and the elapsed time since accident. Clin Imaging 28:334–339
26. Miki T, Ogata S, Uto M et al (2004) Multidetector-row CT findings of colonic perforation: direct visualization of ruptured colonic wall. Abdom Imaging 29:658–662
27. Stuhlfaut JW, Soto JA, Lucey BC et al (2004) Blunt abdominal trauma: performance of CT without oral contrast material. Radiology 233:689–694
28. Yeung KW, Chang MS, Hsiao CP et al (2004) CT evaluation of gastrointestinal tract perforation. Clin Imaging 28:329–333
29. Kunin JR, Korobkin M, Ellis JH et al (1993) Duodenal injuries caused by blunt abdominal trauma: value of CT in differentiating perforation from hematoma. AJR Am J Roentgenol 160:1221–1223
30. Rubesin SE, Levine MS (2003) Radiologic diagnosis of gastrointestinal perforation. Radiol Clin North Am 41:1095–1115
31. Fultz PJ, Skucas J, Weiss SL (1992) CT in upper gastrointestinal tract perforations secondary to peptic ulcer disease. Gastrointest Radiol 17:5–8
32. Smith CH, Gore RM (2000) Postoperative stomach and duodenum. In: Gore RM, Levine MS (eds) Textbook of gastrointestinal radiology, 2nd edn. WB Saunders, Philadelphia, pp 682–697
33. Blachar A, Federle MP (2002) Gastrointestinal complications of laparoscopic Roux-en-Y bypass surgery in patients who are morbidly obese: findings on radiography and CT. AJR Am J Roentgenol 179:1437
34. Blachar A, Federle MP, Pealer KM et al (2002) Gastrointestinal complications of laparoscopic Roux-en-Y gastric bypass surgery: clinical and imaging findings. Radiology 223:625–632

Small Bowel Perforations: Imaging Findings

6

Stefania Romano

6.1 Introduction

Perforation of the gastrointestinal tract is a common surgical presentation [1], may occur spontaneously in various gastrointestinal diseases, or may develop due to an ingested foreign body, iatrogenic complication, and blunt or penetrating injuries [2]. However, perforation of the mesenteric small bowel represents not a frequent cause of an acute abdomen and can be due to different etiologies [3]: in underdeveloped countries, infection is probably the most common cause, while in industrialized nations, perforation may be due to Crohn's disease, diverticulitis, foreign body, trauma, tumor, mechanical obstruction, primary ischemic event, or iatrogenic causes [3]. A prompt diagnosis of hollow viscus perforation is strongly required, in order to avoid significant morbidity and mortality from hemorrhage, peritonitis, or abdominal sepsis [4]. Whereas conventional radiograph still represents in most institutions the first imaging method used in patient with acute abdomen and suspected perforations and detection of extraluminal air on radiographs of the chest or abdomen is often the initial clue to the diagnosis [2], however, this finding may be not visible when the perforation is small, rapidly sealed, or well contained [2].

S. Romano
Department of Radiology, "A. Cardarelli" Hospital, Viale Cardarelli 9, Naples 80131, Italy
e-mail: stefromano@libero.it

Because the clinical signs and symptoms of these injuries are often not specific and usually develop late, a timely diagnosis of damages requiring operative repair depends almost exclusively on their early detection by the radiologist on computed tomography (CT) examination [4]. Actually, CT exam is even more considered as a good initial imaging examination in patients with an acute abdomen [3]. CT findings in the setting of small bowel perforations are often subtle but, when present, may help the radiologist determine a specific cause of perforation and make the correct diagnosis [3]. In fact, in recent years, CT has been shown to be accurate for predicting the site of GI perforation and has become the investigation of choice [1, 3, 4]: differentiating features consequently strongly facilitate the accurate multidisciplinary preoperative evaluation, necessary to plan patient management and potential surgical approach [1].

6.2 Imaging Findings

Perforation of the small intestine represents an emergent medical condition for which the diagnosis is usually not made clinically but by CT, a common imaging modality used for the diagnosis of acute abdomen [5]. A spontaneous pneumoperitoneum usually indicates perforation of a hollow viscus and requires undelayed operative intervention [6].

A plain film examination is often performed before surgery to establish a definitive diagnosis

L. Romano, A. Pinto (eds.), *Imaging of Alimentary Tract Perforation*,
DOI 10.1007/978-3-319-08192-2_6, © Springer International Publishing Switzerland 2015

[6]: with careful attention to technique and localizing anatomic features, it can be a valuable examination, capable of detecting even a very small collection of free air [6], if technically adequate. The presence of free abdominal gas as well as indirect findings of perforation could be appreciable at the conventional radiograph [7]: jejunal and ileal perforations could be diagnosed by direct or indirect findings [7]. It is important to note that jejunal are more rare than ileal perforations and more difficult to identify by conventional radiology [7], which could miss also the presence of free gas signs [7].

Although sonography may not be considered as a first-line investigation of choice in suspected small intestinal perforation [8], identification of free intraperitoneal fluid and intestinal peristalsis alterations may aid the radiologist in the early diagnosis [7, 8].

At CT examinations, direct features that suggest small bowel perforation which are often associated with secondary CT signs of bowel pathology include extraluminal air and oral contrast [5]: whereas the use of i.v. contrast medium could be considered essential in emergency exam, the use of oral endoluminal contrast is more often – if not exclusively – done in elective conditions. CT findings related to intestinal perforation include the presence of free gas or fluid within the supra- and/or inframesocolic compartments, segmental bowel wall thickening, bowel wall discontinuity, free air location, mottled extraluminal air bubbles or micropneumoperitoneum, stranding of the mesenteric fat, and abscess formation [1, 9] (Figs. 6.1, 6.2, 6.3, and 6.4). However, the imaging findings may be also subtle or only indirectly related to the site or etiology of perforation [1]. In order to improve efficient diagnosis, the use of slice thickness around or less than 1 mm could represent a tool to better achieve good quality reformations and related useful informations for the diagnosis of the perforation site in patients with pneumoperitoneum [10].

6.3 Considerations

The etiology of small intestine perforations seems to influence the diagnostic performance also in CT examinations: in blunt small bowel perforation, discontinuity of the bowel wall and extraluminal gas has been reported, respectively, on 19.2 and 74.4 % of examinations [11], attesting a CT diagnosis as highly specific but not sensitive [11].

Inflammatory conditions of the small intestines could be considered in evaluating CT examinations of patients with acute abdomen and suspected hollow viscus perforations. Crohn's disease and other inflammatory conditions and complications with presence of abscesses must be accurately noted in location and distribution. A rare condition causing perforations almost localized and covered is represented by the small bowel diverticulitis [12], in which wall thickening of the small bowel loop and an adjacent inflammatory mass containing air bubbles [12] could be noted. Small bowel diverticula are rare and mostly asymptomatic [12], but they become clinically relevant when complications arise, such as diverticulitis [12]. The symptoms of jejunoileal diverticulitis are nonspecific, and the diagnosis is performed mainly by imaging studies [12], especially CT. Small bowel diverticulitis at CT usually presents as a focal inflammatory lesion, and the differential diagnosis includes perforated neoplasm, foreign body perforation,

Fig. 6.1 A 38-year-old patient with acute abdomen from ileal perforation. CT examination shows the presence of free peritoneal air with falciform ligament sign (**a**, **b**) and some small peritoneal bubble gas; multiplanar reconstructions seem to show the evidence of bowel discontinuity at level of the left colonic flexure (**c**, *arrow* in **d**); however, surgery revealed the presence of an ileal perforation. Small amount of peritoneal fluid and presence of free peritoneal air in the abdomen can be appreciated (**e**, **f**); note some bubbles of gas in the soft tissue of the right abdominal wall (*small arrow* in **g**). Small intestinal loops of jejunum and proximal ileum are collapsed, whereas in the pelvis, free peritoneal air (*longer arrow* in **g**) surrounds an ileal loop distended by fluid with signs of endoluminal stasis (**f**)

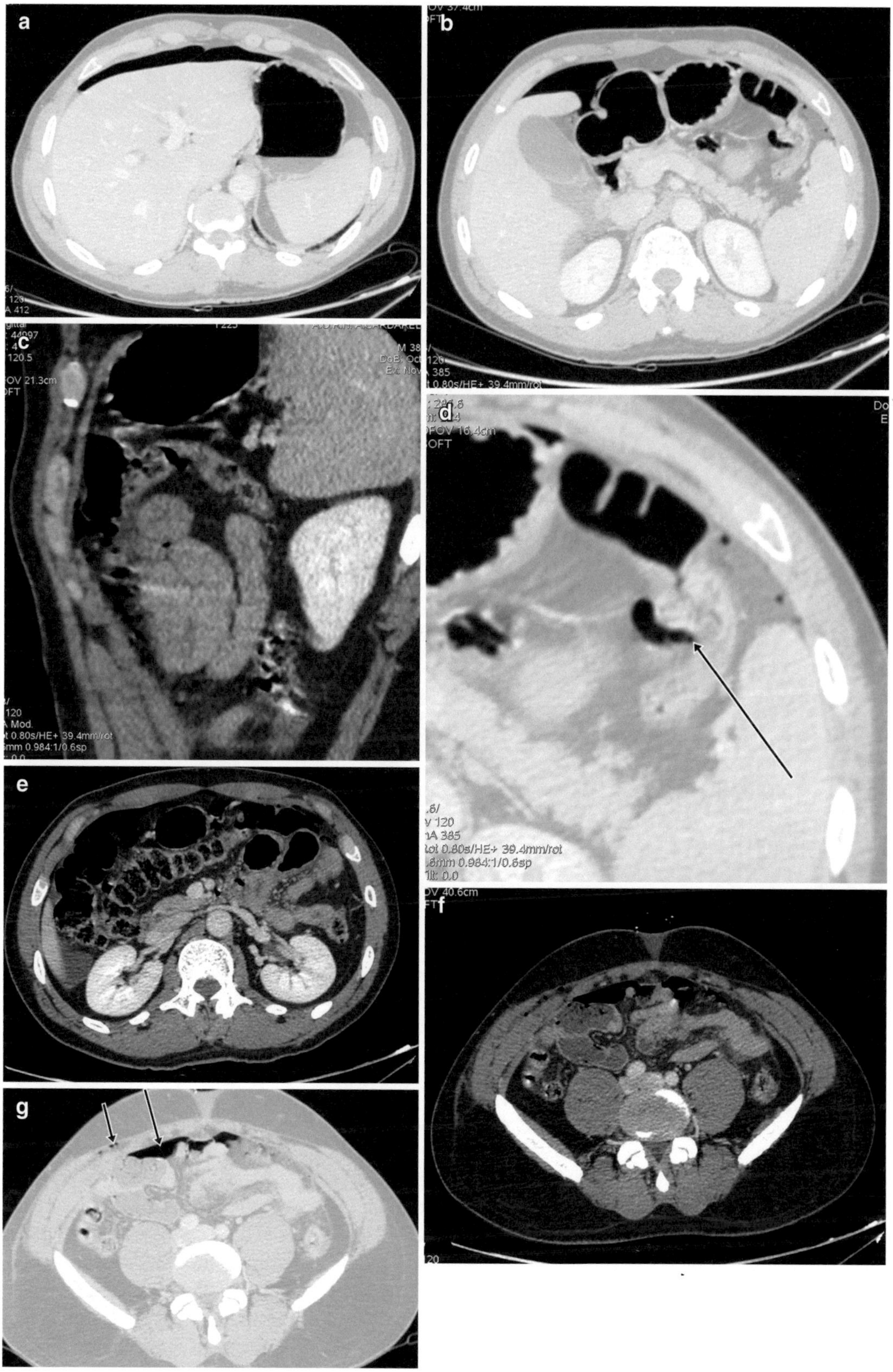
a
b
c
d
e
f
g

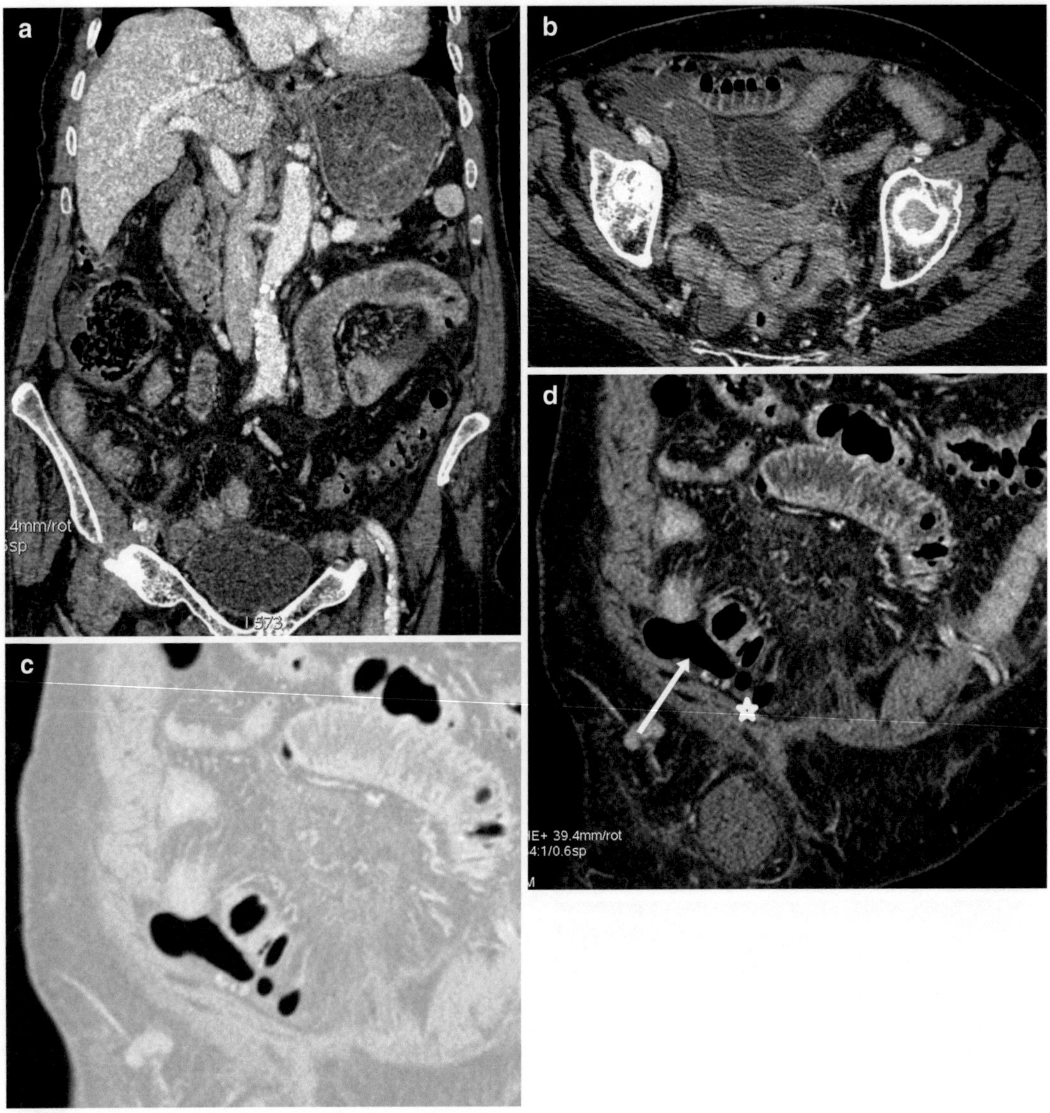

Fig. 6.2 A 90-year-old patient with acute abdomen due to perforation from small bowel complicated obstruction. CT shows the presence of small amount of free peritoneal fluid (**a**, **b**), fluid distension of the stomach, moderate distension of some small intestinal loops at the left abdominal quadrant with parietal thickening (**a**). Note the evidence of bowel segment distended by fluid and with decreased enhancement in the right iliac fossa (**b**). The presence of small amount of free air surrounding a bowel loop in the right iliac fossa is evident (**c**, *arrow* and *star* in **d**)

small bowel ulceration from nonsteroidal anti-inflammatory drug use, Crohn's disease, and diverticulitis [13, 14].

Different and various processes may cause acute peritonitis from perforations: on CT, in addition to the small bowel findings, there is some combination of free intraperitoneal gas or fluid, mesenteric edema, and peritoneal thickening [15]. In the presence of focal perforation of the gastrointestinal tract, the specific site of perforation seems to be identifiable on CT in 85–90 % of cases [11, 16]. Moreover, in addition to directly visualizing the site of perforation, associated CT findings to look for include a cluster of extraluminal gas bubbles close to the suggestive perforation site as well as an abscess

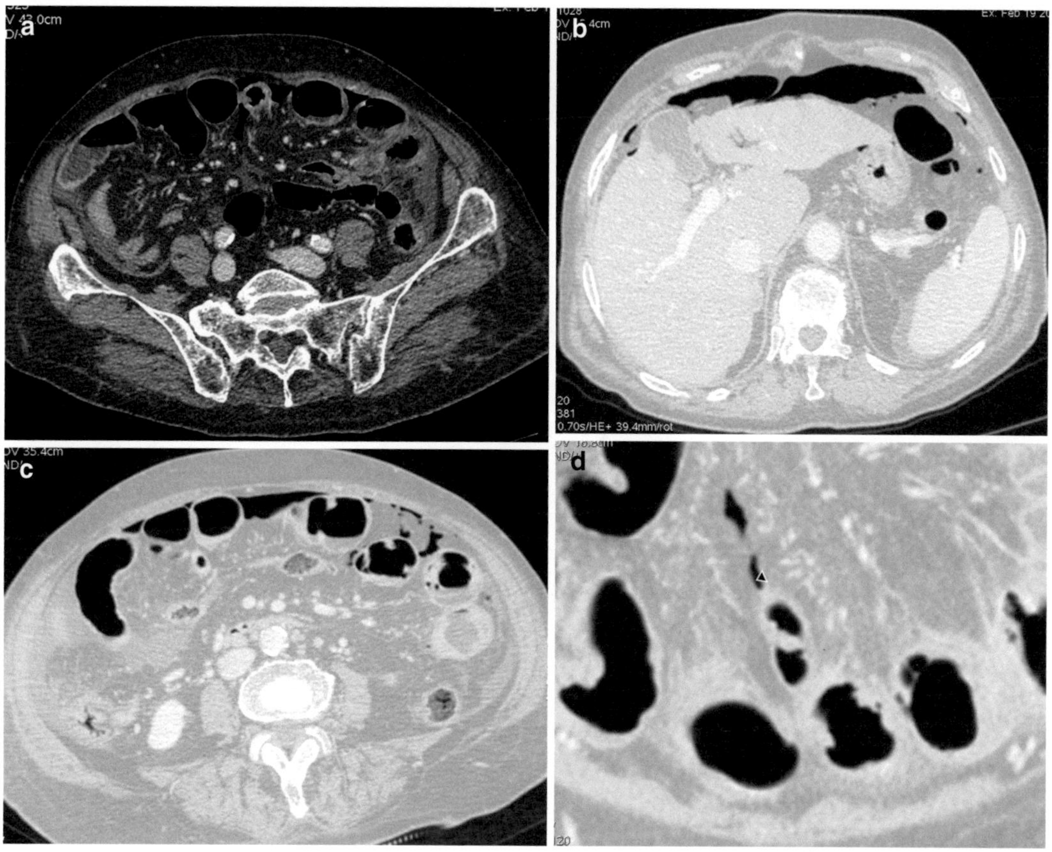

Fig. 6.3 An 88-year-old patient with perforation from small bowel obstruction. CT shows the presence of free peritoneal air (**a–d**), small amount of free fluid, small bowel proximal loops moderately distended, some of them characterized by altered trophism. Multiplanar reformation shows the presence of linear mesenteric gas surrounding a small intestinal loop in the left abdominal quadrant suggestive of fissuration (*arrowhead* in **d**)

formation [11, 16] especially in covered perforations. In patients affected by severe disease and poorer outcome from intestinal perforations, the attenuation of the peritoneum on non-contrast CT has been reported as significantly lower, presumably reflecting a greater degree of edema [17]. The specific air distribution seems to be more frequently present in patients with gastroduodenal perforations than lower gastrointestinal tract perforations [18]; however, the specific air distribution had a less significant role than the strong predictors of the site of bowel perforation [18]. Periportal free air sign has been reported as a useful finding that can help to distinguish upper from lower gastrointestinal tract perforation: when this sign is present, upper gastrointestinal tract perforation is strongly suggested [19]. However, the specific air distribution could be also influenced by the perforation site, the elapsed time after perforation, and the amount of pneumoperitoneum [18]. Therefore, prediction of the perforation site using specific free air distributions could be considered as limited [18].

A correctly performed CT examination represents the basic condition for an efficient diagnosis. Administration of intravenous contrast medium could be considered important for all the acute intestinal conditions in order to evaluate the bowel wall feature and enhancement, essential and useful for all differential diagnoses. In suspected gastrointestinal perforations, the incremental diagnostic value of low-thickened around or less than 1 mm slice reconstructions for direct visualization of the perforation site in patients

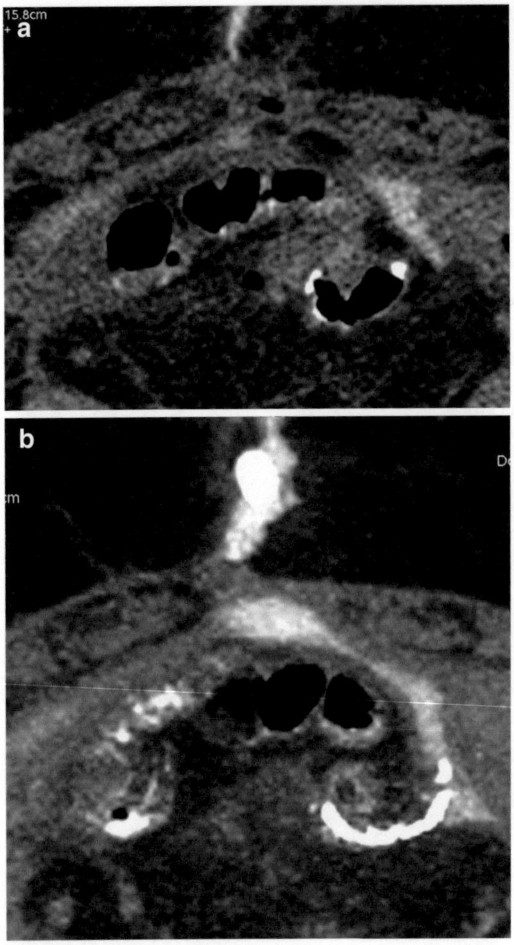

Fig. 6.4 A 56-year-old patient with anastomotic leaks well documented by the endoluminal positive contrast medium (**a**, **b**)

with nontraumatic free pneumoperitoneum has been already assessed [10] as well as the agreement between readers as significantly higher with thin slices and reformatting [10]. Regarding the CT features related to small bowel perforation, the presence of extraluminal air is the first finding to search for, from the CT-falciform ligament sign crossing the midline to scattered pockets of air [20]. Small bowel wall thickening (>3 mm) [20], either segmental or diffuse, could represent the second important finding to note for. All the eventual associated signs such as intestinal fluid or gas distension or collapsed loops, abscess formation, peritoneal, fat stranding evidence [20], they have to be considered as puzzle pieces in order to make a suggestive diagnostic frame (Fig. 6.1). With respect to conventional plain film, CT is able to detect extraluminal air in more cases and could actually represent a good imaging tool to differentiate the various types of gastrointestinal perforations [20]. Among not frequent causes of pneumoperitoneum, there are also the ingested foreign bodies such as generally unconsciously ingested chicken and fish bones [21]. From a clinical point of view, the acute presentations of this intestinal damage are nonspecific, mimicking more common acute abdominal conditions [21]: at CT thickened intestinal segment with localized pneumoperitoneum, surrounded by fatty infiltration and associated with already present or developing obstruction or subobstruction, could represent the most common CT signs; however, the specific diagnosis could be done by the identification of the foreign bodies [21]. The high specificity of the CT diagnosis in making avoidance of surgical exploration possible has been reported not only in the latter case of perforations just reported [21] but also in evaluating postoperative acute abdominal conditions such as post-laparoscopic interventional procedures [22]. In case of evaluation of patients who underwent laparoscopic procedures more frequently such as cholecystectomies, the eventual intestinal perforation due to trocar injury leads to extensive pneumoperitoneum [22]. In fact, small bowel injuries should be suspected when at CT examination a large or an increasing amount of free air is detected following laparoscopic procedures [22].

CT diagnosis of perforation is essentially based on direct findings of extraluminal air or positive oral contrast medium, as well as on indirect findings of an abscess or an inflammatory mass or a bowel wall-related phlegmon or abscess with fluid in the mesentery or surrounding a radiopaque foreign body [23]. The CT sensitivity in intestinal perforations in the emergency setting is high; however, further evaluations by the use of endoluminal positive contrast medium could be required to demonstrate the site and nature of the perforation [2], especially in postoperative intestine to evaluate any eventual anastomotic leaks (Fig. 6.4).

Perforation is also a serious life-threatening complication of lymphomas involving the gastrointestinal tract [24]; although some perforations occur as the initial presentation of gastrointestinal lymphoma, others occur after initiation of chemotherapy [24]. It has been reported that the median day of perforation after initiation of chemotherapy is 46 days and 44 % of perforations occur within the first 4 weeks of treatment [24]; damage to the intestinal microvasculature resulting in ischemia seems to be the common underlying mechanism of this kind of bowel injury [25, 26]. Diffuse large B-cell lymphoma has been reported as the most common lymphoma associated with perforation [24]; compared with indolent B-cell lymphomas, the risk of perforation was higher with aggressive B-cell lymphomas or T-cell/other types [24]. The small intestine has been reported as the most common site of perforation (59 %) in intestinal lymphomas [24], which remains a significant complication more frequently associated with aggressive than indolent lymphomas [24]. Perforation often occurs at tumor sites or surgical anastomoses as well [25]. Tumor rupture and gastrointestinal perforation have been also reported in patients with gastrointestinal stroma tumor treated with imatinib, a tyrosine kinase inhibitor [27]. Intestinal perforations may also result from intraperitoneal chemotherapy for advanced ovarian cancer [28], and the resulting bowel injury may lead to peritonitis [26].

Finally, controversies exist regarding the need for contrast agents for emergency abdominal computed tomography examinations [29]. A survey on the US Academic Emergency Departments to document national practice [29] was recently performed in which respondents were asked about their institutions' use of oral, intravenous (i.v.), and rectal contrast for various abdominal/pelvic CT indications [29]. Intravenous contrast was the most frequently cited contrast [29], with at least 90 % of respondents reported using i.v. contrast in 12/18 indications [29]. Oral contrast was more variably used and rectal contrast was rarely used [29]. Among the most common indications for which no contrast agent has been used, viscus perforation was reported in 19 % [29].

In conclusion, although if CT seems to be able to accurately predict upper gastrointestinal tract perforation with high reliability [9] than for other perforation sites, knowledge of whole CT findings predicting perforation site can overall improve the diagnostic accuracy [9] also in evaluating the small intestine.

References

1. Zissin R, Osadchy A, Gayer G (2009) Abdominal CT findings in small bowel perforation. Br J Radiol 82(974):162–171
2. Macari M, Balthazar EJ (2001) Review: computed tomography of bowel wall thickening: significance and pitfalls of interpretation. AJR Am J Roentgenol 176:1105–1116
3. Hines J, Rosenblat J, Duncan DR et al (2013) Perforation of the mesenteric small bowel: etiologies and CT findings. Emerg Radiol 20(2):155–161
4. LeBedis CA, Anderson SW, Soto JA (2012) CT imaging of blunt traumatic bowel and mesenteric injuries. Radiol Clin North Am 50(1):123–136
5. Cho CK, Baker SR (2005) Manifestations of intraperitoneal air. In: Meyers MA (ed) Dynamic radiology of the abdomen: normal and pathologic anatomy. Springer, New York, pp 309–331
6. Kim HC, Yang DM, Kim SW et al (2014) Gastrointestinal tract perforation: evaluation of MDCT according to perforation site and elapsed time. Eur Radiol 24:1386–1393
7. Broder JF, Amedani AG, Liu SW et al (2013) Emergency department contrast practices for abdominal/pelvic computed tomography – a national survey and comparison with the American College of Radiology appropriateness criteria. J Emerg Med 44(2):423–433
8. Hainaux B, Agneessens E, Bertinotti R et al (2006) Accuracy of MDCT in predicting site of gastrointestinal tract perforation. AJR Am J Roentgenol 187:1179–1183
9. Singh JP, Steward MJ, Booth TC et al (2010) Evolution of imaging for abdominal perforation. Ann R Coll Surg Engl 92(3):182–188
10. Kuzmich S, Burke CJ, Harvey CJ et al (2013) Sonography of small bowel perforations. AJR Am J Roentgenol 201:W283–W291. doi:10.2214/AJR.12.9882
11. Ghahremani GG (1993) Radiologic evaluation of suspected gastrointestinal perforations. Radiol Clin North Am 31(6):1219–1234
12. Grassi R, Pinto A, Rossi G et al (1998) Conventional plain film radiology, ultrasonography and CT in jejuno-ileal perforations. Acta Radiol 39(1):52–56
13. Coulier B, Tancredi MH, Ramboux A (2004) Spiral CT and multidetector-row CT diagnosis of perforation of the small intestine caused by ingested foreign bodies. Eur Radiol 14(10):1918–1925

14. Ho AC, Horton KM, Fishman EK (2000) Perforation of the small bowel as a complication of laparoscopic cholecystectomy: CT findings. Clin Imaging 24(4):204–206
15. Maniatis V, Chryssikopoulos H, Roussakis A et al (2000) Perforation of the alimentary tract: evaluation with computed tomography. Abdom Imaging 25(4):373–379
16. Vaidya R, Habermann TM, Donohue JH et al (2013) Bowel perforation in intestinal lymphoma: incidence and clinical features. Ann Oncol 24(9):2439–2443
17. Liu YI, Jha P, Zhen J et al (2012) Abdominal complications of chemotherapy: findings at computed tomography. Clin Imaging 36:54–60
18. Badgwell BD, Camp ER, Feig B et al (2008) Management of bevacizumab associated bowel perforation: a case series and review of the literature. Ann Oncol 19:577–582
19. Benjamin RS, Blanke CD, Blay JY et al (2006) Management of gastrointestinal stromal tumors in the imatinib era: selected case studies. Oncologist 11:9–20
20. Ghekiere O, Lesnik A, Millet I et al (2007) Direct visualization of perforation sites in patients with a non-traumatic free pneumoperitoneum: added diagnostic value of thin transverse slices and coronal and sagittal reformations for multi-detector CT. Eur Radiol 17(9):2302–2309
21. Park MH, Shin BS, Namgung H (2013) Diagnostic performance of 64-MDCT for blunt small bowel perforation. Clin Imaging 37(5):884–888
22. Graña L, Pedraja I, Mendez R et al (2009) Jejuno-ileal diverticulitis with localized perforation: CT and US findings. Eur J Radiol 71(2):318–323
23. Macari M, Faust M, Liang H et al (2007) CT of jejuna diverticulitis: imaging findings, differential diagnosis, and clinical management. Clin Radiol 62:73–77
24. Katz DS, Scheirey CD, Bordia R et al (2013) Computed tomography of miscellaneous regional and diffuse small bowel disorders. Radiol Clin North Am 51:45–68
25. Tsujimoto H, Yaguchi Y, Hiraki S et al (2011) Peritoneal computed tomography attenuation values reflect the severity of peritonitis caused by gastrointestinal perforations. Am J Surg 202:455–460
26. Choi AL, Jang KM, Kim MJ et al (2011) What determines the periportal free air, and ligamentum teres and falciform ligament signs on CT: can these specific air distributions be valuable predictors of gastroduodenal perforation? Eur J Radiol 77:319–324
27. Cho HS, Yoon SE, Park SH et al (2009) Distinction between upper and lower gastrointestinal perforation: usefulness of the periportal free air sign on computed tomography. Eur J Radiol 69:108–111
28. Yeung KW, Chang MS, Hsiao CP et al (2004) CT evaluation of gastrointestinal tract perforation. Clin Imaging 28(5):329–333
29. Ghekiere O, Lesnik A, Hoa D et al (2007) Value of computed tomography in the diagnosis of the cause of nontraumatic gastrointestinal tract perforation. J Comput Assist Tomogr 31:169–176

7 Acute Perforated Appendicitis: Spectrum of MDCT Findings

Stefania Daniele, Silvana Nicotra, and Carlo Liguori

7.1 Introduction

Acute appendicitis represents one of the most frequent abdominal surgical emergencies. Ready diagnosis of this pathology significantly reduces morbidity and mortality, which can be significantly higher in cases with complications.

Whereas in most patients acute appendicitis can present in a quite easy to diagnose scenario, using clinical and laboratory data, some cases can have a very hazy or atypical manifestation forming a hard to diagnose surgical event. Moreover it is important to consider that many other abdominal pathologies can mimic appendicitis signs and symptoms, increasing the differential diagnosis issue [1]. Since the difficult diagnostic process raises the very high percentage of unnecessary surgical appendicectomy or simple laparotomy, anteriorly to MDCT (*multi-detector computed tomography*) era (14–30 %) [2].

S. Daniele
Department of Radiology, "A. Cardarelli" Hospital, Via Carmine 22, Pozzuoli, NA 80078, Italy
e-mail: cheops@tin.it

S. Nicotra
Department of Radiology, "A. Cardarelli" Hospital, Via Terracina 311, Napoli, NA 80125, Italy
e-mail: sissi.nic@inwind.it

C. Liguori (✉)
Department of Radiology, "A. Cardarelli" Hospital, Via Corcione 116, Aversa, NA 81031, Italy
e-mail: carlo.liguori@gmail.com

In order to lower the probability of useless *laparotomy*, MDCT use has been increased. Thanks to high sensitivity (87–99 %) and specificity (92–99 %), especially among adults, this imaging modality has become the technique of choice for an accurate diagnosis [3]. MDCT availability in the appendicitis diagnostic flow chart dramatically lowered unnecessary laparotomy percentage (2 %) [4].

Nowadays MDCT use is the option of choice in cases of suspected acute appendicitis in patients presenting equivocal symptoms and unclear instrumental data. Nevertheless this is the only modality able to assess pathology severity grade with consequential different therapeutic approaches.

7.2 Normal Anatomy

Vermiform appendix is a blind-ended tube varying 2–20 cm (cm) in length, usually located 2–3 cm below the ileocecal valve and having a 1–2 cm thickened wall. In normal conditions the lumen is occupied by fluid or gas and surrounded by homogeneous fat tissue. According to Wakeley classification, five appendix location varieties can been encountered: sub-cecal, pelvic, pre-ileal, post-ileal and retrocecal [5].

In most cases it has the classical inferomedial or retrocecal position (75 %), less frequent is the sub-cecal or pelvic (20 %) and pre- or post-ileal location (5 %) [6].

L. Romano, A. Pinto (eds.), *Imaging of Alimentary Tract Perforation*,
DOI 10.1007/978-3-319-08192-2_7, © Springer International Publishing Switzerland 2015

7.3 Clinical Presentation

In 80 % of cases acute appendicitis is diagnosed on a clinical presentation basis, and its incidence is slightly higher in males (men, 78–92 %; women, 58–85 %).

Typical presentation (50–60 % of cases) is characterised by abdominal diffuse visceral pain subsequently localised in right quadrants, anorexia, nausea, vomiting, fever, right pelvic mass and laboratory leucocytosis. In 20 % of patients, it can be atypical with a large variety of signs and symptoms [1].

Elderly patients, because of the large number of differential diagnoses taken into account, often represent the most challenging clinical issue. Young females are difficult to diagnose as well considering that gynaecological pathologies can mimic a similar scenario. Finally children, in relation to confused clinical history, are always complicated to diagnose.

Appendix anatomical location can condition clinical presentation of the acute pathology, since it is mandatory to understand well anatomical position variants: in cases of *retrocecal* appendicitis, right lumbar pain can be the first symptom, in the absence of pain under deep abdominal palpation.

In cases of pelvic or *sub-cecal* appendicitis, the only manifestation can be represented by urinary or pelvic pain associated with diarrhoea, because of rectal irritation, in the absence of abdominal discomfort.

Pre- or post-ileal appendicitis can be silent in terms of abdominal manifestation and characterised only by vomiting or diarrhoea caused by secondary ileal loop inflammation.

MDCT is extremely helpful in atypical appendicitis diagnoses [7].

7.4 Aetiology and Pathogenesis

In more than 90 % of cases, acute appendicitis is related to an obstructive cause. Obstruction may be due to:

- Appendicolith presence (more than 50 % of cases)
- Lymphoid hyperplasia of the appendix wall
- Foreign bodies
- Parasitic infection (oxyuriasis)
- Neoplasia (colon adenocarcinoma, carcinoid, Kaposi sarcoma and lymphoma)
- Metastasis (colon and breast)

Obstruction of the ileo-appendicular valve determines an increasing pressure in the lumen of the appendix caused by the mucosal continuous secretion, with consequent distension of the viscera.

Visceral distension leads to bacterial multiplication in the appendix, and increased luminal pressure causes occlusion of the wall veins and capillaries with consequential vascular congestion. Progressive lumen enlargement and increasing wall pressure can subsequently determine arterial blood supply reduction, especially in less vascularised zones, like the antimesenteric portion of the loop, and the process finally ends up into wall infarct and *perforation*.

On the other hand it is important to underline that gas, fluid or a clear *appendicolith* can be present in normal appendix too, and presence cannot be considered an unequivocal sign of acute appendicitis [2].

On the anatomopathological basis acute appendicitis can be classified in three different types accounting for micro- and macroscopic characteristics of the surgical specimen:

- *Catarrhal* appendicitis: inflammation is limited to mucosal layer.
- *Phlegmonous* appendicitis: wall inflammation is more extensive than the previous with parietal microscopic phlegmon presence.
- *Gangrenous* appendicitis: is characterised by parietal extensive necrosis.

7.5 Differential Diagnoses

Acute appendicitis must be differentiated by several other acute abdomen causes. Main factors can affect appendicitis diagnosis: anatomical position of the inflamed appendix, severity of the inflammation (complicated or simple), age of the patient and sex.

Other pathologies potentially can mimic appendicitis scenario and can be grouped into four entities:

- Surgical issues
  - Bowel obstruction
  - Intussusceptions

  - Acute cholecystitis
  - Perforated duodenum ulcer
  - Mesenteric lymphadenitis
  - Meckel's diverticulitis
  - Colonic diverticulitis
  - Pancreatitis
- Urological issues
  - Right renal colic
  - Right pyelonephritis
- Gynaecological issues
  - Ectopic pregnancy
  - Functional ovarian cyst bleeding
  - Ovarian cyst torsion
  - Salpingitis or pelvic inflammatory disease (PID)
- Clinical issues
  - Gastroenteritis
  - Inflammatory bowel disease
  - Diabetic cheto-acidosis
  - Herpetic pain X–XI nerve root

Most frequently seen are mesenteric lymphadenitis, ovarian cyst, Crohn's disease, enterocolitis, bowel obstruction, disease and diverticulitis [8].

7.6 CT Findings

Whereas during the single-slice CT scanner era appendix visualisation was often difficult, introduction of MDCT scanner technology, acquisition protocol standardisation and operator confidence improvement, made normal appendix routinely assessable [7].

A non-pathological appendix finding automatically can exclude appendicitis presence, much easier than the absence of inflammation signs. Consequently surgeons ask for the chance to directly visualise the *appendix*, because in such cases there is a significant implementation of CT examination negative predictive value [9].

Almost never, as a tubular and curved structure, it can be visualised in a single slice, requiring multiple contiguous axial plans. *Multiplanar reconstructions* (MPR) give fundamental help for a correct identification and displaying of the viscera.

In normal condition length can vary between 4 and 25 cm (medium 9 cm) and maximum diameter (wall to wall) can achieve 0.6 cm. In the lumen fluids, faecal material, air, or appendicolith can be found even in non-pathological conditions. Regular appendix wall can measure up to 0.1 cm [7].

In case of inflammation the aspect can be different according to pathology severity and presence of complications. A pathologic appendix shows constantly an enlarged lumen with caliber wider than 0.6 cm. This specific finding has been described as extremely sensitive (sensitivity 100 %) and constantly encountered in all inflammation cases, independently of appendicitis severity. On the other side it has a low specificity, since a normal appendix characterised by a wide caliber can be seen in normal subjects too.

Wall thickness enlargement is another specific characteristic of acute appendicitis with a diameter for each wall wider than 0.2 cm; thickening is usually asymmetric and is coupled with parietal enhancement alteration. Increased enhancement of the wall is a typical sign of inflammation caused by increment of blood supply; it can be seen in 86 % of acute appendicitis and 100 % of cases with catarrhal aetiology [2].

A reduced wall enhancement or a patchy pattern indicates the reduced vascularisation areas, usually achieved in more severe inflammation conditions with subsequent ischemic parietal zone formation; these two signs are usually present in case of gangrenous appendicitis [2].

Inflammation progression in acute appendicitis leads to involvement of the adipose tissue surrounding the viscera. Evaluation of the appendix surrounding fat is mandatory: in cases of missed appendix direct visualisation, the absence of fat alterations can exclude appendicitis presence with same certainty [10]. In 69–100 % of acute appendicitis, an increased density of the *appendicular fat* (dirty fat sign) can be encountered [9]. In a second step, in the course of pathology progression, fluid collections (phlegmon) surrounding the appendix, without a clear wall, can be seen. When the phlegmon acquires a definite thick wall, showing peripheral enhancement after *medium contrast* administration, it is a clear sign of progression into abscess.

In advanced cases appendix inflammation can involve adjacent structures and preliminarily the caecum. In such cases caecal wall thickens just around the site of appendix insertion generates the arrowhead sign (Fig. 7.1), which is assessable in 30 % of acute appendicitis cases with a 100 % specificity [11].

In cases of severe appendicitis, it is important to identify the presence of potential complications and mainly perforation. Presence of perforation significantly increases morbidity and mortality [3] and can condition therapeutic treatment. In some cases when it is present, often associated to abscess formation, surgical treatment is avoided in a first-line choice and medical therapy or percutaneous drainage is preferred. Perforation dramatically increases the risk of complications after surgical period.

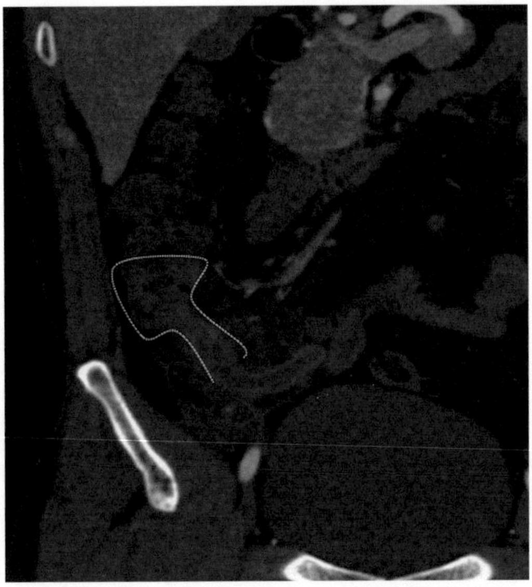

Fig. 7.1 MDCT MPR coronal oblique image shows inflammation of the appendix with fluid-filled lumen, associated to inflammatory thickening of the caecal wall

From this aspect comes the importance of a correct pathology definition in the preoperative setting using a high sensitive and specific technique.

There are five MDCT signs of appendix perforation which are very specific:

- *Enhancing defect foci of the wall*: it has high sensitivity, specificity and accuracy (95, 97 and 96 %, respectively) [3]. Some authors, otherwise, underline the possibility of artefact presence that hampers the utility of the sign in cases of specific technical factors such as peristaltic movement of the surrounding bowel loops or close presence of bony structures. It is mandatory to consider positive the defect only in clear, not equivocal cases (Figs. 7.2 and 7.3).
- *Abscess presence*: abscess is defined as a well-circumscribed fluid collection with thick wall

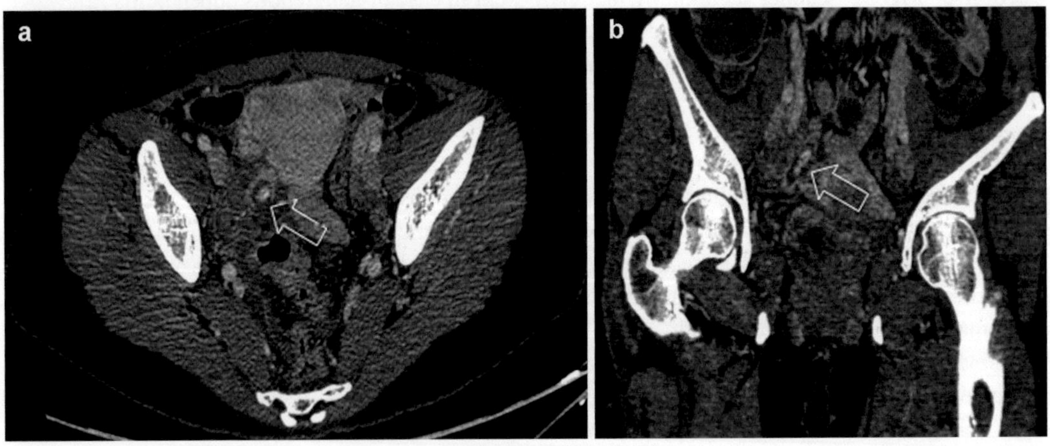

Fig. 7.2 MDCT axial (**a**) and MPR oblique (**b**) images show inflamed appendix with the presence of appendicolith inside and moderate amount of fluid in the lumen. Parietal enhancement defect can be appreciated (*arrows*) as a sign of perforation with associated fluid in the surrounding fat space

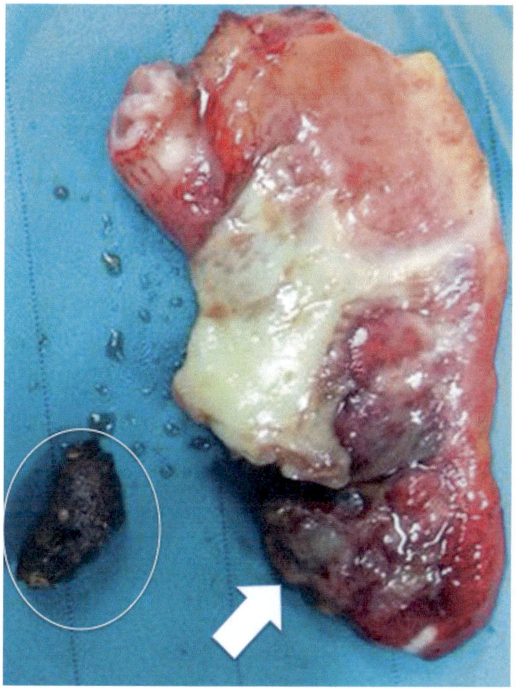

Fig. 7.3 Surgical finding from patient in Fig. 7.1. After appendicectomy wall necrotic area (*arrow*) corresponds exactly to not enhancing portion depicted at MDCT; extracted appendicolith (*circle*) causing appendicitis

showing positive enhancement. Gas can be seen in the context of the collection due to anaerobic bacterial presence or due to a direct communication with appendicular lumen. Many authors consider this sign the most specific for perforation diagnosis [2–12] (Fig. 7.4).

- *Phlegmon presence*: it is defined as a fluid collection without a clear wall associated to an increased fat tissue density. Many authors consider this event as a highly specific sign of perforation (95 %) but with a low sensitivity (40 %) (Fig. 7.5).
- *Extraluminal air*: it is defined as a bubble gas presence outside the appendix showing a high specificity (98 %) but low sensitivity (22–35 %) for perforation assessment. Especially in very skinny subjects, with a poor fat presence in the abdomen, bowel loop gas can sometimes mimic an extraluminal gas collection.
- *Extraluminal appendicolith*: it is the presence of a calcified nucleus outside the appendix, showing a very high specificity for perforation diagnosis (100 %) but poorly sensitive (32 %) (Fig. 7.6).

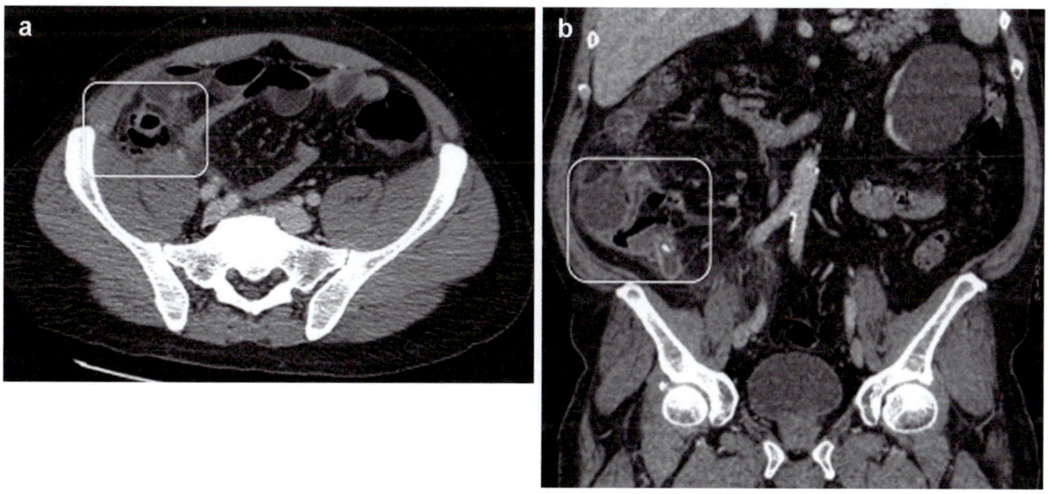

Fig. 7.4 MDCT axial (**a**) and MPR coronal (**b**) images show appendicular abscess with air-fluid level. In the *rectangle* (**a, b**) appendicolith obstructing the appendix valve and thick enhancing wall of the abscess can be appreciated

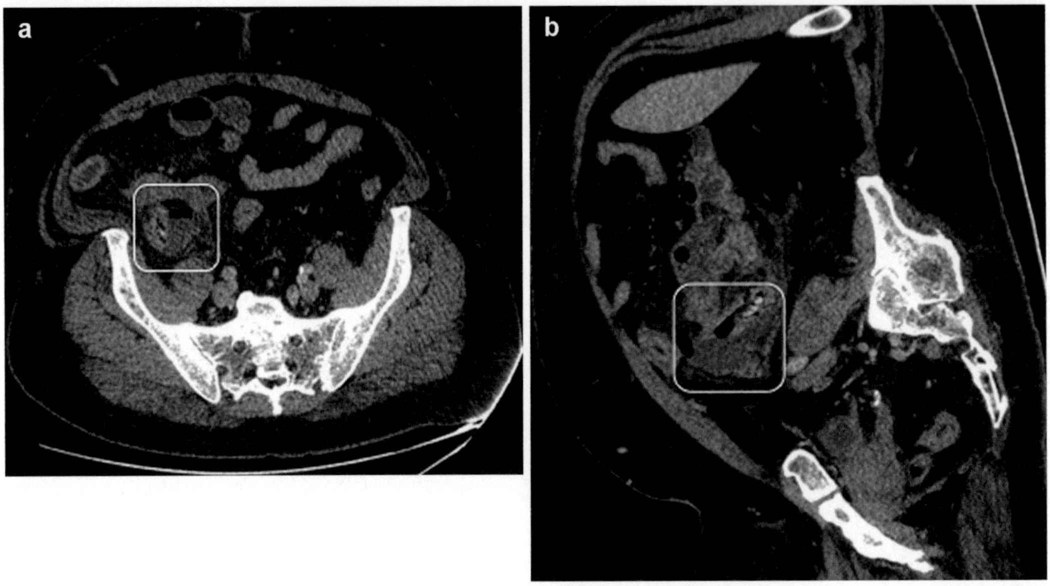

Fig. 7.5 MDCT axial (**a**) and MPR sagittal (**b**) images show fluid collection without enhancing wall surrounding the appendix. In the *rectangle* (**a, b**) the distal inferior portion of the appendix is characterised by not enhancing wall as a sign of perforation

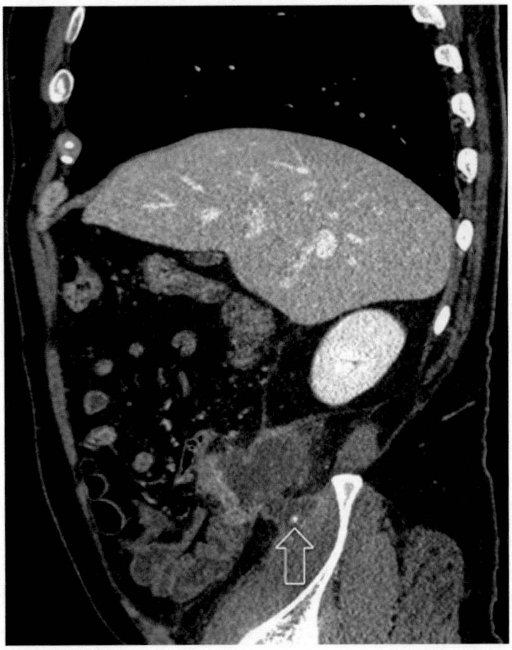

Fig. 7.6 MDCT MPR sagittal image depicts a calcified nucleus (*arrow*) outside the appendix with associated fluid collection as a sign of migrated appendicolith in a perforated appendicitis

References

1. Athanasios NC, Ioanna T et al (2008) CT in appendicitis. Diagn Interv Radiol 13:19–25
2. Miki T, Ogata S et al (2005) Enhanced multidetector-row computed tomography (MDCT) in the diagnosis of acute appendicitis and its severity. Radiat Med 23: 242–255
3. Bixby SD, Lucey BC et al (2006) Perforated versus nonperforated acute appendicitis: accuracy of multidetector CT detection. Radiology 241:780–786
4. Jones K, Peña AA et al (2004) Are negative appendectomies still acceptable? Am J Surg 188: 748–754
5. Wakeley CP (1993) The position of the vermiform appendix as ascertained by an analysis of 10000 cases. J Anat 67:277–283
6. Humes DJ, Simpson J (2006) Acute appendicitis. BMJ 333:530–534
7. Ghiatas AA, Chopra S et al (1997) Computed tomography of the normal appendix and acute appendicitis. Eur Radiol 7:1043–1047
8. Novelline RA, Rhea JT et al (1999) Helical CT in emergency radiology. Radiology 213:321–339
9. Weltman DI, Yu J et al (2000) Diagnosis of acute appendicitis: comparison of 5 and 10 mm CT section in the same patient. Radiology 216:172–177

10. Niholaidis P, Hwang CM et al (2004) The nonvisualized appendix: incidence of acute appendicitis when secondary inflammatory changes are absent. AJR Am J Roentgenol 183:889–892
11. Rao PM, Wittenberg J et al (1997) Appendicitis: use of arrowhead sign for diagnosis at CT. Radiology 202: 363–366
12. Tsuboi M, Takase K et al (2008) Perforated and nonperforated appendicitis: defect in enhancing appendiceal Wall-Depiction with multi-detector Row CT. Radiology 246:142–147

Acute Perforated Diverticulitis: Spectrum of MDCT Findings

8

Maria Giuseppina Scuderi and Teresa Cinque

8.1 Introduction

Colonic perforation is a common complication of diverticulitis that requires early diagnosis and treatment.

MDCT, without bowel preparation, allows high-resolution multiplanar detection of diverticula perforation because it is the most valuable imaging technique for identifying the wall of the colon as well as the surrounding pericolic fat and the presence, the site and the cause of the GI perforations.

The spectrum of MDCT findings of the diverticulum perforation depends on the site of the lesion (if perforation regards the retroperitoneal or the intraperitoneal space) and on the entity of the inflammatory process.

8.2 Diverticular Disease: Diverticulitis

The presence of an uninflamed diverticula (diverticular disease or diverticulosis) occurs more commonly in Western countries, correlated to diet low in fibre and to other causes of increased intracolonic pressure.

M.G. Scuderi (✉) • T. Cinque
Department of Radiology, "A. Cardarelli" Hospital, Largo A. Cardarelli, Naples 80131, Italy
e-mail: margiscuderi@hotmail.com; teresacinque66@gmail.com

The incidence increases with age, and diverticulosis is rather uncommon in people under 40 years of age: in fact it occurs in 10 % of people over age 40, in 50 % of people over 60 and in 70 % in people over 80 years [1].

Diverticula develop from the outpouching of the mucosa and submucosa through the muscular layers of the wall, in the loci of minoris resistentiae where penetrating vessels cross through the wall.

Diverticula can be found anywhere throughout the colon, most frequently in the sigmoid tract [2]. They can be less or more numerous and may have a variable size usually between 2 mm and 2 cm, but giant diverticula (up to 25 cm), usually solitary, have been described in the sigmoid tract [3].

Diverticula usually present as air-filled pockets, but it is not so rare to find spontaneously hyperdense or calcified diverticula from dehydration of faecal material trapped in the diverticular pocket because of the lack of muscular layer in the wall and the narrowing of the neck that prevent clearance from the faecal material.

Occlusion by stool or food particles may lead to bacterial overgrowth and local tissue ischaemia that starts an inflammatory process. Complicated diverticulitis is due to possible microscopic, usually covered, perforation with extension into the pericolic fat and possible formation of an abscess or a phlegmon [4].

The abscess may be confined in the pericolic fat and may spread along the retroperitoneal fat planes

L. Romano, A. Pinto (eds.), *Imaging of Alimentary Tract Perforation*,
DOI 10.1007/978-3-319-08192-2_8, © Springer International Publishing Switzerland 2015

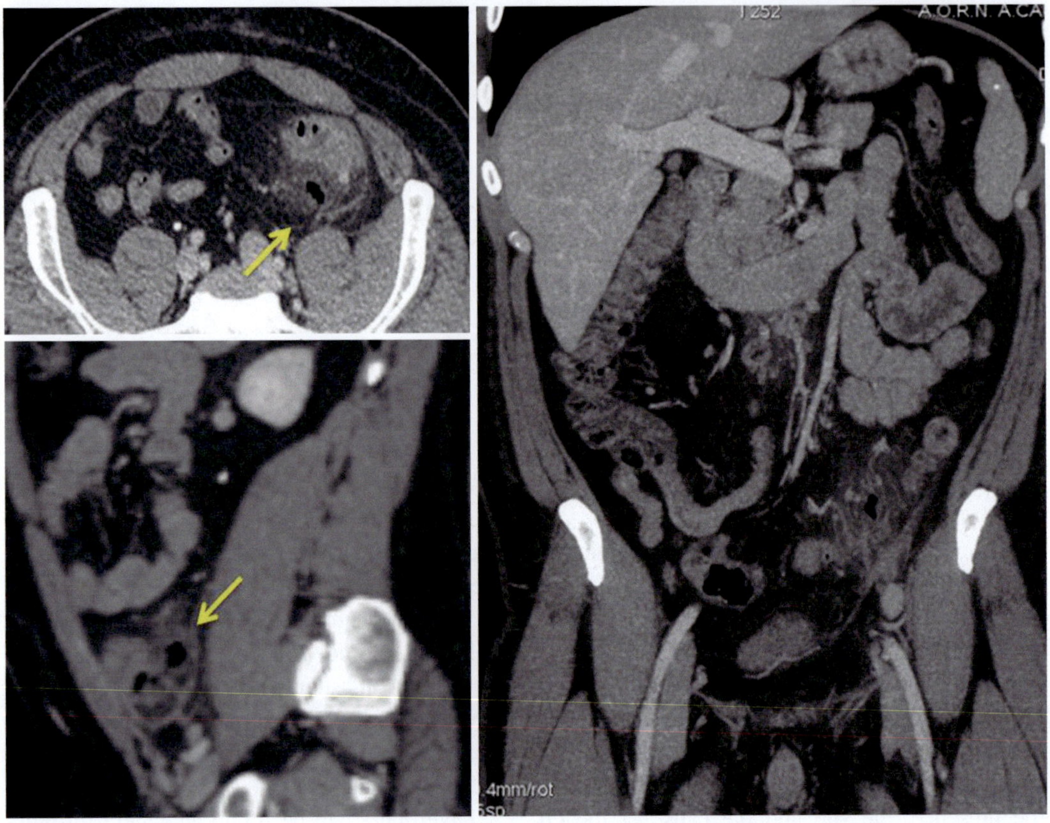

Fig. 8.1 Diverticular microperforation: little amount of free air associated with thickening of the sigmoid wall, diverticular pouch and perivisceral signs (mild, fuzzy hyperdensity and stranding of pericolic tissue, *arrows*)

or the peritoneal recesses or into the adjacent organs as fistulous tract to the small bowel, bladder, vagina, uterus and adnexa or abdominal wall.

Rarely, diverticulitis results in free peritoneal perforations (only 1 or 2 % of diverticulites presenting with acute abdominal pain have free perforation).

The clinical spectrum of diverticular disease varies from asymptomatic diverticulosis to fatal complication such as generalized peritonitis (worse if faecal) from rupture of a peridiverticular abscess or from free rupture of an uninflamed diverticulum (Fig. 8.1) [5].

8.3 Spectrum of MDCT Finding

The diagnosis of acute diverticular perforation requires the presence of the diverticula usually associated with circumferential thickening of a long segment of the colonic wall and with signs related to a cellulitic process into the perivisceral tissue: hyperdensity (sometimes very slight and fuzzy) and increase of perivisceral lymphatics and vessels presenting as hyperaemia and stranding of the pericolic fat are the first signs of inflammation eventually associated with thickening of the retroperitoneal or peritoneal folds [6].

Phlegmon may appear, in proximity of the inflammation site, as a little mass, round or ovular, that is hyperdense (from +15 to +35 HU), enhanced after MDCT and surrounded by slightly dense tissue (Fig. 8.2).

A fluid, hypodense, collection with surrounding thickened, hyperdense inflammatory wall due to an abscess may be more frequently found. Small air-bubble or air-fluid levels may be contained in the centre of the collection (Fig. 8.3).

The presence, the grade of thickness and of post-contrastographic density and the presence of septa and air-bubble levels are related to the grade of the abscess maturation.

The spectrum of MDCT findings of diverticulum perforation depends on the site of the lesion and on the involvement of the retroperitoneal or peritoneal spaces.

The most frequent perforation site is the sigmoid colon; the transverse colon accounts for approximately 18 % of perforations, whereas perforation of the cecum and the right colon is rare (only 5 % of perforations). The sigmoid mesocolon and thus the subperitoneal space are most frequently involved but, due to the continuity of the spaces beneath the posterior parietal peritoneum and abdominal pelvic walls with the root of the sigmoid mesentery and pelvic ligaments, a retroperitoneal or peritoneal extension of the process may happen.

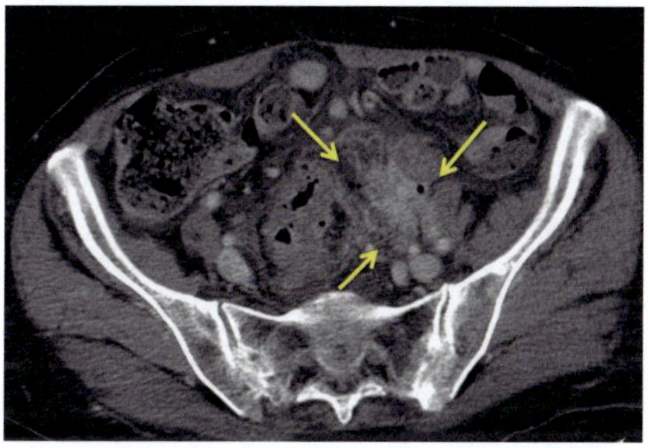

Fig. 8.2 Phlegmon, (*arrows*): hyperdense tissue (from +15 to +35 HU), enhanced after MDCT contiguous to a diverticulitis site and microbubbles of free air

When perforation is associated with an abscess formation, the abscess can be confined to the pelvis or can extend far into the abdomen.

When the peritoneal cavity is involved, the abscessual collection is always well delimited by thickened peritoneal folds presenting as a dense and uniform capsule.

In the sigmoid perforation MDCT has excellent contrast resolution to detect the presence of small amounts of free extraluminal air in close proximity to the intestinal wall thickening or centred within paracolic inflammatory tissue in the pericolic space. Extraluminal air can always be detected with adequate window setting even if there are only small bubbles [7].

In sigmoid free perforation a greater amount of air can diffuse into the subperitoneal space, the retroperitoneal space of the pelvis, of the abdomen and also, through the diaphragmatic hiatus, of the thorax and of the neck resulting in pneumomediastinum and cervical emphysema [8] (Fig. 8.4).

In case of colonic perforation (left and right colon), air bubbles are preferentially located in the pericolic fat (contained perforation) (Fig. 8.5) [7].

In case of free perforation into the peritoneal cavity, the air rapidly reaches the most antideclive position usually in the anterosuperior part of the involved peritoneal recess (Fig. 8.4).

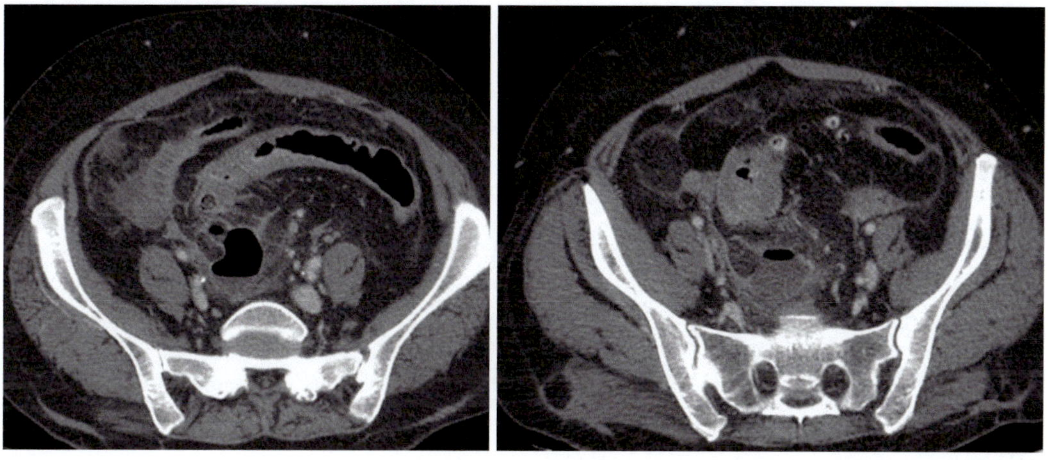

Fig. 8.3 Parasigmoid abscess: hypodense fluid collection, contained in the mesosigma, with an air-fluid level, and delineated by thickened, hyperdense inflammatory rim

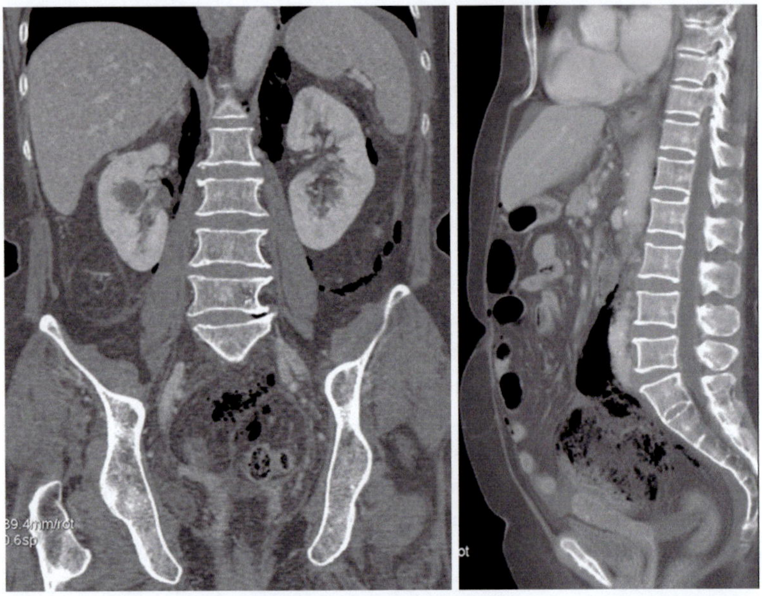

Fig. 8.4 Retroperitoneum from diverticular perforation: free air in the mesosigma and perirenal space

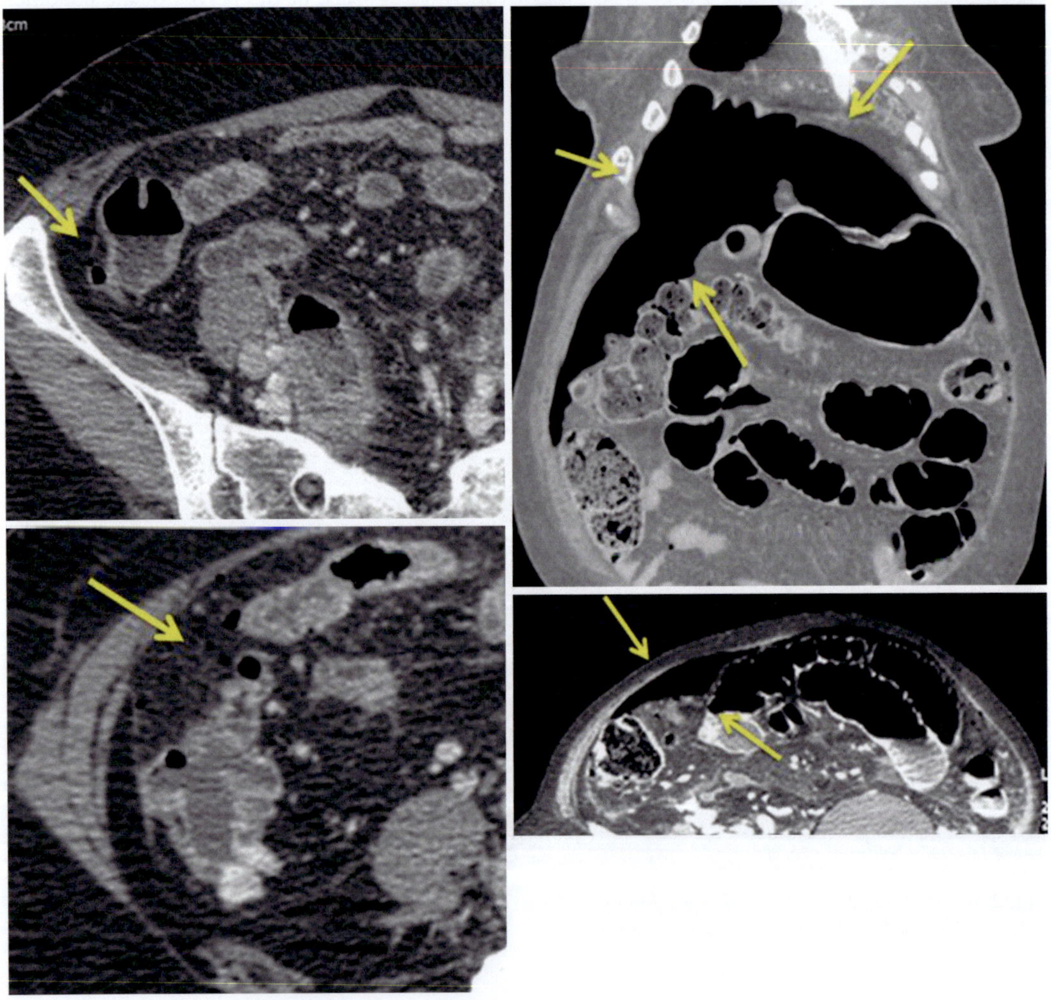

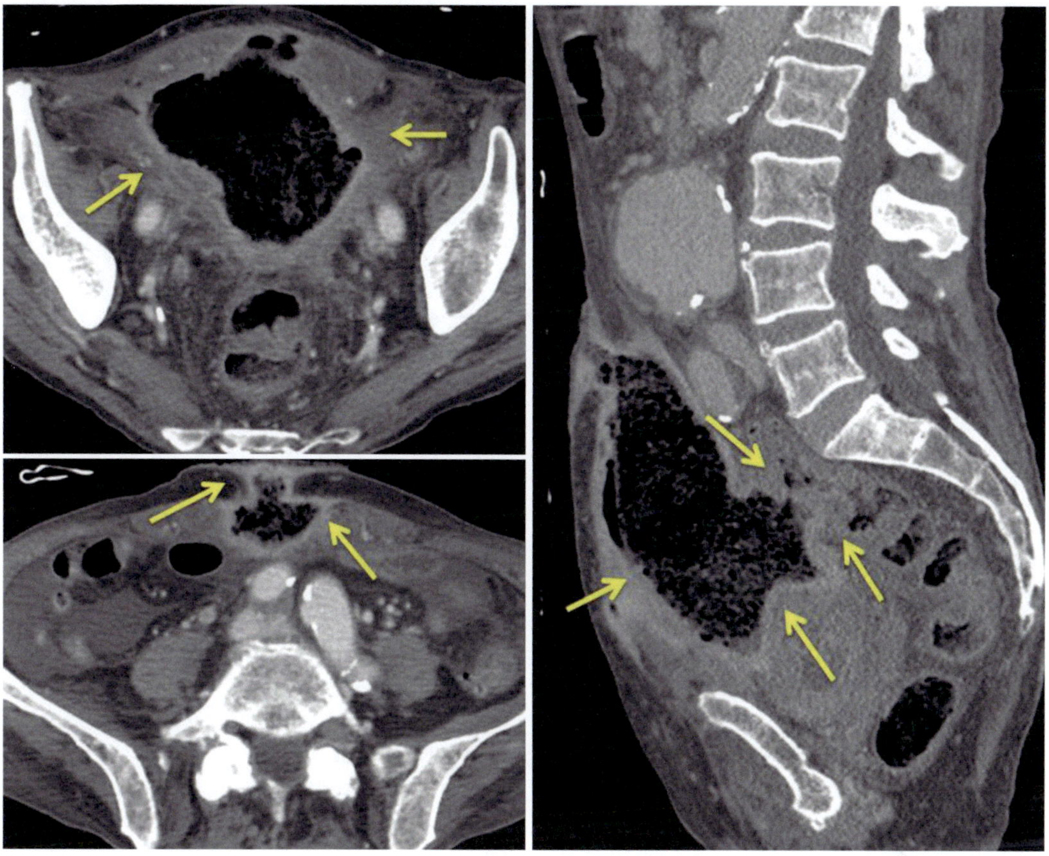

Fig. 8.6 Dirty mass (faecal abscess, *arrows*) fistulized to the abdominal wall

The risk of an adverse outcome is highest if the perforation of the diverticular or of the abscess wall allows faecal discharge in the peritoneum. The presence of spilled faeces or "dirty mass" in the lower abdomen is a specific indicator of colonic perforation [9].

A CT features an extravasated faeces that is a low-attenuation soft tissue mass containing small air bubbles (Fig. 8.6).

The spread of the inflammatory process into adjacent organs may have several clinical presentations such as hydronephrosis, psoas abscess, abdominal wall abscess [10] and spondylodiscitis.

Fistulization more frequently can involve small bowel loops (Fig. 8.7) or the bladder, especially in men. In women, uterine, adnexal or vaginal fistulization can occur.

In the absence of bladder catheterization, air in the bladder associated with signs of sigmoid diverticulitis and thickening of the bladder wall, usually in a posterolateral site, suggests a fistula. Bladder collection of the stool and faecaluria may be observed (Fig. 8.8).

8.4 Diagnostic Findings for Adequate Management

The traditional, surgical, Hinchey classification has been used, before the advent of MDCT imaging, to verify the extent and the degree of the pelvic and abdominal disease at the time of surgery.

It is a four-graded classification with a pericolic abscess confined by the mesentery of the

Fig. 8.5 Colonic perforation: evidence of pneumoperitoneum and air bubbles preferentially located in the pericolic fat (*arrows*)

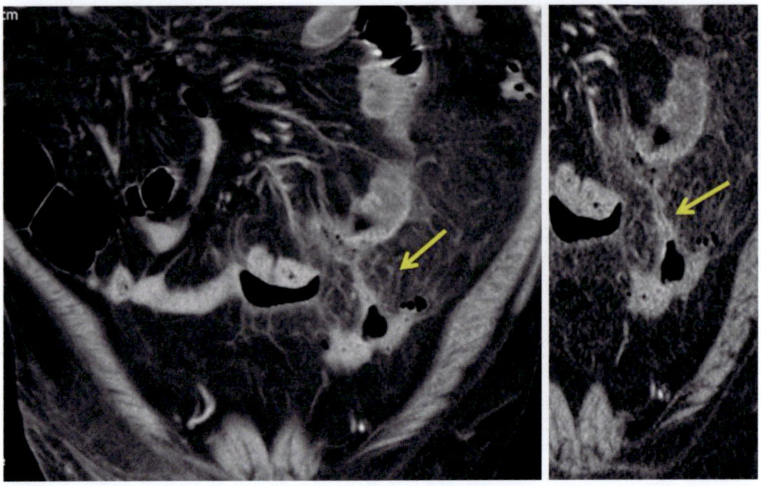

Fig. 8.7 Ileocolic fistula in diverticulitis: long fistulous track (*arrow*) between the colonic wall and an ileal loop

colon in grade I, pelvic abscess resulting from a local perforation of a pericolic abscess in grade II, generalized purulent peritonitis from rupture of a pericolic or pelvic abscess into the general peritoneal cavity in grade III and faecal peritonitis from free perforation of a diverticulum or abscess with faecal discharge in grade IV [1].

Nowadays the surgical treatment and the management of diverticulitis have changed, and a CT-guided classification (Ambrosetti) is preferred [11–15].

In mild diverticulitis the thickening of the colonic wall is <3 mm and is associated with perivisceral signs.

Moderate diverticulitis has significant wall thickening (>3 mm) determining segmental lumen narrowing in association with phlegmon or small abscess.

Severe diverticulitis is defined as parietal thickening >5 mm with abscess greater than 5 cm or perforation.

These findings help to discriminate those patients with mild diverticulitis or with an abscess less than 3 cm, which are generally treated with antibiotics, from those in whom an abscess greater than 3 cm may be percutaneously drained [12].

In some cases of complicated diverticulitis, the ureter may be trapped in the inflammatory phlegmon and may require a presurgical stenting or a careful legation at the time of intervention.

8.5 Differential Diagnosis

The typical clinical signs of an acute diverticulitis are represented by localized pain and guarding in the left lower quadrant, fever and leucocytosis. However clinical signs may be atypical, and a CT differential diagnosis becomes necessary.

The CT diagnosis of acute diverticulitis is based on the assessment of the diverticula associated with inflammatory signs and on the exclusion of other pathological conditions.

From a clinical point of view, in the acute right lower quadrant, a differential diagnosis may be required from an appendicitis and a right-sided or a redundant sigmoid colon diverticulitis. In this case multiplanar reconstructions are very helpful to individuate the anatomical structure involved and the perivisceral signs. It is not so rare, in fact, to find a very elongated sigma with inflamed diverticular pouches in the right lower quadrant in close relationship with the cecum and normal appendix; or otherwise an inflamed appendix, eventually related to an ectopic, pelvic cecum, goes in close contact to an uninflamed sigmoid diverticula [16].

More frequently in the acute left lower quadrant, the main pathology in differential diagnosis with diverticulitis perforation is colon carcinoma. In perforated colon carcinoma the pericolic fat stranding and vascular engorgement can mimic diverticulitis. But greater wall thickening, often eccentric, of a short segment of the colon and local lymphadenopathy are more indicative of carcinoma.

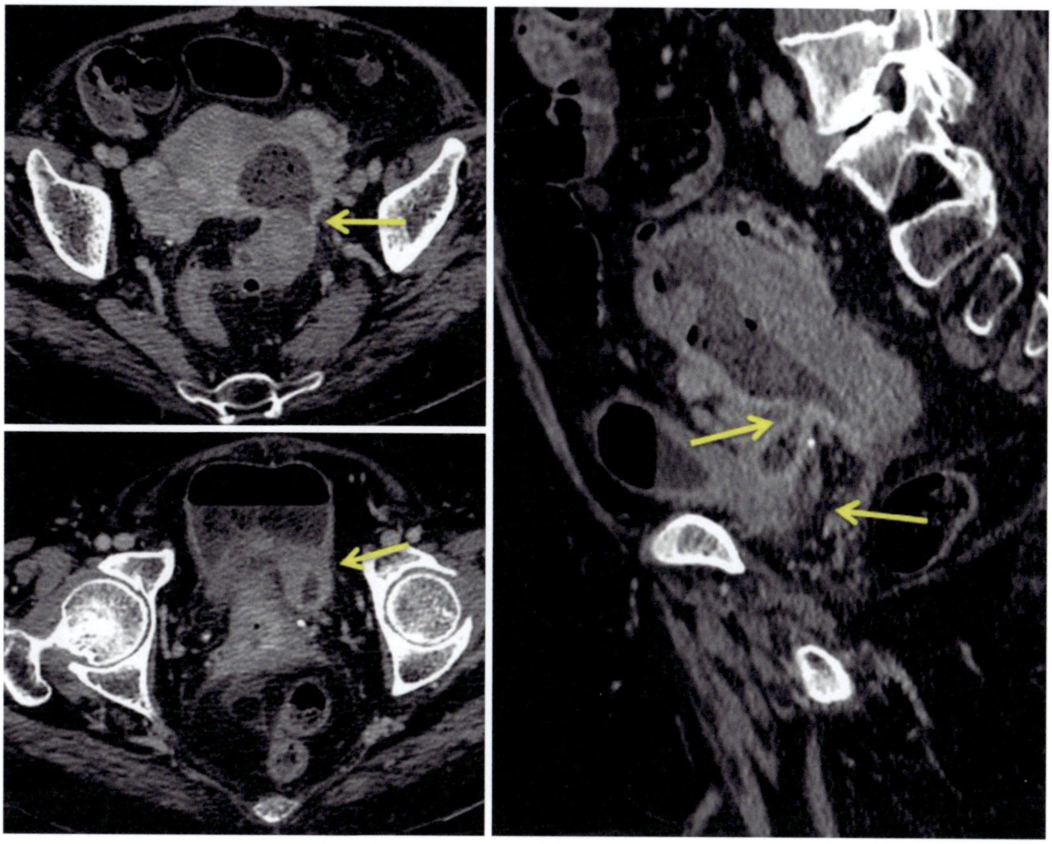

Fig. 8.8 Colovesical fistula: faecal abscess contiguous to the thickened sigmoid wall and fistulous track to the bladder wall (thickened and hyperdense, *arrows*); faecal material in the catheterized bladder

Other colonic inflammatory conditions, such as Crohn's disease or ulcerative colitis and pelvic inflammatory disease, may require a differential diagnosis.

In diverticulitis, a colovesical fistula is suggested by the endoluminal air and by the thickening of the bladder wall usually in a posterolateral site, whereas a colovesical fistula from a Crohn's disease usually involves the terminal ileum and the right anterior surface of the bladder.

References

1. Jacobs DO (2007) Diverticulitis. N Engl J Med 357:2057–2066
2. Horton KM, Corl FM, Fishman EK (2000) CT evaluation of the colon: inflammatory disease. Radiographics 20:399–418
3. Thomas S, Pee RL, Evans LE, Haarer KA (2006) Best cases from AFIP: giant colonic diverticulum. Radiographics 26:1869–1872
4. Werner A, Diehl SJ, Farag-Soliman M, Duber C (2003) Multi-slice spiral CT in routine diagnosis of suspected acute left-sided colonic diverticulitis: a prospective study of 120 patients. Eur Radiol 13:2596–2603
5. Stoker J, vanRanden A, Lameris W, Boermeester MA (2009) Imaging patients with acute abdominal pain. Radiology 253:31–46
6. DeStiger K, Keating D (2009) Imaging update: acute colonic diverticulitis. Clin Colon Rectal Surg 22(3):147–155
7. Pinto A, Scaglione M, Giovine S (2004) Comparison between the site of multislice CT signs of gastrointestinal perforation and the site of perforation detected at surgery in forty perforated patients. Radiol Med 108(3):208–217
8. Pyong WCJ (2011) Pneumomediastinum caused by colonic diverticulitis perforation. J Korean Surg Soc 80:S17–S20
9. Saeky M, Hoshikawa Y, Miyazaki O (1998) Emergency computed tomographic analysis of colonic perforation: dirty mass, a new CT finding. Radiology 5:140–145

10. Vasileios R, Anna G, Christos L (2013) Abdominal wall abscess due to acute perforated sigmoid diverticulitis: a case report with MDCT and US findings. Case Rep Radiol 2013:565928. doi: 10.1155/2013/565928
11. Ambrosetti P, Becker C, Terrier F (2002) Colonic diverticulitis: impact of imaging on surgical management- a prospective study of 42 patients. Eur Radiol 12:1145–1149
12. Siewert B, Tye G, Kruskal J, Sosna J, Opelka F (2006) Impact of CT-guided drainage in the treatment of diverticular abscess: size matters. AJR Am J Roentgenol 186:680–686
13. Stocchi L (2010) Current indications and role of surgery in the management of sigmoid diverticulitis. World J Gastroenterol 16(7):804–817
14. Biondo S, Lopez Borao J, Millan M (2012) Current status of the treatment of acute colonic diverticulitis: a systematic review. Colorectal Dis 14(1):1–11
15. Moore F, Catena F, Moore E (2013) Management of perforated sigmoid diverticulitis. Position paper. World J Emerg Surg 8:55
16. Yaacoub IB, Boulay I, Jullès MC (2011) CT findings of misleading features of colonic diverticulitis. Insights Imaging 2(1):69–84

Colorectal Perforation: Assessment with MDCT

9

Gianluca Ponticiello, Loredana Di Nuzzo, and Pietro Paolo Saturnino

9.1 Introduction

Colorectal perforation represents a medical condition where CT plays an important role for diagnosis and identifies the etiology of acute abdomen. Colorectal perforations are severe conditions with a high rate of mortality. This is due to the fact that patients afflicted with these perforations are often the elderly, with various coexisting morbidities [1]. The frequency of colorectal perforation in the general population is not well known because many cases of minor colorectal perforations are probably missed as the condition resolves itself before the patient goes to the specialist or because studies are not performed early enough in the course of the disease. Sometimes, many colorectal perforations are misdiagnosed as other colonic infection or inflammatory diseases. The clinical manifestations depend on a number of factors, including the size of the perforation, the level of extra colonic contamination, and the body's ability to contain this contamination [2]. Colorectal perforation presents different clinical features from peridiverticulitis and small pericolic abscesses to large intra-abdominal or pelvic abscesses and purulent or fecal peritonitis [3]. Today the mortality rates of colorectal perforation have remained unchanged over the last two decades, even with the many improvements in medical therapy, intensive care, and surgical techniques [4]. This situation may reflect a lack of knowledge about the condition and strategies to prevent it [5].

9.2 Causes of Colorectal Perforation

Nontraumatic colorectal perforation can be caused by inflammatory, neoplastic, or ischemic etiology as well as by iatrogenic injuries and as a postoperative complication. The perforation sites of the large intestine can frequently be correlated with their causes [6]. Malignant neoplasm, diverticulitis (in Western countries), blunt trauma, and ischemia are common causes of perforation on the left side of colonic loops. Inflammatory bowel disease, diverticulitis (in eastern countries), and penetrating trauma tend to be observed on the right side of the colonic loops. The cecum can be perforated in patients with mechanical colonic obstruction. Iatrogenic injuries usually involve the rectum and sigmoid colon. Penetration of the serosal layer of the colon may lead to either a covered perforation, with phlegmon and abscess formation and localized peritonitis, or less

G. Ponticiello (✉) • L. Di Nuzzo • P.P. Saturnino
Department of Radiology, "A. Cardarelli" Hospital, Via A. Cardarelli, 9, Naples 80131, Italy
e-mail: gponticiel@sirm.org; loredanadinuzzo@yahoo.it; pietropsaturnino@libero.it

L. Romano, A. Pinto (eds.), *Imaging of Alimentary Tract Perforation*,
DOI 10.1007/978-3-319-08192-2_9,

frequently to free perforation into the retroperitoneum or the intraperitoneal cavity, depending on the involved colonic segment. The clinical and laboratory data can help in establishing the cause of the perforation [7, 8].

9.3 CT Technique

The entire abdomen from the dome of the diaphragm to the pelvic floor should be scanned. Contiguous axial images at 2.5 mm thickness are obtained, and multiplanar reformations may be applied when necessary. After the precontrast images have been acquired, CT scanning is initiated 70–80 s after the intravenous injection of contrast media (iodine) at high concentration (400 mgl/mL), at a rate of 3–4 mL/s. Sometimes it can be useful, especially when we suspect iatrogenic perforation, to use hydrosoluble iodine contrast by retrograde way (rectum).

9.4 Gas Localization and General CT Findings

Computed tomography (CT) is helpful in detecting extraluminal gas.

Multi-detector CT (MDCT) is superior to single helical or conventional CT as it is able to provide rapid, high-volume coverage and diagnostic images even in patients unable to perform prolonged breath-holds. A study of MDCT showed 86 % accuracy in predicting the site of perforation. The diagnosis of gastrointestinal (GI) tract perforation is based on direct CT findings, such as discontinuity of the bowel wall and the presence of extraluminal air, and on indirect CT findings [9–13].

9.5 Direct CT Findings

9.5.1 Discontinuity of the Bowel Wall

Direct visualization of the discontinuity of the bowel wall can identify the presence and site of GI tract perforation, which is marked by a low-attenuating cleft that usually runs perpendicular to the bowel wall on CT. However, this cleft is observed less frequently than free air on CT, and a cleft is usually seen in less than 50 % of the patients with GI tract perforation. This is related to the small size of the lesion. MDCT with post-processing images can be helpful in identifying discontinuity of the bowel wall [9–13].

9.5.2 Extraluminal Air

Free air localization depending on the perforation site can detected in intraperitoneal or retroperitoneal spaces. Colonic perforation, like gastroduodenal perforation, can appear as massive pneumoperitoneum with free gas all over the abdomen and pelvis. If free gas is present only in the pelvis, the colon, and not the small bowel, is the usual site of perforation. The reverse is true for supramesocolic free gas. However, during sigmoid perforation we can have free air only in the supramesocolic compartment; in this case we must find focal signs such as wall thickening and pericolonic stranding to identify the site of perforation [9–13].

9.6 Indirect CT Findings

Indirect CT findings are represented by bowel wall thickening, abnormal bowel wall enhancement (includes interruption or lack of bowel wall enhancement on enhanced scan), abscess, and an inflammatory mass adjacent to the bowel [13].

9.7 Colonic Neoplasm and Perforation

Perforation related to colonic tumors has a reported incidence of 1.2–9 %. The perforation related to tumor mostly occurs at the cecum, secondary to marked prestenotic dilatation with a competent ileocecal valve, or at the site of the tumor, due to tumor necrosis.

On CT, both the perforation and the colonic tumor can be seen; colonic carcinoma results in diffuse or focal bowel wall thickening and pericolonic stranding (Fig. 9.1). Once the tumor invades the serosal fat, there is increased possibility of perforation with abscess formation and gas leak (Fig. 9.2) [7, 14].

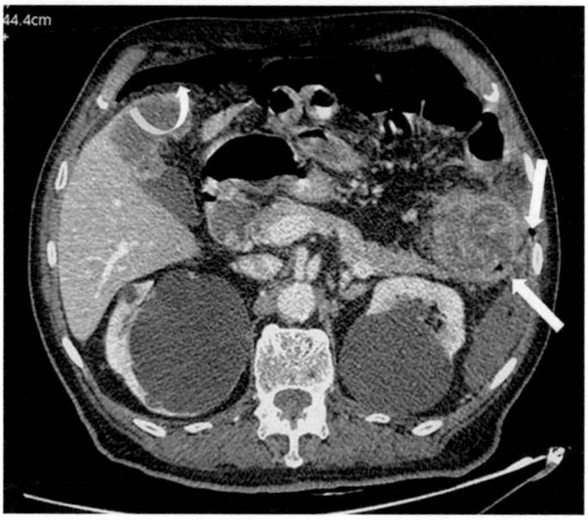

Fig. 9.1 Expansive solid lesion of the descending colon with free small air bubbles near the lesion (*arrow*) and pneumoperitoneum (*curved arrow*)

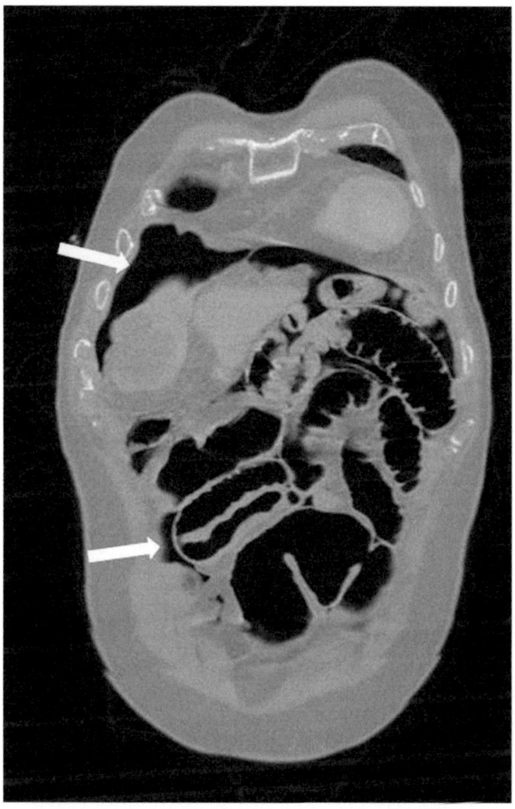

Fig. 9.2 Modest quote of pneumoperitoneum between intestinal loops and below the diaphragm (*arrows*)

9.8 Colonic Ischemia and Stercoral Perforation

Stercoral perforation is related to a localized mucosal ulceration and ischemic pressure necrosis of the bowel wall for vascular occlusion, caused by a stercoraceous mass, most often involving the sigmoid or rectosigmoid.

Risk factors include conditions leading to longstanding constipation, often in bedridden patients, such as drug-induced constipation (narcotics, nonsteroidal anti-inflammatory drugs, postoperative analgesia, and methadone), scleroderma, and an underlying obstructing colonic lesion such as neoplasm or stricture [15].

The most useful tool for diagnosis of stercoral perforation is abdominopelvic CT [16]. The main specific CT finding of vascular impairment of the colonic wall (ischemia) is lack or poor enhancement of its wall and often, in relation to focal fecal distension of the colonic lumen, is indicative of stercoral perforation (Fig. 9.3) [8]. Other CT findings are free intraperitoneal air (Fig. 9.4), colonic mural thickening, and adjacent fat stranding [17].

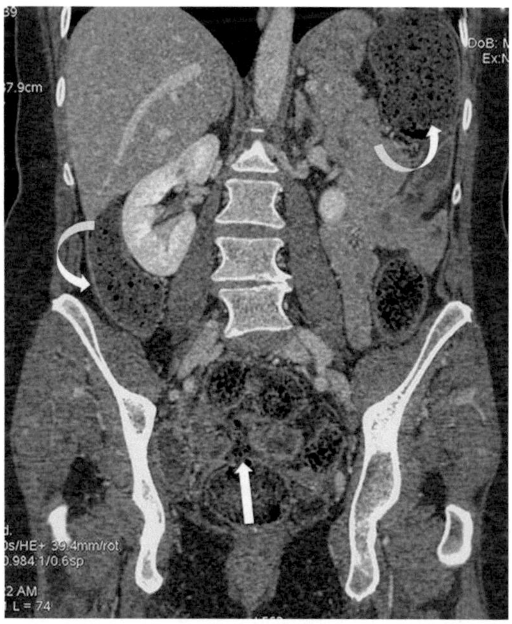

Fig. 9.3 Stercoraceous mass of rectal-sigma (*curved arrow*) and lack of wall contrast enhancement (*arrows*)

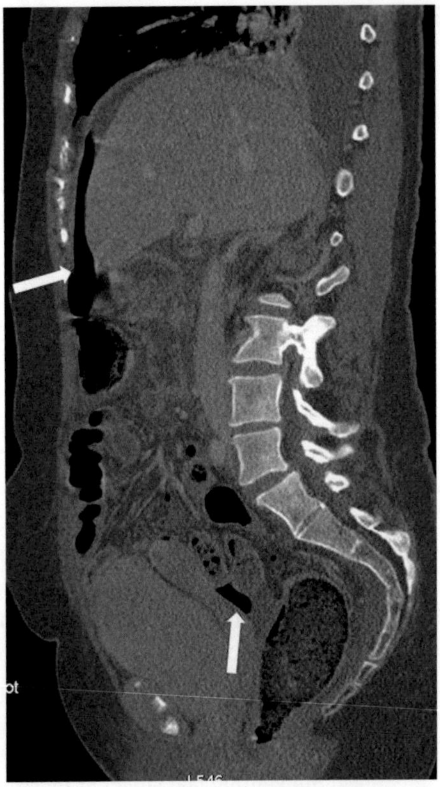

Fig. 9.4 Supramesecolic and undermesocolic free intraperitoneal air (*arrows*)

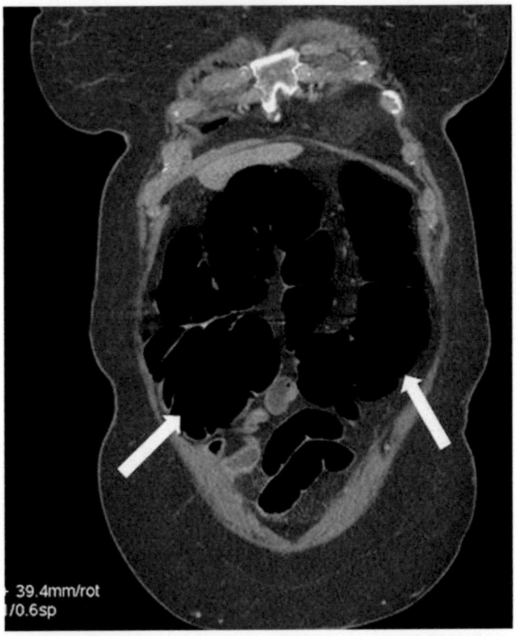

Fig. 9.5 Gaseous distention of the colon due to recent colonoscopy (*arrows*)

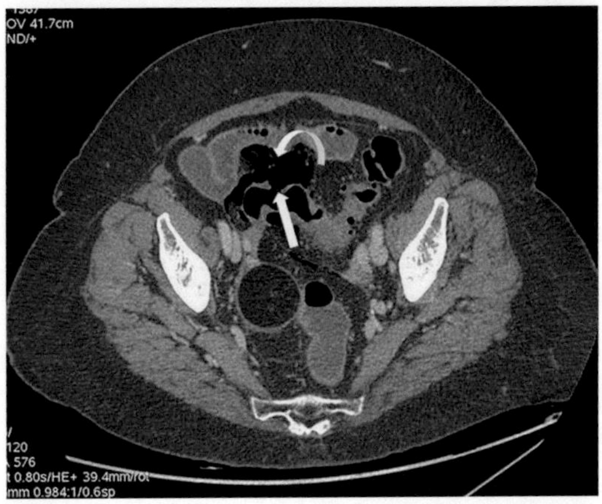

Fig. 9.6 Discontinuity of the anterior sigma wall (*arrow*) with modest quote of perivisceral free air (*curved arrow*)

9.9 Iatrogenic Injury: Perforation During Colonoscopy

Post-colonoscopic perforation is rare. These iatrogenic perforations occur in approximately 1 in 1,000 patients. The clinical presentation varies from acute abdomen to subtle clinical findings.

In diagnostic colonoscopy the rectosigmoid is the most common site of perforation followed by the cecum, while post-polypectomy perforation, in therapeutic colonoscopy, occurs at the site of the excised polyp. A perforated site is typically a large anti-mesenteric tear of colonic wall if it is caused by the shaft of the endoscope. Furthermore, a smaller perforation can be found in an injury from the tip of the endoscope. If a perforation is clinically suspected and conventional chest and abdominal X-ray exclude free abdominal or subdiaphragmatic air, air within the colonic wall, subcutaneous emphysema, or pneumomediastinum or pneumothorax, a CT is recommended [7, 18]. As we said before, about direct findings, in iatrogenic perforation, we can find free retroperitoneal gas in the anterior pararenal space caused by perforation of the posterior walls of the sigmoid, ascending, and descending colon.

When we have anterior wall sigmoid perforation, the direct sign is discontinuity of the bowel wall with free extraluminal air near the lesion and eventually in the intraperitoneal spaces (Figs. 9.5 and 9.6).

9.10 Perforation After Colon: Rectal Surgery (Anastomotic Dehiscence)

The most alarming complication following colorectal surgery is anastomotic leakage which is associated with a high mortality rate.

Different factors are involved: the type of surgery (higher risk after restorative proctocolectomy or rectal resection), the extraperitoneal site of the anastomosis, the type of the anastomosis (higher risk after coloanal or ileal-anal pouch or colorectal), the stapled anastomosis, and the intraoperative complications.

The risk of leakage has become gradually higher for low and ultralow coloanal anastomosis [19–21].

CT represents the modality of choice for the optimal recognition of postoperative complications and for the assessment of patients with postoperative sepsis. Most postoperative CT features overlap between patients with and without clinically important anastomotic leak (CIAL). The only feature seen statistically more frequently with CIAL is peri-anastomotic loculated fluid containing air.

Evident anastomotic leak is suspected on the basis of a large hydropneumoperitoneum or if pneumoperitoneum enlarges on successive examinations. Usually the collection is situated between the rectum and the sacrum, and the rectum is anteriorly displaced by the collection. Sometimes we can find the fluid collections around the anastomotic site also in patients without anastomotic leakage. The key point for suspicion of a leakage is visualization of air or contrast into the fluid collection (Figs. 9.7 and 9.8) [22, 23].

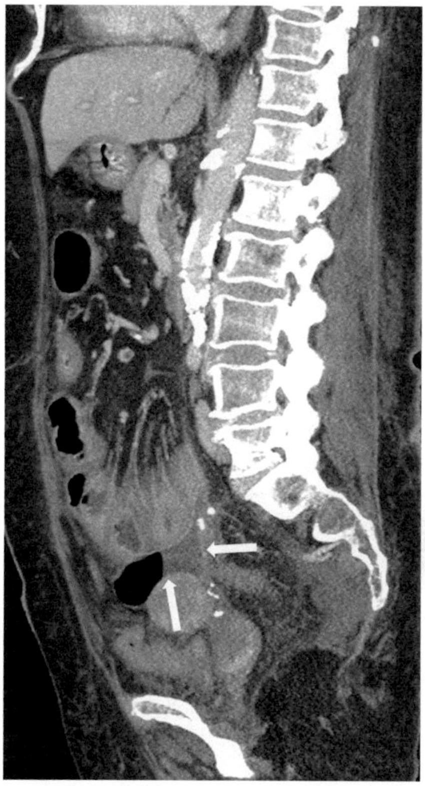

Fig. 9.7 Sigma resection with air-fluid collections around the colon – rectal anastomosis (*arrows*)

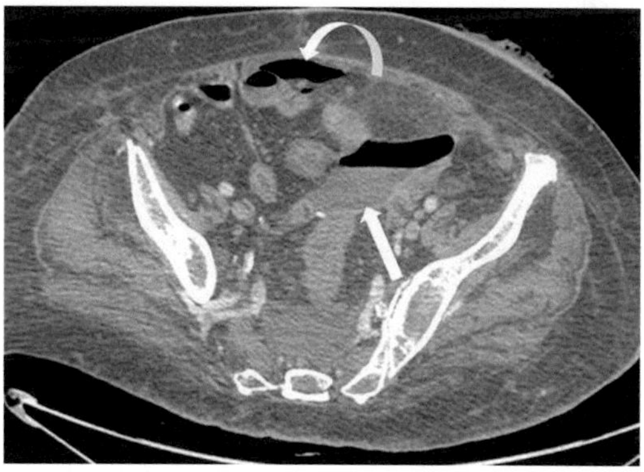

Fig. 9.8 Air-fluid collections around the anastomotic site (*arrow*) with free air along the anterior abdominal wall (*curved arrow*)

9.11 Inflammatory Bowel Disease (IBD)

Perforating complications in IBD are rare. In ulcerative colitis (UC), free perforation, occurring in about 2 %, is often associated with toxic megacolon, caused by marked colonic dilatation in acute presentation. In UC when perforation involves the sigmoid, we can have free air only in the supramesocolic compartment; in this case, we must find focal signs such as wall thickening and pericolonic stranding to identify the site of perforation (Figs. 9.9 and 9.10). Free perforation in Crohn's disease (CD) is not so common (3 %), often it occurs during exacerbation of toxic colitis, while sealed-off perforations are more frequent in CD, related to the transmural inflammatory process and inter-loop adhesions, leading to phlegmon and abscess formation with localized peritonitis [24].

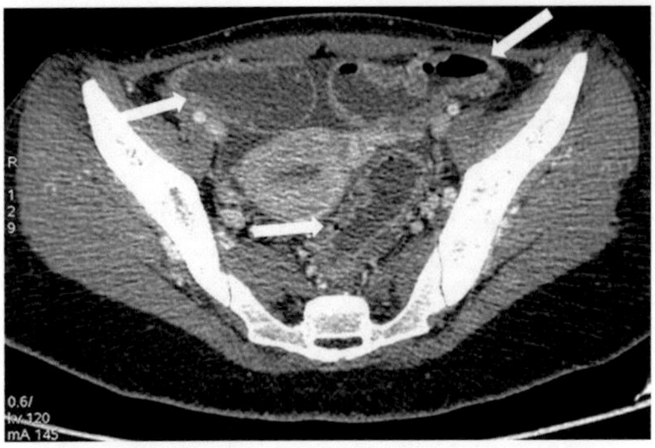

Fig. 9.9 Widespread wall colon and sigma thickening with transmural ulceration and fluid collection in the pelvic cavity (*arrows*)

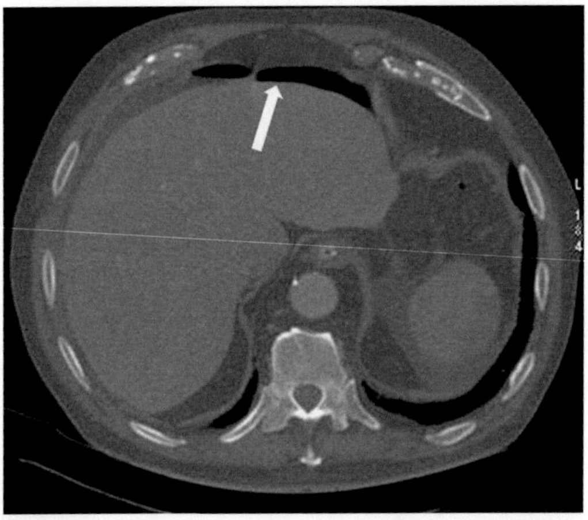

Fig. 9.10 Modest quote of pneumoperitoneum below the diaphragm (*arrow*)

References

1. Bohnen J, Boulanger M, Meakins JL (1983) Progress in generalized peritonitis. Relation to cause and risk factors. Arch Surg 118:285–290
2. Michael RBK, Norman SW (1999) Surgery of the anus, rectum and colon, 2nd edn. Bailliere Tindall, London, p 2434
3. Morris CR, Harvey IM, Stebbings WS et al (2002) Epidemiology of perforated colonic diverticular disease. Postgrad Med J 78:654–658
4. Imperiali G, Meucci G, Alvisi C et al (2000) Segmental colitis associated with diverticula: a prospective study. Am J Gastroenterol 95:1014–1016
5. Hsu CW, King TM, Wang JH et al (2007) Colorectal perforation: spectrum of the disease and its mortality. J Soc Colon Rectal Surg (Taiwan) 18:81–88
6. Ghahremani GG (1993) Radiologic evaluation of suspected gastrointestinal perforations. Radiol Clin North Am 31:1219–1234
7. Rubesin SE, Levine MS (2003) Radiologic diagnosis of gastrointestinal perforation. Radiol Clin North Am 41:1095–1115
8. Zissin R, Hertz M, Osadchy A et al (2008) Abdominal CT findings in nontraumatic colorectal perforation. Eur J Radiol 65:125–132
9. Sung HK, Sang SS, Jeong YY et al (2009) Gastrointestinal tract perforation: MDCT findings according to the Perforation Sites Korean. J Radiol 10:63–70
10. Ghekiere O, Lesnik A, Hoa D et al (2007) Value of computed tomography in the diagnosis of the cause of nontraumatic gastrointestinal tract perforation. J Comput Assist Tomogr 31:169–176
11. Maniatis V, Chryssikopoulos H, Roussakis A et al (2000) Perforation of the alimentary tract: evaluation with computed tomography. Abdom Imaging 25: 373–379
12. Stuhlfaut JW, Soto JA, Lucey BC et al (2004) Blunt abdominal trauma: performance of CT without oral contrast material. Radiology 233:689–694
13. Singh JP, Steward MJ, Booth TC (2010) Evolution of imaging for abdominal perforation. Ann R Coll Surg Engl 92:182–188
14. Zissin R, Hertz M, Osadchy A (2008) Abdominal CT findings in nontraumatic colorectal perforation. Eur J Radiol 65:125–132
15. Heffernan C, Pachter HL, Megibow AJ et al (2005) Stercoral colitis leading to fatal peritonitis: CT findings. Am J Roentgenol 184:1189–1193
16. Kumar P, Pearce O, Higginson A (2011) Imaging manifestations of faecal impaction and stercoral perforation. Clin Radiol 66:83–88
17. Jeonghyun Kang, Min Chung (2012) A stercoral perforation of the descending colon. J Korean Surg Soc 82:125–127
18. Zissin R, Konikoff F, Gayer G (2006) CT findings of iatrogenic complications following gastrointestinal endoluminal procedures. Semin Ultrasound CT MR 27:126–138
19. Pronio A, Di Filippo A, Narilli P et al (2007) Anastomotic dehiscence in colorectal surgery. Analysis of 1290 patients. Chir Ital 59:599–609
20. Nicksa GA, Dring RV, Johnson KH et al (2007) Anastomotic leaks: what is the best diagnostic imaging study? Dis Colon Rectum 50:197–203
21. Power N, Atri M, Ryan S (2007) CT assessment of anastomotic bowel leak. Clin Radiol 62:37–42, Computed tomography (CT) is the most readily available imaging tool for diagnosis of postoperative lower gastrointestinal tract (LGIT) leak
22. Danse E, Goncette L, Kartheuser A (2007) Optimal diagnosis of anastomotic colorectal leak by combination of conventional colonic enema and CT. JBR–BTR 90:526–527
23. Khoury W, Ben-Yehuda A, Ben-Haim M et al (2009) Abdominal computed tomography for diagnosing postoperative lower gastrointestinal tract leaks. J Gastrointest Surg 13:1454–1458
24. Berg DF, Bahadursingh AM, Kaminski DL et al (2002) Acute surgical emergencies in inflammatory bowel disease. Am J Surg 184:45–51

MDCT Imaging of Blunt Traumatic Bowel and Colonic Perforation

10

Francesco Iaselli, Isabella Iadevito, Franco Guida, Giacomo Sica, Giorgio Bocchini, and Mariano Scaglione

10.1 Epidemiology and Etiopathogenesis

The intestine represents the third most frequently involved structure in blunt abdominal trauma (BAT) after the liver and the spleen. Injuries of the small bowel and of the colon are relatively uncommon, being found in approximately 3–5 % of patients undergoing laparotomy and in about 1 % of patients evaluated with computed tomography (CT) [1–3].

Pathogenic mechanisms at the basis of small bowel and colonic traumatic perforations are substantially three, acting isolated or combined:

- A direct force may crush the gastrointestinal tract between the vertebrae and the anterior abdominal wall.
- A rapid deceleration may produce a shearing force between fixed and mobile portions of the involved tract.
- A sudden increase in intraluminal pressure may result in bursting injuries [1, 2, 4].

The leading cause of small bowel and colonic perforations in BAT is represented by road traffic accidents (RTA, 70–85 %), followed by aggressions and falls from heights. The incidence of these conditions is significantly higher in childhood in relation to the incomplete maturation of the muscles of the abdominal wall (in this age group, one of the most common causes is represented by impact of the handlebar of bicycle against the abdominal wall) [5–7].

With regard to intestinal perforations from RTA, an increase of the incidence of these conditions has been registered after the introduction of seat belts, which compress the intestinal loops at impact creating a "closed" hollow viscus; the subsequent increase of the intraluminal pressure exposes to the risk of bursting injuries. The presence of a "seat belt mark" sign is not surprisingly considered a reliable predictor of bowel injury [8].

The effect of a traumatic force applied to the intestinal wall is determined by the type and the severity of the traumatic insult, the anatomical features of the segments involved, the degree of distension of the intestinal lumen, and the characteristics of the intestinal content (a high content of fibers makes the loop more susceptible to "bursting" injuries) [9].

The most common site of traumatic intestinal perforation is the small intestine (70 %). In particular are more exposed to damage the loops close to points of anatomical or constituted fixity, where mobile and fixed portions of the gut are contiguous and therefore susceptible to shearing force: proximal jejunum near the ligament of Treitz, distal ileum near the ileocecal valve, and

F. Iaselli (✉) • I. Iadevito • F. Guida • G. Sica
G. Bocchini • M. Scaglione
Dipartimento di Diagnostica per Immagini, Clinica "Pineta Grande",
Via Domitiana, Km 30, Castel Volturno, Caserta 81100, Italy
e-mail: francescoiaselli@hotmail.it; isa.iadevito@hotmail.it; fraguida@hotmail.com; sicagf@libero.it; giorgio.bocchini@gmail.com; mscaglione@tiscali.it

L. Romano, A. Pinto (eds.), *Imaging of Alimentary Tract Perforation*,
DOI 10.1007/978-3-319-08192-2_10, © Springer International Publishing Switzerland 2015

intestinal segments close to bridles and adhesions [2, 9]. Rapid deceleration represents the primary mechanism of blunt duodenal injury causing tearing at the junction of the intraperitoneal (free) and retroperitoneal (fixed) portions of the duodenum, such as between the third and fourth portions. Associated signs of pancreatic injury should be sought in all cases, considering the very low incidence of isolated duodenal lesions in adults [10].

When perforation occurred at mobile segments of the small bowel, predicting the exact perforation site may be difficult [11].

Colon injury from BAT is uncommon, being diagnosed in about 0.5 % of all major blunt traumas and in 10.6 % of patients undergoing laparotomy. Most of these lesions are of partial thickness, and only 3 % of patients undergoing laparotomy have full-thickness colonic tears [7, 12].

Small bowel and colonic injuries from BAT can be divided into major and minor according to a prognostic criterion: "minor" intestinal lesions include incomplete lacerations of the intestinal wall, intramural hematomas, and parietal contusions; the only intestinal "major" injury in BAT is the full-thickness parietal tear resulting in small bowel or colonic perforation.

In the broad spectrum of intestinal injuries from BAT, small bowel and colonic perforations represent a significant condition for several reasons:

- The interruption of the intestinal wall creates a continuity between the septic intraluminal ambient and the peritoneum. The risk of chemical peritonitis and contamination of the peritoneal cavity by enteric pathogens imposes to perform proper therapeutic interventions in the quickest time possible [9].
- A direct traumatic force involving vascular structures afferent to the affected loops may lead to coexisting active bleeding or ischemic sufferance of the intestine, deprived of its vascular supply [13]. Both conditions result in a worse prognosis with respect to the cases of isolated involvement of the loop.
- Perforation may occur several hours after the traumatic event, as a consequence of structural primary alterations of the intestinal wall induced by trauma or, more frequently, as a result of the associated vascular lesions [2, 11].

10.2 Limits of Clinical and Laboratoristic Assessment

Tenderness is the most common sign of peritoneal irritation at physical examination of the abdomen in patients with small bowel or colonic perforation from BAT: these patients, in fact, have significantly higher rates of abdominal tenderness than patients with non-perforative small bowel and colonic injuries, and the presence of this clinical finding should always raise the suspicion of a severe intra-abdominal injury [3, 14].

Signs observed less frequently are decrease of bowel sounds, markings, and distention appearance.

Clinical diagnosis of small bowel and colonic perforation in BAT is often challenging for several reasons:

- Objective data are often nonspecific, and symptoms of peritoneal irritation are found in only half of the alert, non-comatose patients.
- Clear clinical signs of peritonitis have late onset (may not appear for hours), especially in the cases of perforations of the small intestine, whose content is characterized by neutral pH, low bacterial charge, and weak enzymatic activity.
- Symptoms can be hidden or attenuated by concomitant injuries, as in the case of major trauma or neurological impairment due to involvement of the head or spinal cord, or by medications which can mask pain and guarding,
- The attention for suspicious signs from the gastrointestinal tract can be reduced by coexisting, distracting lesions, such as femur fractures [9, 15, 16].

Previous studies reported that using clinical assessment alone as the indication for laparotomy to treat bowel or mesenteric injuries is associated with a negative laparotomy rate that may be as high as 40 % [17, 18].

Low values of specificity have been also described for laboratory parameters used in the assessment of patients with BAT [17, 18].

Diagnostic peritoneal lavage (DPL), according to different authors, is more sensitive than CT (even if performed with oral and endovenous contrast medium, slice thickness, and multidetector scanners) in identifying small bowel or colonic perforations and is limited, by practical factors, excessive sensitivity (even minor, self-limiting injuries may be emphasized), low specificity in assessing the site and the extent of the intraperitoneal damage, and lack of sensitivity for traumatic perforations of retroperitoneal viscera [14].

10.3 Minor Diagnostic Tools

Although ultrasonography (US) can identify peritoneal fluid collections, its sensitivity and specificity rates in diagnosing traumatic small bowel and colonic perforations are discouraging; moreover, same way as the DPL, US is "blind" towards lesions of retroperitoneal tract of the intestine because of its deep position [7, 15, 18].

Abdominal radiograms may reveal antideclivous air collections from a perforated hollow viscus or signs of impaired canalization due to the effects of BAT on the intestinal tract or the afferent blood vessels. In the era of multidetector CT, however, the role of conventional radiography is limited to particular situations, evaluated case by case [14, 16, 18].

10.4 Multidetector Computed Tomography

Multidetector computed tomography (MDCT) has been shown to be extremely accurate in diagnosing small bowel and colonic perforations from BAT, being the diagnostic test of choice in the hemodynamically stable and semi-stable patient [15, 18–21].

The diagnostic accuracy of MDCT in the detection of traumatic bowel perforation has significantly increased in the last decade due to the considerable availability of performing scanners and the consequent reduction of motion artifacts [2, 19, 21].

In the era of MDCT, all exams must be performed with a high-resolution protocol, with slice thickness, and a reconstruction interval values equals to 1 mm and completed by multiplanar reconstructions [19, 21].

Basal scans may be useful to detect free peritoneal air and to highlight the spontaneous hyperdensity of fluid collections [2]. A biphasic, arterial, and venous assessment after the intravenous infusion of 120–150 ml of iodinated contrast material at sufficient rate (≥3 ml/s) is recommended in order to detect active bleeding and to identify perfusion abnormalities of the walls of the intestinal loops. According to the "whole body" CT protocol for trauma, an acquisition in the late phase, 3–5 min after starting the infusion, may be useful in order to rule out low-flow active bleeding [13, 18, 21].

The radiologist is asked not only to identify the signs of trauma but also to provide an indication of the clinical significance of the detected lesions, focusing on conditions which, requiring immediate operative treatment, may change the management of the ill patient [15, 20–22].

10.5 CT Signs of Small Bowel and Colonic Traumatic Perforations

According to the kind and the degree of lesion, the CT signs of traumatic intestinal perforation are commonly divided into specific and nonspecific [9, 15, 20, 23].

Direct visualization of a bowel wall discontinuity and extraluminal spillage of enteric contents (such as fluid, oral contrast material, solid ingests, feces) represent the only specific signs of traumatic small bowel or colonic perforation. However, these signs are very uncommon [14, 22].

Nonspecific signs of perforation include acute intestinal behaviors, extraluminal air collections, intraperitoneal free fluid, and infiltration of the mesentery.

Bowel wall discontinuity, extraluminal spillage of enteric contents, and extraluminal air represent signs of major lesion, while infiltration of the mesentery and intraperitoneal fluid may be associated with both minor and major lesions [20, 23].

Intramural hematoma, wall thickening, and abnormal bowel wall enhancement are ancillary signs, not directly addressing to perforation but often coexisting with the abovementioned [20, 24].

10.5.1 Specific CT Signs of Small Bowel and Colonic Traumatic Perforation

10.5.1.1 Bowel Wall Discontinuity or Transection of the Wall with Focal Discontinuity of the Bowel Wall

Although this sign is 100 % specific, its sensitivity is low (approximately 7 %) [20, 24, 25] because, in most of the cases, bowel perforation is small and cannot be directly identified at CT but only with a meticulous surgical exploration.

10.5.1.2 Extraluminal Spillage of Enteric Contents

Similarly to the above-described sign, extraluminal spillage of enteric contents is highly specific but is affected by low sensitivity values (12 %) [24, 25] even if the study is conducted with previously oral contrast medium administration.

In this regard, it should be noted that most of the evidences in the literature discourage the administration of oral contrast material before the execution of the CT exam as well as it is time-consuming (time required for its preparation, its administration per os or using a nasoenteric probe, and its progression along the intestine may significantly affect the patient's prognosis by retarding the identification of traumatic injuries – e.g., active bleeding – requiring urgent interventions) [20, 26]. Moreover, the administration of oral contrast material in emergency patients with BAT does not seem to be diagnostically essential, especially in conditions of limited bowel distension [3, 14].

10.5.2 Nonspecific CT Signs of Small Bowel and Colonic Traumatic Perforation

10.5.2.1 Acute Intestinal Behaviors

Variations in tone, motility, shape, and location of the intestinal loops may represent the first hint of a small bowel or colonic perforation even in the absence of small amounts of free fluid and air [9, 27].

In most of the cases, reflex spastic ileus (RSI) due to persistent contracture of the bowel with a complete absence of intestinal gas is the first sign in order of appearance. When hypertonic spastic reaction ends, the bowel loops relaxes and the tone decreases leading to reflex hypotonic ileus (RHI) [23, 27].

RSI and RHI are characterized by an "intrinsic evolutivity" and should not be considered as separate entities, being possible the transition of each of these in the other at any time in response to internal or external stimuli [28].

10.5.2.2 Intraperitoneal Fluid

In most of the cases, intraperitoneal fluid may be the only sign of a significant bowel injury at the first CT evaluation: pneumoperitoneum or retropneumoperitoneum, in fact, may not be visible immediately after the trauma, taking some hours to appear (Fig. 10.1) [11, 24]. Management of patients with intraperitoneal fluid as the sole finding on CT scans includes laparotomy, diagnostic peritoneal lavage, or conservative management with follow-up CT [14, 21].

Nonphysiologic amounts of free intraperitoneal fluid (>75 ml in minimally resuscitated

Fig. 10.1 A 24-year-old male patient admitted to the emergency department after a blunt abdominal trauma (motor vehicle accident). (**a**) Plain film radiograph, upright view, shows scarce amount of air within the small bowel, with clear evidence of the psoas muscle's outline consistent with reflex spastic ileus. (**b**, **c**) Contrast-enhanced axial scan shows small amount of free fluid within the peritoneal cavity and absence of air. (**d–f**) Contrast-enhanced follow-up CT study (wide window) performed 24 h later depicts evidence of small amount of free air and fluid. The patient was sent to the operating room. At surgery, a traumatic small bowel perforation was found

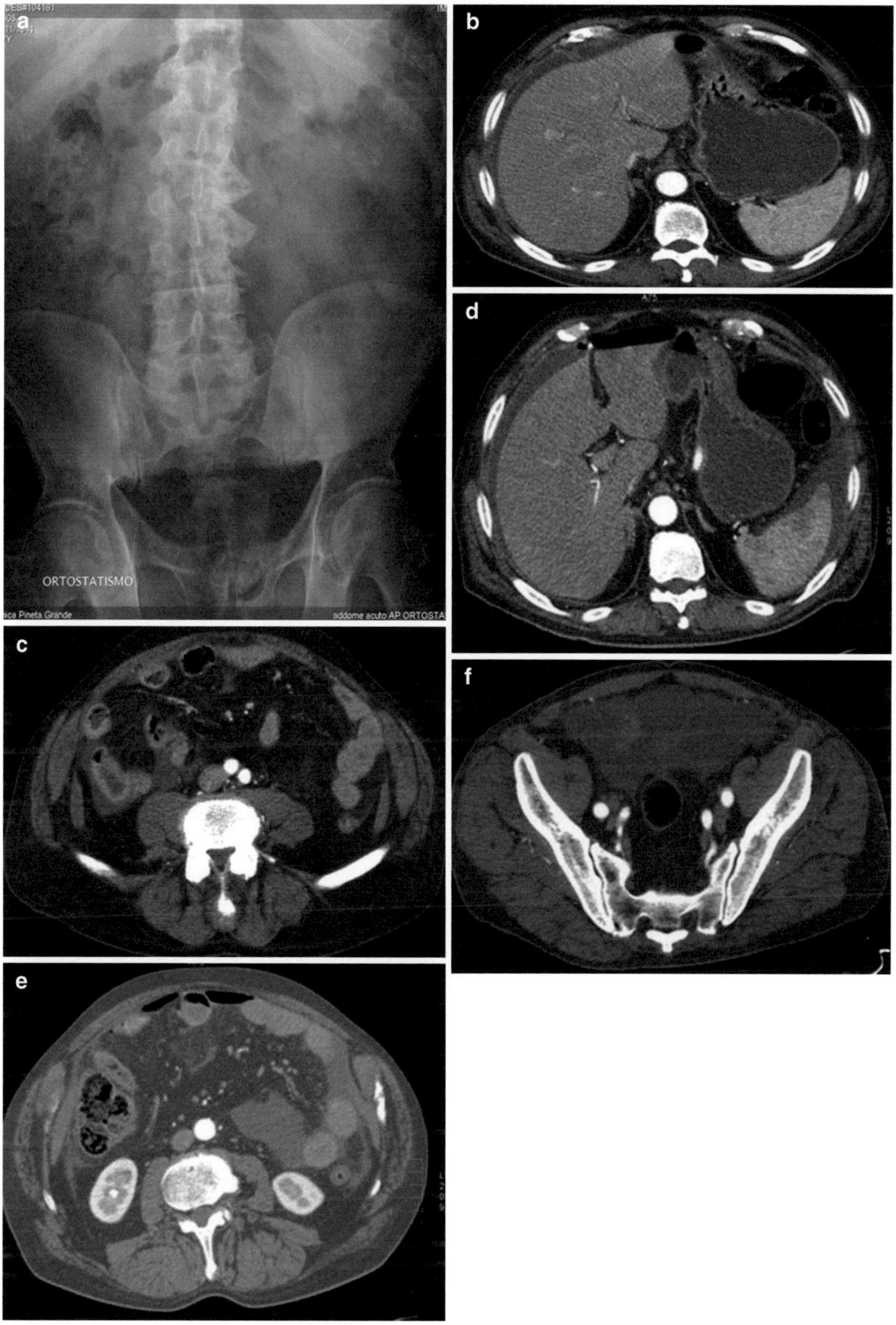
a
b
d
c
f
e
ORTOSTATISMO
ica Pineta Grande
addome acuto AP ORTOSTA

women of child bearing age, >25 ml in minimally resuscitated adult males, and >25 ml in children) without evidence for intraperitoneal solid organ injury suggest occult hollow viscus injury [28].

The distribution of fluid collections may indicate the injured structure [28]: while the hemoperitoneum from laceration of the liver or spleen is classically distributed in the subphrenic spaces, along the parieto-colic gutters and in the pelvis, in the case of a mesenteric or intestinal injury, fluid is more frequently observed among the loops and within the mesenteric folds, forming typical polygonal-shaped collections. In the case of a serosal laceration, in fact, the blood spreads through the mesenteric folds with a V-shaped morphology, with the base corresponding to the loop and the apex to the mesenteric root [23]. Fluid from laceration of a retroperitoneal hollow viscus tends to remain localized close to the site of injury [3, 29].

Origin of a peritoneal fluid may be also deduced from its densitometric characteristics: a low-density collection (average values of density lower than 20 HU, comparable to those of the bile inside the gallbladder or of the urine in the bladder) suggests the spillage of fluid from the intestine; a medium-density collection (>25 HU) is generally consisting largely of extravasated blood; a high-density collection (>120 HU) is attributable to the extravasation of contrast medium from damaged vessels or to the spillage of oral contrast material through bowel wall tears [28]. Notwithstanding these general assumptions, densitometric values do not have an absolute diagnostic value: a blood collection, for example, can appear with reduced density because of decreased hematocrit or the admixture with other fluids of lesser density (e.g., ascites, bile, urine) [20].

10.5.2.3 Extraluminal Air Collection (Intraperitoneal, Mesenteric, or Retroperitoneal)

Free extraluminal air represents a nonspecific but highly suggestive sign of intestinal injury from BAT; when observed, even in the absence of specific signs (interrupted intestinal wall, extraluminal spillage of enteric contents, intramural hematoma), the diagnostic hypothesis bowel injury should always be sought [9, 24]. Coexistent ancillary signs

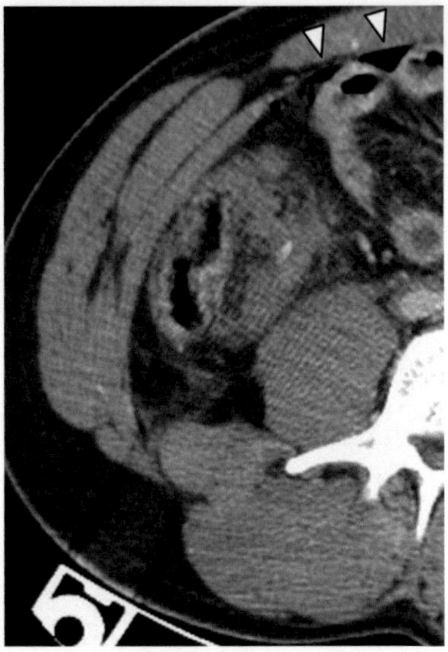

Fig. 10.2 Contrast-enhanced axial CT scan in a patient with blunt thoracoabdominal trauma shows asymmetric wall thickening of the medial aspect of the cecal wall associated with perivisceral soft tissue haziness. Note also the presence of free air with a typical triangular appearance (*arrows*). CT findings consisting with cecal perforated hematoma, confirmed at surgery

such as bowel wall thickening, abnormalities of parietal enhancement, free peritoneal fluid, and mesenteric infiltration may strengthen the diagnostic suspicion (Fig. 10.2) [25].

Extraluminal air collection is subdivided into free floating air (pneumoperitoneum and retroperitoneum) and mottled air bubbles (air entrapped within mesenteric layers).

Free floating peritoneal air is typically localized right off of the anterior abdominal wall or along the anterior surface of the liver and spleen, being easily identifiable even in small quantities [3, 23].

Mottled air bubbles indicate air nuclei confined inside the mesenteric sheets, into the lumen of the mesenteric and portal veins, in the thickness of the intestinal wall, or right off of a gas-filled hollow viscus. Their detection is more challenging and time-consuming, justifying the limited overall sensitivity reported in the literature for free air at computed tomography (44–55 %) [23, 24]. In these cases, detection of the small air bubbles may be difficult and time-consuming.

Mottled air bubbles, especially if adjacent to a bowel loop, have higher positive predictive value

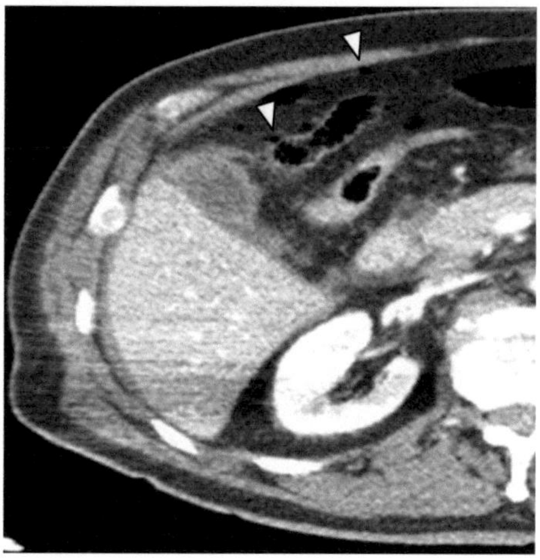

Fig. 10.3 Contrast-enhanced axial CT scan shows very small gas bubbles (*arrow heads*) in the peritoneal cavity, consisting with traumatic perforation of the adjacent bowel loop. This case outlines the importance of a careful assessment of the peritoneal cavity with a wide window setting

for intestinal lesion than free floating peritoneal air. This sign may suggest the location of bowel injury (Fig. 10.3) [4, 28].

A traumatic perforation of the duodenum and of the dorsal sides of the ascending and descending colon causes a pneumoretroperitoneum: extraluminal air extends through the fascial planes and may dissect them, being so detectable even at a great distance from the site of perforation [10, 29].

In all patients with blunt trauma who have any CT finding that could potentially be associated with a hollow viscus injury, images should be reviewed with lung or bone window settings, in addition to the routine soft tissue ones, in order to assess even small amounts of free abdominal air [9, 23].

10.5.2.4 Associated Mesenteric Anomalies

This minor CT sign of combined intestinal and mesenteric traumatic injury, represented by striae of inhomogeneous increase of the density of mesenteric fat, is caused by small hemorrhages within the mesentery.

Low specificity is reported for this finding, since it may be associated with both major and minor mesenteric lesions or bowel isolated lesion [30].

10.5.3 Ancillary Signs

10.5.3.1 Intramural Hematoma

Intramural hematoma represents a specific finding, difficult to detect in most of the cases, being recognized only after a careful retrospective analysis of the cases as an abnormal parietal mass [25].

Identification is more frequent in duodenal injuries (for its peculiar anatomical position, a direct force may crush the viscus against the vertebrae, as frequently happens in childhood traumas from bicycle's handlebars [5, 6] or in adults in traumas from steering wheels), rare in colonic lesions [10].

Flexion-distraction fractures of L1–L2 (Chance fracture) have been reported in association with duodenal intramural hematomas [10].

In the case of duodenal involvement, bowel thickening may be observed in association with fluid in the anterior pararenal space, making it challenging to differentiate a wall hematoma from a traumatic duodenal perforation in the absence of a frank perforation. Only the detection of free air in the anterior pararenal space addresses the diagnosis of perforation of the duodenum [10, 29].

Treatment is usually conservative: the hematoma resolves spontaneously within 3 weeks. In a limited percentage of cases, complications are observed at a medium to long term, most often in the form of luminal stenosis or obstruction [2].

10.5.3.2 Segmental/Focal Bowel Wall Thickening

Disproportionate circumferential thickening compared with the normal bowel segment and bowel wall thickness >3 mm is considered a nonspecific but significantly more sensitive sign of bowel traumatic injury compared to free air and extravasated oral contrast medium, being appreciable in approximately 75 % of full-thickness lacerations [24, 28, 31]. The associated finding of intramural air makes increases the specificity of wall thickening, making also likely the possibility of a full-thickness laceration [29].

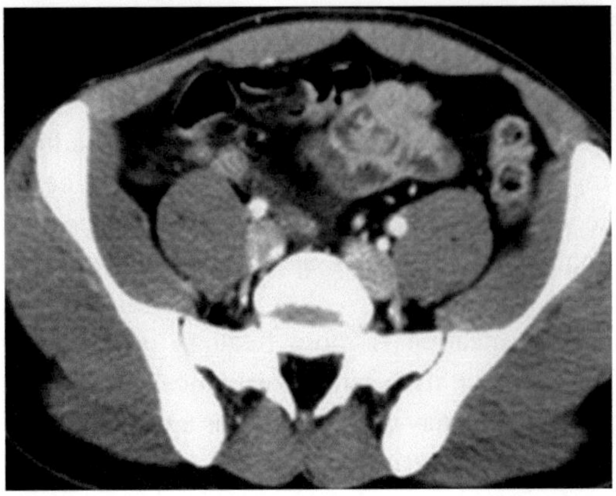

Fig. 10.4 Contrast-enhanced axial CT scan shows focal hyper-enhancement of the distal ileum. This CT finding is nonspecific and requires clinical correlation

10.5.3.3 Abnormal Bowel Wall Enhancement

Unequivocal focal abnormal enhancement (decreased or increased) of a segment of the bowel is a highly suspicious finding often associated with a significant injury especially if associated with a pocket of fluid in the adjacent mesentery or free fluid in the peritoneal cavity (Fig. 10.4) [20].

Vascular supply to a loop may be compromised by traumatic intestinal or mesenteric lesions: consequent hypoperfusion can paradoxically manifest itself as increased wall enhancement in the early stages due to the passage of molecules of the contrast medium through the more permeable damaged vascular endothelium.

Bowel wall density may be evaluated compared to that of the psoas muscle or of the contiguous vessels [32]. Patchy, irregular areas of increased impregnation of contrast medium represent a nonspecific sign of full-thickness laceration. Conversely, areas of decreased or absent bowel wall enhancement indicate traumatic bowel ischemia due to mesenteric vascular laceration [20].

10.6 CT Signs of Major Primary Mesenteric Injuries in BAT

Spectrum of primary mesenteric traumatic injuries includes conditions potentially associated with bowel primary or secondary involvement. Avulsion of the meso, active contrast medium extravasation, and mesenteric hematoma represent specific CT signs of mesenteric bowel injury. Nonspecific signs include mesenteric infarction and fluid collections [24, 30].

10.6.1 Mesenteric Avulsion

Peritoneal folds may be damaged at their insertion on the loop. In CT a triangular-shaped collection is observed, with the base oriented parallel to the loop and apex facing towards the meso; signs of loop sufferance from ischemia are generally associated [30, 32].

10.6.2 Active Hemorrhagic Extravasation

Traumatic laceration of the meso associated with mesenteric vessel rupture leads to hemorrhage and subsequent necrosis of the intestine, deprived of its vascular supply. The discontinuity of the vessel wall is demonstrated by the appearance of a blush of contrast medium along the course of the vessel circumscribed by a halo of tenuous hyperdensity, corresponding to the hematoma. This CT sign is characterized by 100 % specificity [30], representing an absolute indication for urgent operative treatment and frequently associating with major traumatic lesions of the bowel walls.

10.6.3 Mesenteric Hematoma

Contained vascular lesions usually lead to the formation of mesenteric hematomas. In the absence of an active bleeding, the treatment of such entities is conservative. However, large hematomas may compress vascular structures leading to ischemic changes of the intestine [30, 32].

CT density of a not-supplied hematoma is usually closer to that of soft tissues to that of the fluid, being the blood in large part coagulated. Basal scans may reveal a circumscribed, inhomogeneously hyperdense hematoma close to the site of active blood extravasation "the sentinel clot sign."

10.7 Pitfalls, Mimic, and Masks

- The administration of oral contrast material in emergency patients with BAT represents a potential source of pitfalls and misdiagnoses [26, 32]: the spread of the iodine-based, endovenous contrast medium from an intraperitoneal traumatic rupture of the bladder, for example, may mimic the spillage of previously administered oral contrast material from intestinal loops. Extraluminal oral contrast material from injured bowel loops, then, may mimic extravasated contrast medium from ruptured vessels [33, 34].
- Unsatisfactory specificity rates are reported for intraperitoneal fluid as a sign of mesenteric or intestinal lesion: its presence may be related to other coexisting lesions (e.g., hepatic, splenic). As already written, analysis of qualitative (e.g., density, locations) and quantitative characteristics of fluid collections may help in identifying the injured structure. As a general rule, the presence of intraperitoneal fluid without clear evidence of splenic or hepatic lesions should always address towards the suspicion of intestinal injury [29, 33, 34].
- In patients with history of BAT, before attributing with certainty the presence of free air in the peritoneum to the trauma itself, it is necessary to exclude other potential causes of pneumoperitoneum: previous execution of a diagnostic peritoneal lavage, diffusion of air from the mediastinum, mechanical ventilation, pulmonary barotrauma, pneumothorax, chest and diaphragmatic injury (Fig. 10.5), provenience of the air from the apparatus female genital tract, and laceration of the peritoneal side of the bladder [34].
- The so-called pseudo-pneumoperitoneum (air entrapped between the abdominal wall and the parietal peritoneal layer) represents a diagnostic pitfall, mimicking true pneumoperitoneum [9].
- A non-circumferential parietal thickening, limited to the declivous side of the loop, should not be interpreted as a sign of intestinal traumatic injury, being only apparent, caused by the stratification of the intestinal contents [24, 34].

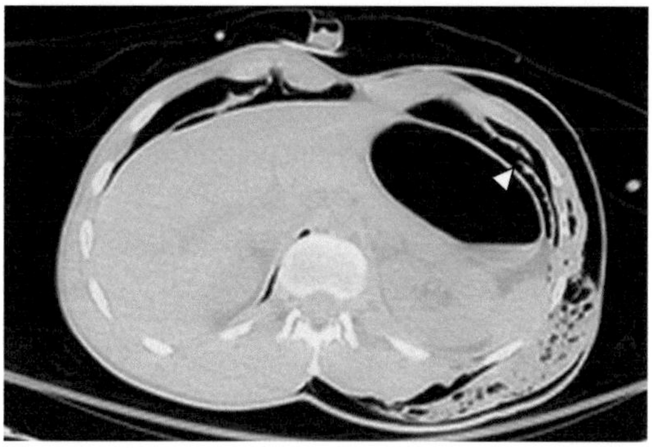

Fig. 10.5 Axial CT scan in a patient with severe blunt trauma (lung window) shows subcutaneous and properitoneal air tracking into the peritoneal cavity through a diaphragmatic tear (*arrow*)

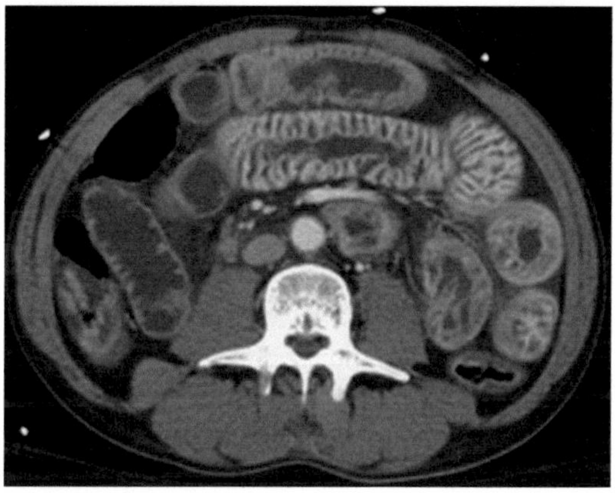

Fig. 10.6 Contrast-enhanced axial CT scan shows diffuse parietal thickening, fluid distension of the loops, and increased bowel wall enhancement secondary to profound hypotension with hypoperfusion complex in a male patient after blunt abdominal trauma: "shock bowel"

- "Shock bowel" represents a transient condition source of false positivity for posttraumatic bowel wall thickening in patients with BAT: diffuse parietal thickening, fluid distension of the loops, and increased bowel wall enhancement (Fig. 10.6) may be secondary to profound hypotension with hypoperfusion complex. Probably during hypoperfusion, vascular permeability increases with a preferential shift of blood flow to the mucosa [35]. The identification of the hypoperfusion complex (flat inferior vena cava, increased enhancement of the adrenal glands, bowel, pancreatic and retroperitoneal edema, "nutmeg liver" appearance, or periportal edema, with concentric halo of low attenuation around the portal vein) may help in the differential diagnosis between "shock bowel" and segmental/focal bowel wall thickening from bowel injury [34, 35].

- A reversible, diffuse bowel wall thickening may also be associated with hyperhydration and volume overload; edematous imbibitions of the mesentery and fluid film in the periportal and pericholecystic spaces are often observed, while the increased wall enhancement and the signs of systemic hypotension are absent.
- Further possible sources of false positivity for bowel wall thickening from trauma are the lack of bowel distension, coexisting inflammatory infectious diseases, isolated tear of the mesentery, interruption of the vascular arterial supply, or venous drainage and nontraumatic hematoma [24, 25, 34].

Conclusions

Clinical assessment alone of patients with suspected intestinal injury from BAT is associated with unacceptable diagnostic delays. Prompt identification and proper classification of small bowel and colonic injuries represent crucial issues in the management of patients with BAT. Their prognosis is significantly influenced by a timely diagnosis in the cases requiring immediate surgical interventions. The radiologist, moreover, may suggest the opportunity of conservative treatment in the cases of mild and moderate, noncomplicated, or self-limiting injuries.

References

1. Watts DD, Fakhry SM (2003) Incidence of hollow viscus injury in blunt trauma: an analysis from 275,557 trauma admissions from the East multi-institutional trial. J Trauma 54(2):289–294
2. Romano S, Scaglione M, Tortora G, Martino A, Di Pietto F, Romano L, Grassi R (2006) MDCT in blunt intestinal trauma. Eur J Radiol 59(3):359–366
3. Shanmuganathan K (2004) Multi-detector row CT imaging of blunt abdominal trauma. Semin Ultrasound CT MR 25(2):180–204
4. Scaglione M, Linsenmaier U, Schueller G (2012) Emergency radiology of the abdomen. Springer, Heidelberg, New York, Dordrecht, London
5. Cox TD, Kuhn JP (1996) CT scan of bowel trauma in the pediatric patient. Radiol Clin North Am 34(4):807–818
6. Bruny JL, Bensard DD (2004) Hollow viscous injury in the pediatric patient. Semin Pediatr Surg 13(2): 112–118
7. Bondia JM, Anderson SW, Rhea JT, Soto J (2009) Imaging colorectal trauma using 64-MDCT technology. Emerg Radiol 16(6):433–440
8. Appleby JP, Nagy AG (1989) Abdominal injuries associated with the use of seatbelts. Am J Surg 157(5):457–458
9. Hines J, Rosenblat J, Duncan DR, Friedman B, Katz DS (2013) Perforation of the mesenteric small bowel: etiologies and CT findings. Emerg Radiol 20(2): 155–161
10. Daly KP, Ho CP, Persson DL, Gay SB (2008) Traumatic retroperitoneal injuries: review of multidetector CT findings. Radiographics 28(6):1571–1590
11. Matsushima K, Mangel PS, Schaefer EW, Frankel HL (2013) Blunt hollow viscus and mesenteric injury: still underrecognized. World J Surg 37(4):759–765
12. Williams MD, Watts D, Fakhry S (2003) Colon injury after blunt abdominal trauma: results of the EAST Multi-Institutional Hollow Viscus Injury Study. J Trauma 55(5):906–912
13. Hamilton JD, Kumaravel M, Censullo ML, Cohen AM, Kievlan DS, West OC (2008) Multidetector CT evaluation of active extravasation in blunt abdominal and pelvic trauma patients. Radiographics 28(6):1603–1616
14. LeBedis CA, Anderson SW, Soto JA (2012) CT imaging of blunt traumatic bowel and mesenteric injuries. Radiol Clin North Am 50(1):123–136
15. Tan KK, Liu JZ, Go TS, Vijayan A, Chiu MT (2010) Computed tomography has an important role in hollow viscus and mesenteric injuries after blunt abdominal trauma. Injury 41(5):475–478
16. Fakhry SM, Brownstein M, Watts DD, Baker CC, Oller D (2000) Relatively short diagnostic delays (<8 hours) produce morbidity and mortality in blunt small bowel injury: an analysis of time to operative intervention in 198 patients from a multicenter experience. J Trauma 48(3):408–415
17. Malinoski DJ, Patel MS, Yakar DO, Green D, Qureshi F, Inaba K, Brown CV, Salim A (2010) A diagnostic delay of 5 hours increases the risk of death after blunt hollow viscus injury. J Trauma 69(1):84–87
18. Stuhlfaut JW, Anderson SW, Soto JA (2007) Blunt abdominal trauma: current imaging techniques and CT findings in patients with solid organ, bowel, and mesenteric injury. Semin Ultrasound CT MR 28(2):115–129
19. Hanks PW, Brody JM (2003) Blunt injury to mesentery and small bowel: CT evaluation. Radiol Clin North Am 41(6):1171–1182
20. Soto JA, Anderson SW (2012) Multidetector CT of blunt abdominal trauma. Radiology 265(3):678–693
21. Pinto A, Magliocca M, Grassi R, Scaglione M, Romano L, Angelelli G (2001) Role of computerized tomography in the diagnosis of peritoneo-intestinal lesions resulting from closed trauma.

Experience at 2 emergency departments. Radiol Med 101(3):177–182
22. Joseph DK, Kunac A, Kinler RL, Staff I, Butler KL (2013) Diagnosing blunt hollow viscus injury: is computed tomography the answer? Am J Surg 205(4): 414–418
23. Brofman N, Atri M, Hanson JM, Grinblat L, Chughtai T, Brenneman F (2006) Evaluation of bowel and mesenteric blunt trauma with multidetector CT. Radiographics 26(4):1119–1131
24. Breen DJ, Janzen DL, Zwirewich CV, Nagy AG (1997) Blunt bowel and mesenteric injury: diagnostic performance of CT signs. J Comput Assist Tomogr 21(5):706–712
25. Levine CD, Gonzales RN, Wachsberg RH, Ghanekar D (1997) CT findings of bowel and mesenteric injury. J Comput Assist Tomogr 21(6):974–979
26. Allen TL, Mueller MT, Bonk RT, Harker CP, Duffy OH, Stevens MH (2004) Computed tomographic scanning without oral contrast solution for blunt bowel and mesenteric injuries in abdominal trauma. J Trauma 56(2):314–322
27. Grassi R, Di Mizio R, Pinto A, Romano L, Rotondo A (2004) Serial plain abdominal film findings in the assessment of acute abdomen: spastic ileus, hypotonic ileus, mechanical ileus and paralytic ileus. Radiol Med 108(1–2):56–70
28. Levine CD, Patel UJ, Wachsberg RH, Simmons MZ, Baker SR, Cho KC (1995) CT in patients with blunt abdominal trauma: clinical significance of intraperitoneal fluid detected on a scan with otherwise normal findings. AJR Am J Roentgenol 164(6):1381–1385
29. Rodriguez C, Barone JE, Wilbanks TO, Rha CK, Miller K (2002) Isolated free fluid on computed tomographic scan in blunt abdominal trauma: a systematic review of incidence and management. J Trauma 53(1):79–85
30. Dowe MF, Shanmuganathan K, Mirvis SE, Steiner RC, Cooper C (1997) CT findings of mesenteric injury after blunt trauma: implications for surgical intervention. AJR Am J Roentgenol 168(2):425–428
31. Macari M, Balthazar EJ (2001) CT of bowel wall thickening: significance and pitfalls of interpretation. AJR Am J Roentgenol 176(5):1105–1116
32. Scaglione M, Romano L, Bocchini G, Sica G, Guida F, Pinto A, Grassi R (2012) Multidetector computed tomography of pancreatic, small bowel, and mesenteric traumas. Semin Roentgenol 47(4):362–370
33. Killeen KL, Shanmuganathan K, Poletti PA, Cooper C, Mirvis SE (2001) Helical computed tomography of bowel and mesenteric injuries. J Trauma 51(1): 26–36
34. Brody JM, Leighton DB, Murphy BL, Abbott GF, Vaccaro JP, Jagminas L, Cioffi WG (2000) CT of blunt trauma bowel and mesenteric injury: typical findings and pitfalls in diagnosis. Radiographics 20(6):1525–1536
35. Mirvis SE, Shanmuganathan K, Erb R (1994) Diffuse small-bowel ischemia in hypotensive adults after blunt trauma (shock bowel): CT findings and clinical significance. AJR Am J Roentgenol 163(6):1375–1377

MDCT Imaging of Gastrointestinal Tract Perforation Due to Foreign Body Ingestion

11

Roberta Cianci, Valentina Bianco, Gianluigi Esposito, Andrea Delli Pizzi, and Antonella Filippone

11.1 Etiology and Clinical Scenario

The ingestion of alimentary *foreign bodies* (FBs) is relatively common, but most of them pass through the *gastrointestinal* (*GI*) *tract* uneventfully within 1 week [1], and perforation is rare, occurring in less than 1 % of patients [1, 2]. FBs that complicate with *perforation* are usually sharp, hard, pointed, or elongated; they can be calcified (such as *fish or chicken bones*), metallic, or wooden (such as toothpicks, skewers, chopsticks) [2–5].

Injury may occur anywhere from the mouth to the anus, but the most common sites of perforation include less fixed segments or those with acute angulation, such as the ileum, the ileocecal, and rectosigmoid segments [2, 4].

Voluntary ingestion of FBs is most common among prisoners or in people who attempt suicide [2]. In the majority, FB ingestion is unconscious and/or accidental and is most common in the extremities of life (children and elderly), in patients with mental disorders, in alcohol and drug abusers, in subjects who eat rapidly, and in professionally exposed people (carpenters, dressmakers, upholsterers). Subjects who wear dentures are particularly susceptible, because they lack the sensitivity of the soft palate that is crucial for the recognition of small, sharp, or hard items that may be included in the food bolus [1–3].

Usually, nonmetallic dietary FB accidental ingestion is forgotten as it does not significantly impress patient's memory. Moreover, there may be a considerable time lag of weeks or months between the time of ingestion and the onset of symptoms [1, 3].

FB perforation of the GI tract has a wide spectrum of clinical presentations, which can be acute or chronic. Patients occasionally present with unusual or even bizarre manifestation, including hemorrhage, obstruction, and even ureteral colic [1, 3].

As the clinical suspicion is low and the clinical presentation is varied and nonspecific, imaging plays an important role in the diagnosis [4]. The prompt recognition of the presence, level, and cause of perforation is important for appropriate patient management and surgical planning [6].

11.2 MDCT Technique

The introduction of *multidetector CT* (MDCT) has allowed high-speed acquisition, thin slice collimation, and high spatial resolution, making this technique particularly suitable for the

R. Cianci • V. Bianco • G. Esposito • A.D. Pizzi • A. Filippone (✉)
Section of Diagnostic Imaging, Department of Neurosciences and Imaging, "G. d'Annunzio" University, Via dei Vestini, Chieti 66100, Italy
e-mail: r.cianci@rad.unich.it; valbianco@yahoo.it; gianluigiesposito84@libero.it; andrea.dellipizzi@yahoo.it; a.filippone@rad.unich.it

L. Romano, A. Pinto (eds.), *Imaging of Alimentary Tract Perforation*, DOI 10.1007/978-3-319-08192-2_11, © Springer International Publishing Switzerland 2015 assessment of patients with abdominal pain from GI disease [7].

We suggest to acquire data with a thin collimation (≤1 mm) and to reconstruct the axial images with a thickness of ≤3 mm. The use of these parameters provides a better spatial resolution of both axial and reformatted images.

Intravenous contrast administration (300–400 mgI/mL) is mandatory when not contraindicated, because it aids in depicting abnormalities of the GI wall and surroundings [4, 6, 8]. Usually a delay of 70 s after contrast injection provides a good quality enhancement of both bowel wall and abdominal organs.

The acquisition of non-enhanced phase should be recommended, mainly for less experienced radiologists, since the majority FBs appear as hyperdense objects.

Although extraluminal leakage of oral contrast material has been described as specific of GI perforation, the reported sensitivity of this sign is low, mainly in the presence of FBs [6, 7]. As a matter of fact, the extraluminal passage of the oral contrast material may be precluded by the rapid sealing of the perforation site and by the slow progression due to paralytic ileus, from which these patients may suffer. Moreover, the major limit of positive oral contrast agent is to obscure subtle bowel wall changes or intraluminal high-density foreign objects [5, 7, 8]. Therefore, in our opinion, oral contrast agent is not indicated in patients suspected of having a GI perforation from FBs.

The use of reformatted images, such as multiplanar (*MPR*) and thin-slab maximum intensity projection (*MIP*), is advocated since it may increase the diagnostic confidence. As a matter of fact, these images are very useful when the orientation of an FB with respect to the axial CT scan affects the perception of the viewer [1, 5]. Furthermore, scrolling MPR may help to recognize and follow the bowel loops along their course. In this way it is possible to increase the detection rate of subtle findings, such as small extraluminal fluid or air collections, adjacent to the bowel wall.

Assessment of lung window setting in addition to the standard abdominal window setting increases the sensitivity for detection of small free air pockets [4, 6, 8].

11.3 MDCT Findings

The diagnosis of GI tract perforation on CT is generally based on identification of extraluminal leakage and consequent inflammatory reaction around the perforation site [6]. Extraluminal air is the major specific sign of GI tract perforation [4, 7, 9], and MDCT is the most reliable imaging modality for detecting even small amounts of free air [2, 4, 6–8, 10]. Rarely abundant free pneumoperitoneum occurs in the setting of GI tract *perforation* related to FB ingestion, especially when small bowel is involved [5]. The passage of large amounts of intraluminal air into the peritoneal cavity is limited by the fact that the FB produces a gradual erosion of the intestinal wall which results to being covered by fibrin, omentum, or adjacent bowel loops [1, 3]. Therefore, tiny bubbles of free air embedded in the omentum and mesenteric folds or located along the anterior aspect of the abdominal cavity should be carefully evaluated.

So far, we described all the MDCT findings indicative of the presence of perforation. But since the management may depend on the location of bowel defect, the next step is to identify the site of perforation. The first CT feature to this aim is the focal thickening of the GI wall (>8 mm in stomach and duodenum, > 3 mm in jejunum and ileum, >5 mm in colon and rectum) in close proximity to *extraluminal air bubbles*, with adjacent regional *mesenteric fat stranding* [2, 7, 9].

In other cases, localized perienteric gas or fluid collections and *abscesses* lying on the perforated bowel wall represent an indirect clue of site perforation. Therefore, we recommend to carefully assess both axial and reformatted images for detection of localized interloop collections of extraluminal gas or fluid.

Sometimes the site of *perforation* may be specified by the direct visualization of discontinuity of the GI wall, which appears as a low-attenuating cleft. Although MPR may be useful to identify the focal defect on the GI wall when axial images are indeterminate, this finding is not commonly detected, owing to the small size of the lesion [2, 7, 8].

When the perforation or directly the FB itself causes a local inflammatory reaction which involves the adjacent loops, the main finding is an occlusive pattern. In these cases, the recognition of *obstruction* level may indicate the perforation site [1, 2].

Ultimately, a definitive CT diagnosis is established by identifying the FB. Calcified and metallic FBs are easily detected on CT, and the use of a bone window setting [4, 10] allows to better appreciate their morphology and edges. Also in presence of less radiodense FB, such as *fish bones*, CT provides good contrast resolution, showing a thin and linear hyperdensity [10] (Fig. 11.1).

To be able to detect the FB, the radiologist has to keep in mind that besides an intraluminal or partial extraluminal location (Fig. 11.2) at the level of the perforated loop, it may lie free in the peritoneal cavity passing through the bowel wall. It means that we can find the FB far from the perforation site [3, 5].

We have to underline that, unfortunately, non-calcified wooden FBs, e.g., toothpicks, skewers,

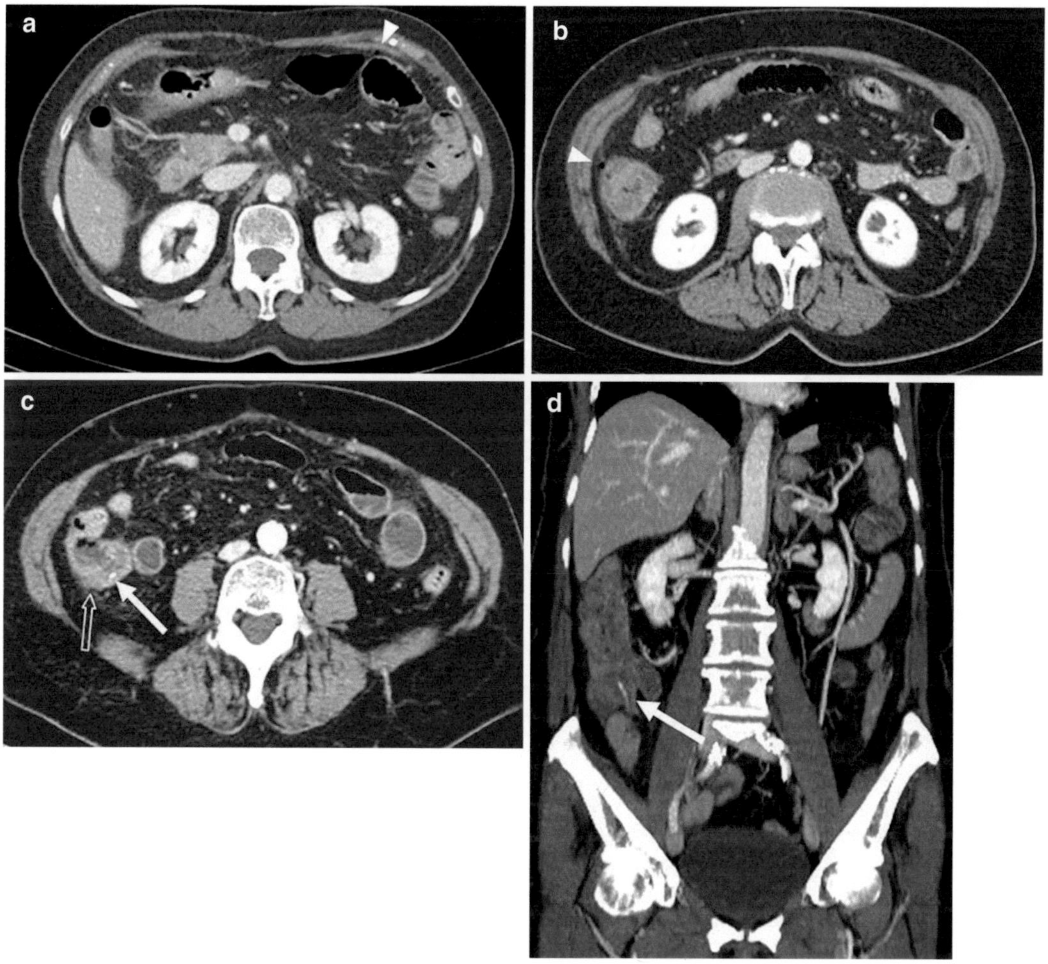

Fig. 11.1 Surgically confirmed right colon perforation caused by a salted codfish bone in a 56-year-old woman complaining with vague abdominal pain. Contrast-enhanced images (**a–c**: axial views, **d**: coronal thin-slab MIP) show tiny free air bubbles (*arrowheads* in **a** and **b**), thickening of the right colon wall with surrounding fat stranding (*open arrow* in **c**), and an endoluminal linear hyperdense structure indicative of foreign body (*arrow* in **c**), better appreciable on MIP reconstruction (*arrow* in **d**)

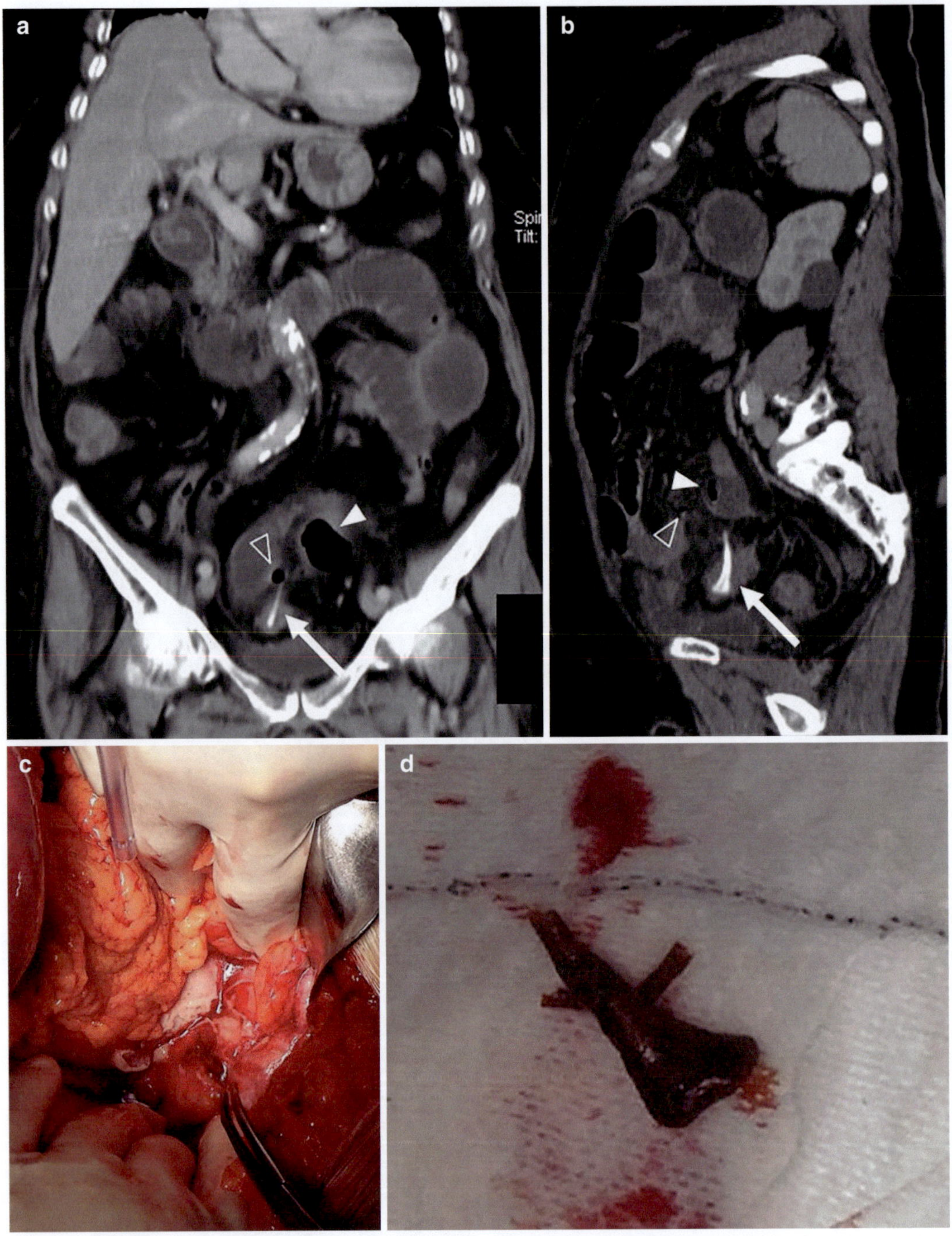

Fig. 11.2 Sigmoid colon perforation caused by a chicken bone in an 84-year-old woman with Alzheimer disease. CT images (**a**: coronal MIP; **b**: sagittal oblique MIP) show free air bubbles (*open arrowheads* in **a** and **b**) and a localized abscess (*arrowheads* in **a** and **b**) with a hyperdense foreign body through the sigmoid colon wall (*arrows* in **a** and **b**). These findings were confirmed by surgery (**c**, **d**: Courtesy of Prof. Felice Mucilli, Department of Biomedical Sciences, "G. d'Annunzio" University of Chieti, Italy)

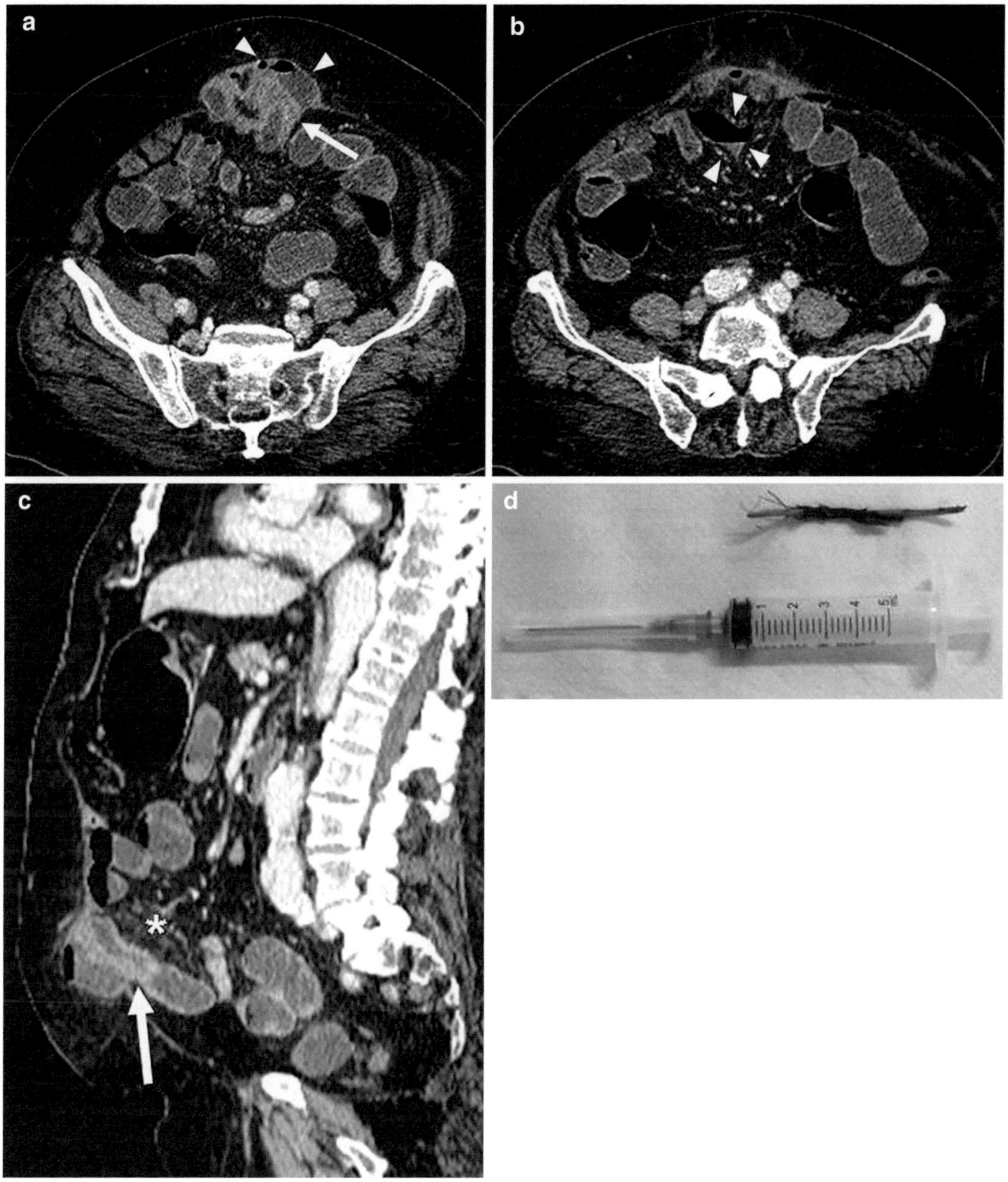

Fig. 11.3 An 81-year-old man presenting at the emergency department with acute abdominal pain and leukocytosis. Contrast-enhanced images (**a**, **b**: axial views, **c**: sagittal MPR) demonstrate dilated fluid filled small bowel loops and a postoperative ventral hernia including a small bowel loop that shows mural thickening (*arrows* in **a** and **c**) with adjacent mesenteric fat stranding (*asterisk* in **c**) and localized air/fluid collections (*arrowhead* in **a** and **b**). These findings were indicative of small bowel obstruction caused by the abdominal hernia, complicated with perforation. At surgery, a fragment of a wood skewer (**d**: Courtesy of Prof. Felice Mucilli, Department of Biomedical Sciences, "G. d'Annunzio" University of Chieti, Italy) was found within the perforated loop. The foreign body was not detectable on MDCT examination owing to its nature

and chopsticks, may be missed even at an accurate inspection, owing to their isoattenuating appearance. Dry and fresh wood may respectively show air and water components, which are hardly distinguishable from the normal GI tract content (Fig. 11.3).

Conclusions

In conclusion, GI tract perforation caused by FB is rarely clinically suspected, owing to the frequent lack of awareness of ingestion [9]. The diagnosis should always be considered at CT, particularly in the elderly patients, when other causes of abdominal pain have been excluded.

The accurate MDCT image analysis performed with a high index of suspicion allows to identify subtle findings and to achieve the correct diagnosis, with obvious advantage for patient's prognosis.

References

1. Goh BK, Tan YM, Lin SE et al (2006) CT in the preoperative diagnosis of fish bone perforation of the gastrointestinal tract. AJR Am J Roentgenol 187(3):710–714
2. Coulier B, Tancredi MH, Ramboux A (2004) Spiral CT and multidetector-row CT diagnosis of perforation of the small intestine caused by ingested foreign bodies. Eur Radiol 14(10):1918–1925
3. Goh BK, Chow PK, Quah HM et al (2006) Perforation of the gastrointestinal tract secondary to ingestion of foreign bodies. World J Surg 30(3):372–377
4. Zissin R, Hertz M, Osadchy A et al (2008) Abdominal CT findings in nontraumatic colorectal perforation. Eur J Radiol 65(1):125–132
5. Hines J, Rosenblat J, Duncan DR et al (2013) Perforation of the mesenteric small bowel: etiologies and CT findings. Emerg Radiol 20(2):155–161
6. Furukawa A, Sakoda M, Yamasaki M et al (2005) Gastrointestinal tract perforation: CT diagnosis of presence, site, and cause. Abdom Imaging 30(5): 524–534
7. Hainaux B, Agneessens E, Bertinotti R et al (2006) Accuracy of MDCT in predicting site of gastrointestinal tract perforation. AJR Am J Roentgenol 187(5): 1179–1183
8. Kim SH, Shin SS, Jeong YY et al (2009) Gastrointestinal tract perforation: MDCT findings according to the perforation sites. Korean J Radiol 10(1):63–70
9. Yeung KW, Chang MS, Hsiao CP, Huang JF (2004) CT evaluation of gastrointestinal tract perforation. Clin Imaging 28(5):329–333
10. Zissin R, Osadchy A, Gayer G (2009) Abdominal CT findings in small bowel perforation. Br J Radiol 82(974):162–171

12 Pneumoretroperitoneum: Imaging Findings

Antonio Pinto, Carlo Muzj, and Giuseppe Ruggiero

12.1 Introduction

Pneumoretroperitoneum is defined by the presence of free air within the retroperitoneal space. The retroperitoneum is the compartmentalized space bounded anteriorly by the posterior parietal peritoneum and posteriorly by the transversalis fascia. It extends from the diaphragm superiorly to the pelvic brim inferiorly [1].

Most often, air is seen surrounding the kidneys and overlying the contour of the iliopsoas muscles. Free air can accumulate in the retroperitoneal space after perforation of a retroperitoneal bowel segment, or air can spread below the diaphragm from a pneumomediastinum.

12.2 Etiology

Common causes of pneumoretroperitoneum are reported in Table 12.1.

Duodenal perforation is an acute illness whose major causes are peptic ulcer disease, endoscopic complication of endoscopic retrograde cholangiopancreatography or sphincterotomy, and blunt abdominal trauma [2].

A. Pinto (✉) • C. Muzj • G. Ruggiero
Department of Radiology,
"A. Cardarelli" Hospital,
Via Cardarelli 9, Naples I-80131, Italy
e-mail: antopin1968@libero.it; cmuzj@sirm.org; gruggiero1@sirm.org

Perforation of the duodenum caused by blunt trauma to the abdomen is now being encountered as an automobile lap belt deceleration injury. In duodenal injuries, mural hematoma, laceration, or complete transection of the duodenum is usually encountered, attributable to the following mechanisms: (1) tearing during deceleration, (2) crushing between the abdominal wall and the spine, and (3) blowout [3].

Rupture usually occurs at the junction of the second and third portions, which are retroperitoneal, resulting in a local accumulation of gas in the right perirenal or anterior pararenal space; multiple perforations are possible, and there may be accompanying traumatic pancreatitis. Duodenal perforation may also be secondary to leukemia and penetrating foreign body. Severe pelvic fractures, dislodging bony fragments, can perforate the rectum, allowing intestinal gas to migrate into the retroperitoneal spaces. Rectal perforations can also result from iatrogenic procedures, infection, or colorectal cancer. Self-induced colorectal perforations are rare and can

Table 12.1 Common causes of pneumoretroperitoneum

Common causes of pneumoretroperitoneum
Penetrating trauma
Blunt traumatic rupture of the duodenum
Pelvic trauma with perforation of the rectum
Postoperative
Post-diagnostic procedure
Spontaneous colon perforation
Extension from pneumomediastinum
Gas-containing retroperitoneal abscess

L. Romano, A. Pinto (eds.), *Imaging of Alimentary Tract Perforation*,
DOI 10.1007/978-3-319-08192-2_12, © Springer International Publishing Switzerland 2015

result from foreign body or accidental impalement. Distinction between injuries to the intraperitoneal and extraperitoneal segments of the rectum is an important consideration in patients with rectal injury given the differences in their subsequent management. The anterior and lateral sidewalls of the upper two-thirds of the rectum are covered with peritoneum, and injuries to these segments are considered intraperitoneal. The distal one-third of the rectum circumferentially and the upper two-thirds of the rectum posteriorly are not covered with peritoneum and are considered extraperitoneal [4].

Spontaneous pneumoretroperitoneum is commonly a consequence of perforations of colonic diverticula or carcinomas. The thorax and the extraperitoneal spaces communicate directly through the mediastinum posteriorly and, to a lesser extent, across small midline openings in the diaphragm anteriorly. Thus, any cause of pneumomediastinum may also determine the presence of pneumoretroperitoneum.

Other causes of pneumoretroperitoneum include superinfected necrotizing pancreatitis, necrotizing fasciitis, abscess formation, percutaneous biopsy, epidural anesthesia, extracorporeal shock-wave lithotripsy, and hydrogen peroxide wound irrigation [1].

Pneumoretroperitoneum following endoscopic procedures is extensive, however, because of the high pressure gradient generated and the large volume of air insufflated; it is thus sometimes associated with pneumoperitoneum and pneumothorax [5]. Pneumoretroperitoneum can be also a possible finding of bowel infarction [6].

12.3 Pneumoretroperitoneum: Plain Abdominal Film and CT Findings

Conventional radiography is commonly the initial imaging examination performed in the diagnostic workup of patients who present with acute abdominal pain to the emergency department.

Conventional radiography includes supine and upright conventional abdominal radiography and upright chest radiography [7]. On plain film, beneath the diaphragm, it is often difficult to differentiate retroperitoneal from intraperitoneal air: retroperitoneal air is usually crescentic, with curvilinear upper and lower borders. Free air rises to the peak of the diaphragmatic dome, whereas retroperitoneal air is usually positioned more inferiorly. Retroperitoneal air generally accumulates either medially or laterally rather than directly beneath the apex of the diaphragmatic leaf [8].

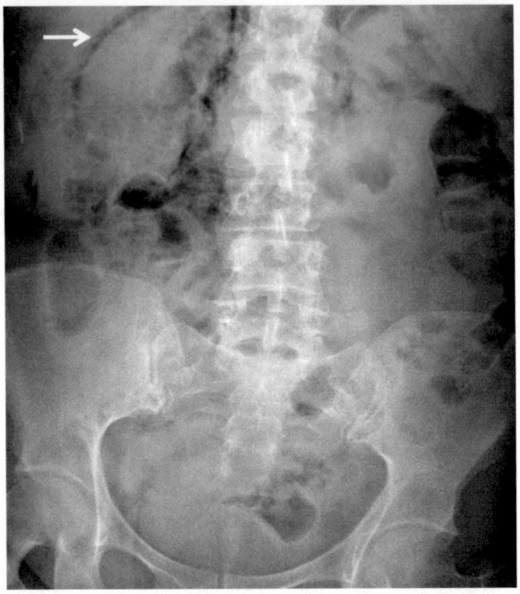

Fig. 12.1 Supine abdominal radiography showing retroperitoneal air (*arrow*) dissecting around the right kidney

Supine abdominal radiographs can show areas of mottled air or collection of air in the left or right upper quadrant (Fig. 12.1), indicating pneumoretroperitoneum, with lack of left psoas muscle shadow, suggesting potentially retroperitoneal illness [9]. Similar findings can be observed on scout CT images (Fig. 12.2).

While confirming the presence of a perforation is critical, clinical management and surgical technique also depend on localizing the perforation site. Multidetector-row computed tomography (MDCT) is accurate in detecting the site of perforation. If the gas is isolated to the extraperitoneum, a retroperitoneal perforation is more likely, including the second or third segments of the duodenum, ascending colon (Fig. 12.3), descending colon (Fig. 12.4), or distal third of the rectum [10].

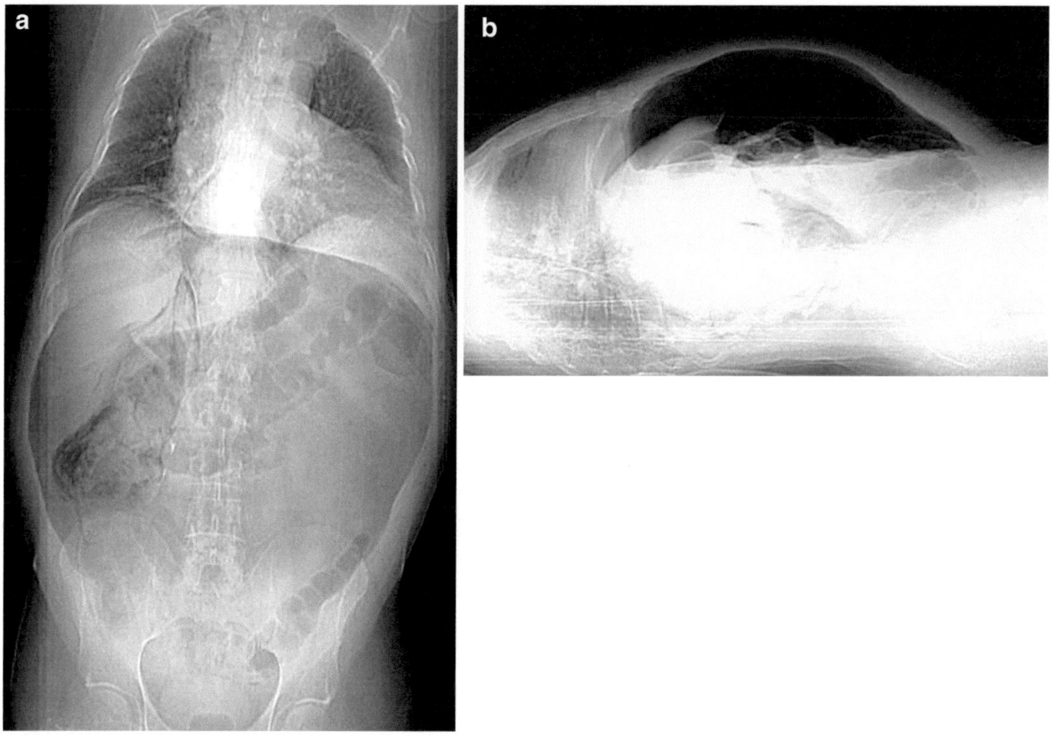

Fig. 12.2 Scout CT images (**a**, AP view; **b**, lateral view) demonstrating the presence of pneumoperitoneum and retropneumoperitoneum

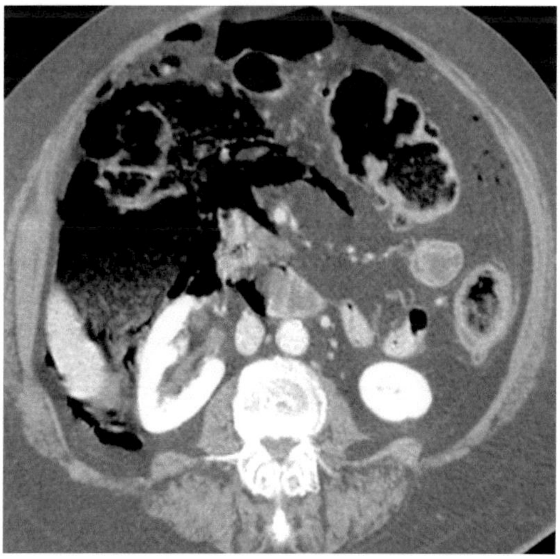

Fig. 12.3 Contrast-enhanced MDCT shows right pneumoretroperitoneum caused by ascending colon perforation. Pneumoperitoneum is also evident

As the duodenum distal to the bulb is retroperitoneal, extraluminal gas in the right anterior pararenal space is a reliable CT finding for diagnosing a distal duodenal perforation. Sensitive, though less-specific findings overlap with perforations elsewhere and include focal bowel wall thickening, perigastric or periduodenal fluid, and adjacent mesenteric fat stranding. Perforation of the descending duodenum is confined to the right anterior pararenal space, but less often the perirenal space is breached and air may dissect into it.

Perforated diverticulitis represents the most serious complication of diverticular disease and can occur at any site along the colon. MDCT has a high sensitivity for detecting complications (Fig. 12.5) secondary to diverticulitis including abscess formation and focal contained perforations. Contained perforations present as small extraluminal pockets of gas. Less often, diffuse pneumoperitoneum and even retroperitoneal and mediastinal gas can occur via subperitoneal communications [11]. MDCT is very useful in order to demonstrate the presence of pneumoperitoneum associated with pneumoretroperitoneum and pneumomediastinum (Fig. 12.6).

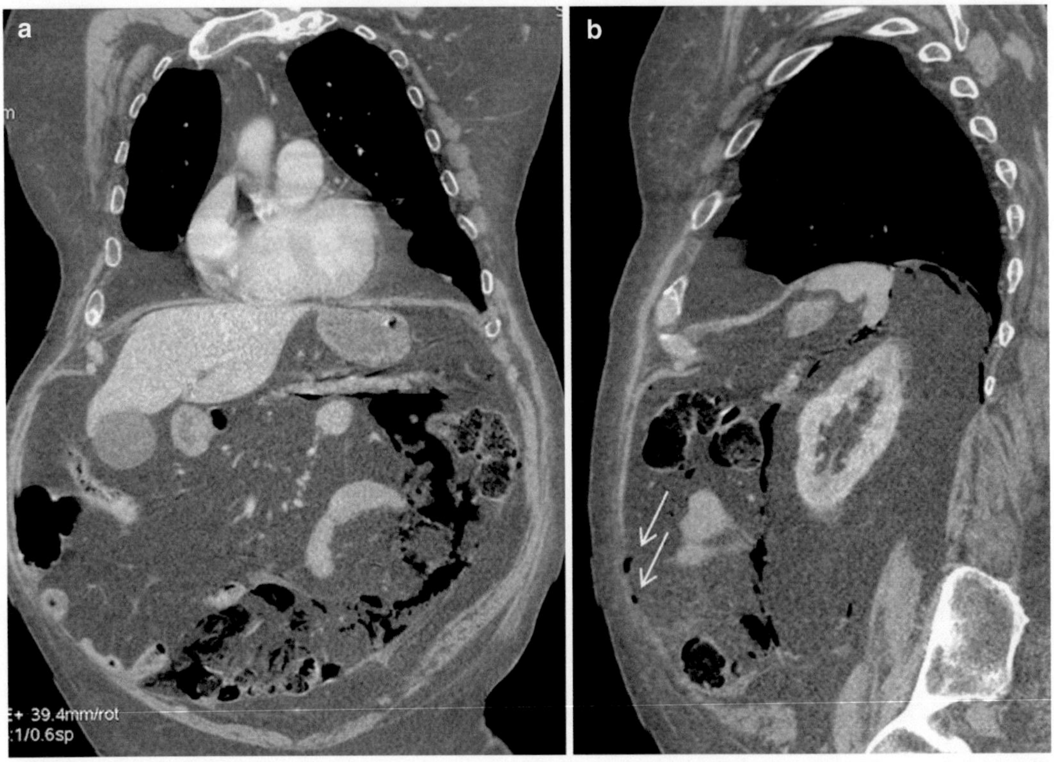

Fig. 12.4 Contrast-enhanced MDCT (**a**, coronal reconstruction; **b**, sagittal reconstruction) shows left pneumoretroperitoneum caused by descending colon perforation. Small amount of pneumoperitoneum (**b**, *arrows*) is also evident

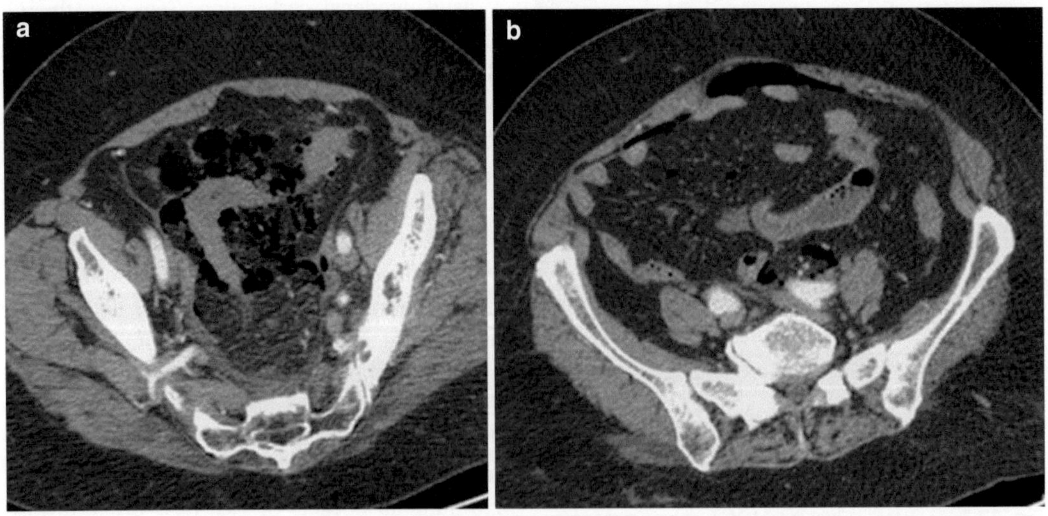

Fig. 12.5 Contrast-enhanced MDCT (**a**) demonstrating pericolic fat stranding, small peritoneal fluid, diverticular outpouching, and multiple extraluminal collections of air adjacent to the sigmoid wall due to perforated sigmoid colon diverticulitis. A more cranial image shows the presence of pneumoretroperitoneum and pneumoperitoneum (**b**)

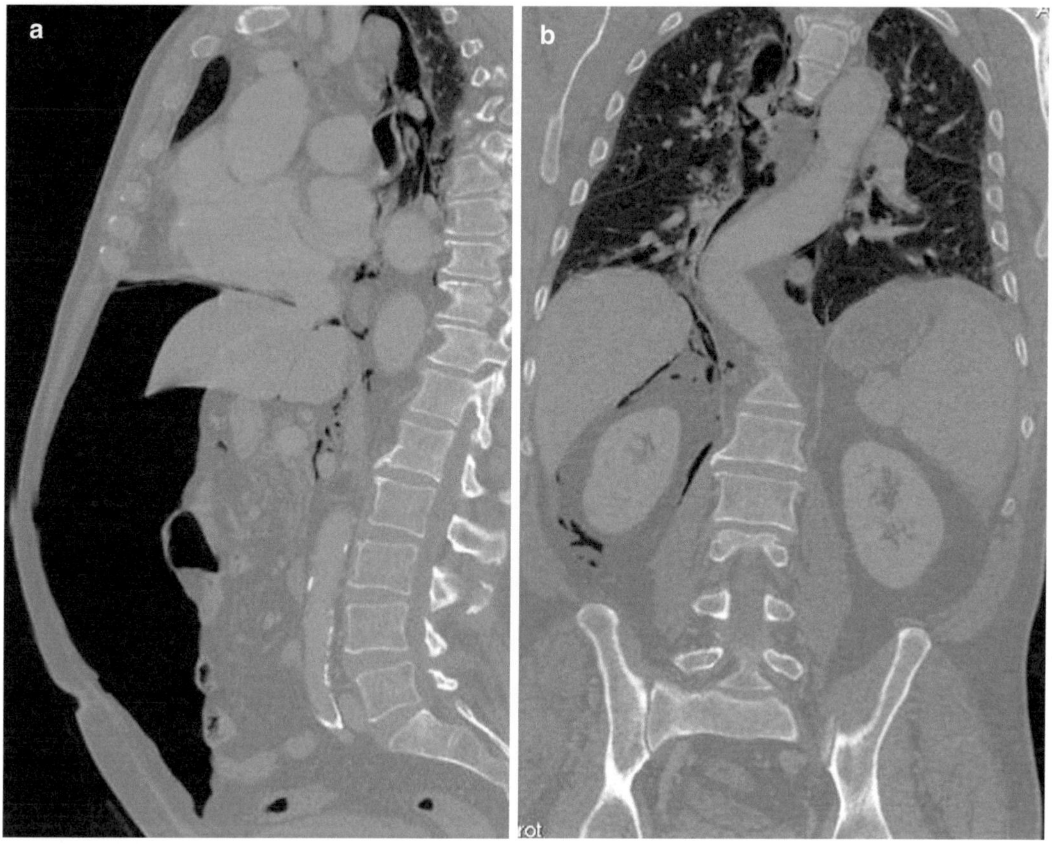

Fig. 12.6 Contrast-enhanced MDCT (**a**, sagittal reconstruction; **b**, coronal reconstruction) shows the presence of massive pneumoperitoneum associated with pneumoretroperitoneum and pneumomediastinum

Typically, rectal perforations are bilateral and displace the properitoneal fat lines on both sides [8].

Conclusions

The importance of discerning between pneumoperitoneum and pneumoretroperitoneum on plain abdominal films cannot be minimized because retroperitoneal air differs markedly from pneumoperitoneum in etiology, clinical course, and patient's treatment.

Besides the awareness of intraperitoneal free air signs, radiologists should take a careful look at the particularly retroperitoneal radiolucency during abdominal radiographic evaluation in cases with high index of suspicion for retroperitoneal infection or bowel perforation.

Recognition of pneumoretroperitoneum is important since rupture of a segment of the gastrointestinal tract is frequently involved. While such air is not in itself dangerous, prompt recognition of its origin is essential as serious septic conditions may be involved.

MDCT is an excellent resource in detecting the presence of pneumoretroperitoneum.

References

1. Goenka AH, Shah SN, Remer EM (2012) Imaging of the retroperitoneum. Radiol Clin North Am 50:333–355
2. Yagan N, Auh YH, Fisher A (2009) Extension of air into the right perirenal space after duodenal perforation: CT findings. Radiology 250:740–748
3. Motateanu M, Mirescu D, Schwieger A-F et al (1992) Computed tomography of retroperitoneal duodenal rupturc in blunt abdominal trauma. Eur J Radiol 15:163–165
4. LeBedis CA, Anderson SW, Soto JA (2012) CT imaging of blunt traumatic bowel and mesenteric injuries. Radiol Clin North Am 50:123–136

5. Pretre R, Robert J, Mirescu D et al (1993) Pathophysiology, recognition and management of pneumoretroperitoneum. Br J Surg 80:1138–1140
6. Grassi R, Pinto A, Rossi G (2000) Isolated pneumoretroperitoneum secondary to acute bowel infarction. Clin Radiol 55:321–323
7. Stoker J, van Randen A, Laméris W et al (2009) Imaging patients with acute abdominal pain. Radiology 253:31–46
8. Baker SR (1990) Plain film radiology of the peritoneal and retroperitoneal spaces. In: Baker SR (ed) The abdominal plain film. Appleton & Lange, Norwalk/San Mateo, pp 71–125
9. Wang YC, Lin CM, Chen SK (2010) Intraperitoneal versus retroperitoneal air signs in abdominal radiographs. Am J Emerg Med 28:109–110
10. Ghekiere O, Lesnik A, Hoa D et al (2007) Value of computed tomography in the diagnosis of the cause of nontraumatic gastrointestinal tract perforation. J Comput Assist Tomogr 31:169–176
11. Oliphant M, Berne AS, Meyers MA (1996) The subperitoneal space of the abdomen and pelvis: planes of continuity. AJR Am J Roentgenol 167:1433–1439

Imaging of Gastrointestinal Tract Perforation in the Pediatric Patient

13

Cecilia Lanza, Elisabetta Panfili, and Andrea Giovagnoni

There are multiple etiologies of gastrointestinal perforation in children. It occurs most frequently in the newborn. The most common causes of perforation include necrotizing enterocolitis (NEC), gastric perforation, Hirschsprung's disease, meconium ileus, imperforate anus, and neonatal small left colon syndrome. Other causes of intestinal perforation are intussusception, volvulus/malrotation, appendicitis, inflammatory bowel disease, and foreign object.

Diagnosis requires a combination of clinical, laboratory, and radiological findings.

The radiological criteria evaluated as predictors of perforation are pneumoperitoneum, intestinal distension, peritoneal fluid, air fluid levels, pneumatosis intestinalis, and gas in the portal venous system.

C. Lanza (✉) • A. Giovagnoni
Dipartimento di Scienze Radiologiche, SOD Radiologia Pediatrica e Specialistica, Azienda Ospedaliero-Universitaria Ospedali Riuniti di Ancona, Via Conca, 71, Ancona 60126, Italy
e-mail: lanzacecilia@hotmail.com; a.giovagnoni@univpm.it

E. Panfili
Dipartimento di Scienze Radiologiche, Scuola di Specializzazione in Radiodiagnostica, Università Politecnica delle Marche, Azienda Ospedaliero-Universitaria Ospedali Riuniti di Ancona, Via Conca, 71, Ancona 60126, Italy
e-mail: ellisbi83@gmail.com

13.1 Suggestive Signs of Perforation

The presence of *pneumoperitoneum* on the abdominal radiograph is widely accepted as an absolute indication for perforation; free air can be seen above the liver in upright films or below the anterior abdominal wall on supine lateral abdominal radiograph with horizontal beam. Various radiological descriptions are used for specific distribution of free intraperitoneal gas, such as the Rigler sign (gas outlining both sides of the bowel), football sign (oval–shaped peritoneal gas, Fig. 13.1), increased lucency in the right upper quadrant (gas accumulating anterior to the liver), and triangle sign (triangular gas pocket between the three loops of bowel, Fig. 13.2). Although conventional radiography is a common method for detecting small amount of intraperitoneal free air [1, 2], imaging may not detect pneumoperitoneum or retroperitoneum in up to 49 % of patients [3]. Intestinal *distention* is the most frequently encountered radiological sign especially in patients with necrotizing enterocolitis, Hirschsprung's disease, volvulus, and meconium ileus. In patients with small-bowel obstruction, supine views show dilation of multiple loops of small bowel, with a paucity of air in the large bowel. Those with large-bowel obstruction may have dilation of the colon, with decompressed small bowel in the setting of a competent ileocecal valve.

L. Romano, A. Pinto (eds.), *Imaging of Alimentary Tract Perforation*,
DOI 10.1007/978-3-319-08192-2_13, © Springer International Publishing Switzerland 2015

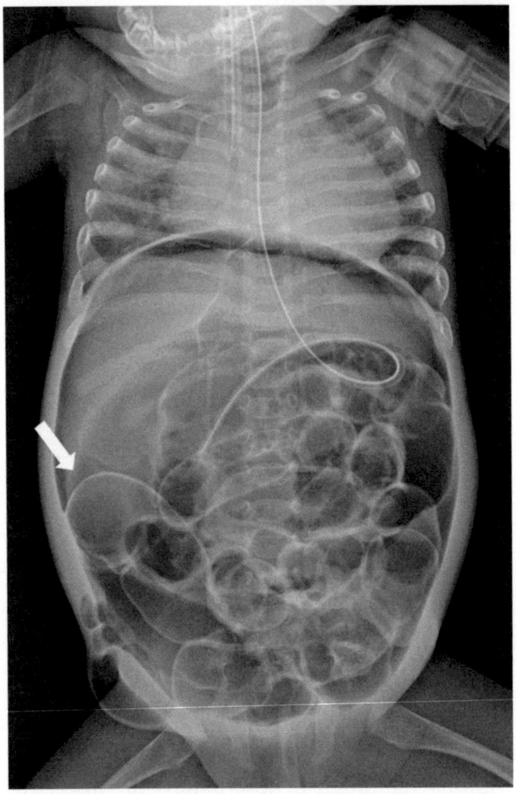

Fig. 13.1 The radiography shows both football sign, as oval-shaped peritoneal gas, and Rigler sign (*arrow*)

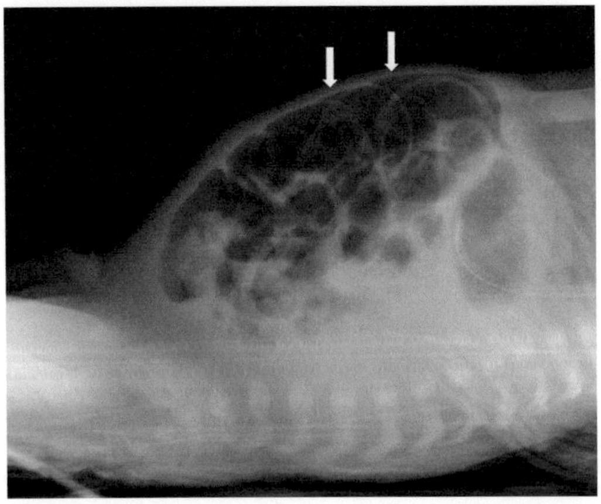

Fig. 13.2 Triangle sign: triangular gas pockets between loops of bowel (*arrows*) are seen in small amount of peritoneal gas

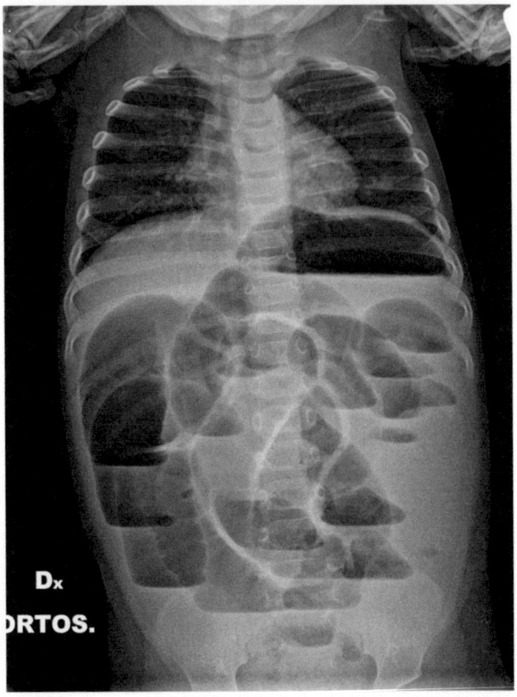

Fig. 13.3 Multiple air fluid levels and bowel parietal thickening in intussusception

Another suggestive sign of perforation is *peritoneal fluid* that is associated with high mortality rate.

Gas in the intestinal wall and portal venous system in infant is invariably associated with enteritis or enterocolitis, except when the gas has been introduced accidentally through an indwelling umbilical catheter.

Upright or cross-table lateral radiograph films may show laddering *air fluid levels*. These findings, in conjunction with a lack of air and stool in the distal colon and rectum, are highly suggestive of mechanical intestinal obstruction (Fig. 13.3).

In some cases of perforation of hollow viscera, the clinical and plain film findings may be inconclusive. In such circumstances, examination with contrast material may be indicated. The site of perforation may be demonstrated if extravasation of contrast medium occurs.

If a perforation is suspected, barium is contraindicated, and water-soluble agents should be used [4, 5].

Therefore, the use of Gastrografin, which contains a wetting agent, was used when looking for a gastrointestinal perforation. However, Gastrografin may cause dehydration secondary to the hyperosmolarity. Recently Iopamidol has been preferred to Gastrografin for its lower osmotic pressure, with the same rate of success.

13.2 US Examination

Ultrasound may be particularly useful in children where radiation burden should be limited. Ultrasonography could be useful as an initial diagnostic test to determine, in various cases, the presence and, sometimes, the cause of the pneumoperitoneum. Ultrasound has lower sensitivity than radiography (76 % vs. 92 %, respectively) and should be used in selected cases only (clinical conditions preventing radiographs from being performed correctly, persisting clinical suspicion with negative or questionable radiographic findings, the exclusion of other acute abdominal conditions) [6].

The main sonographic sign of perforation is free intraperitoneal air, resulting in an increased echogenicity of a peritoneal stripe associated with multiple reflection artifacts and characteristic comet-tail appearance. It is best detected using linear probes in the right upper quadrant between the anterior abdominal wall, in the prehepatic space.

Direct sign of perforation may be detectable, particularly if they are associated with other sonographic abnormalities, called indirect signs, like thickened bowel loop and air bubbles in ascitic fluid or, in a localized fluid collection, bowel thickened wall associated with decreased bowel motility or ileus.

Nevertheless, this exam has its own pitfalls. It is strongly operator dependant; some machines have low-quality images that may not able to detect intraperitoneal free air; furthermore, children are uncooperative; sonography is also difficult in patients with subcutaneous emphysema.

13.2.1 Necrotizing Enterocolitis

Necrotizing enterocolitis (NEC) is an often fatal inflammatory disease involving the intestinal tract of premature infants in which intestinal perforation is common. The condition may mimic obstruction both clinically and radiologically. NEC is considered primarily a pathology related to prematurity. Over 90 % of cases occur in preterm infants [7]. NEC can develop in any portion of the gastrointestinal tract, with the small bowel and proximal large bowel being most frequently affected [8, 9]. NEC diagnosis requires a combination of clinical, laboratory, and radiological findings.

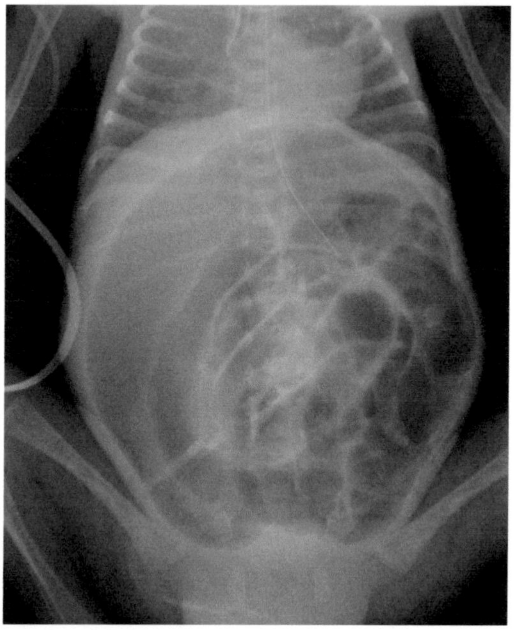

Fig. 13.4 Intestinal distension in NEC may mimic Rigler sign (see Figure), due to air inside two near intestinal loops with near bowel walls

Early diagnosis is critical to the institution of proper therapy in premature infants with necrotizing enterocolitis. In order to make the early diagnosis of NEC, plain abdominal radiographs must be taken of all premature infants with abdominal distension, vomiting, apneic spells, jaundice, or bloody stools. If the radiographs are negative, but symptoms continue, they should be repeated.

Radiological signs play an important part in making the diagnosis of NEC. [10]. Intestinal distension (Fig. 13.4) is the most frequently encountered radiological sign in patients with NEC (55–100 % of cases) [8, 11].

Previous studies have reported the presence of radiological signs suggestive of peritoneal fluid

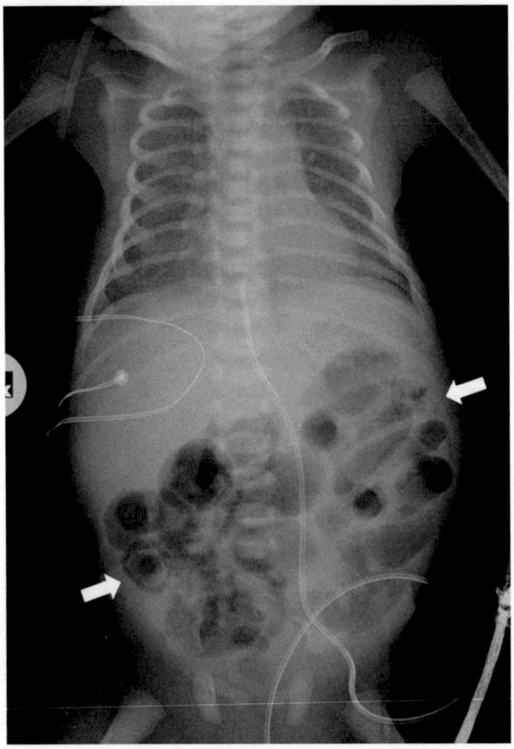

Fig. 13.5 Intramural gas (*arrows*) in severe pneumatosis in NEC

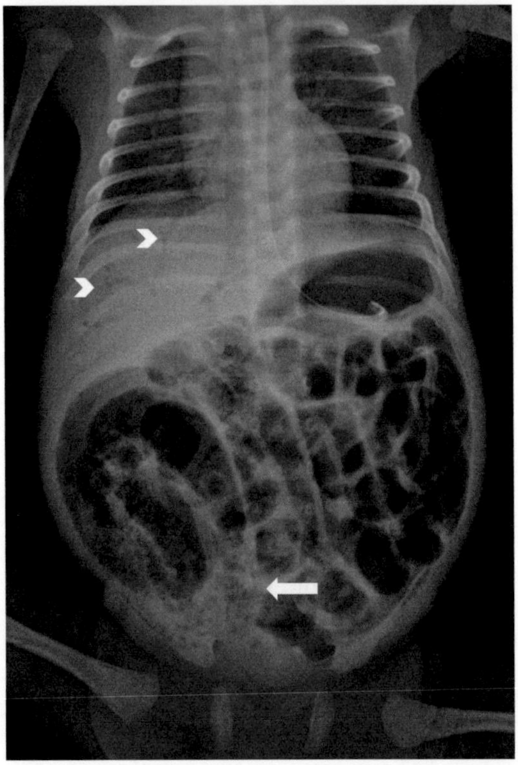

Fig. 13.6 Pneumatosis intestinalis, seen as lucency inside the bowel wall and bubbly appearance of bowel (*arrow*), and gas in the portal venous system (*arrowheads*) in a case of necrotizing enterocolitis

in 11 % of cases and have shown a higher incidence of patient mortality in these patients. Common radiographic features included increased intraluminal gas and fluid, a "bubbly" or "frothy" appearance to the bowel, intramural gas (Fig. 13.5), hepatic portal venous gas, and pneumoperitoneum. Gas in the wall of the intestine, mesentery and retroperitoneum, and portal vein gas are the most important and useful radiographic features (Fig. 13.6). Neither is pathognomonic; both features have been observed in patients afflicted with such entities as Hirshsprung's disease, imperforate anus, meconium ileus, small-bowel atresia, and following surgical repair of coarctation of the aorta. Portal vein gas can be introduced inadvertently through umbilical vein catheters. The sonographic appearance of free intraperitoneal air results in an increased echogenicity of a peritoneal stripe associated with multiple reflection artifacts and characteristic comet-tail appearance that can be changed by changing the patient's position.

Direct sign, such as localized gas collections related to bowel perforations, may be detectable, particularly if they are associated with other sonographic abnormalities, called indirect signs (thickened bowel loop and air bubbles in ascitic fluid or, in a localized fluid collection, bowel thickened wall associated with decreased bowel motility or ileus).

13.2.2 Gastric Pneumatosis in Infancy

Gastric pneumatosis in infancy (defined as gas within the wall of the stomach) may be easily detected by radiography. It presents as a fine lucent stripe conforming to the contour of the stomach and enveloping any intraluminal gas and fluid content. The finding, though quite rare, is of almost clinical importance.

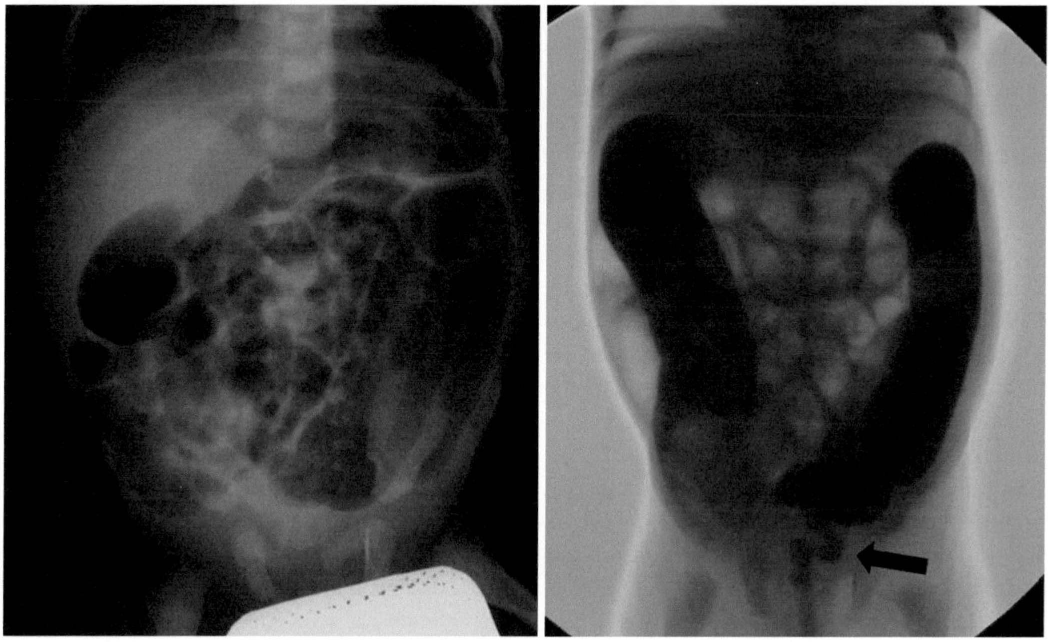

Fig. 13.7 Hirschsprung's disease: radiography shows dilated large bowel without evidence of gas in rectum; fluoroscopic examination with contrast medium enema confirms narrowing segment of aganglionic rectum. The *arrow* indicates transition zone.

In infancy, isolated gastric pneumatosis has been seen very rarely in gastric outlet obstruction. It has also been reported in neonatal necrotizing enterocolitis, in association with intestinal pneumatosis or after perinatal stress though it may rarely be isolated.

Thus, radiographic detection of gastric pneumatosis indicates serious underlying disease, and determination of its cause will depend on the associated clinical findings.

13.2.3 Hirschsprung's Disease

Hirschsprung's disease is a major differential consideration in a neonate or young infant with radiographic evidence of distal bowel obstruction and clinical signs of abdominal distension, vomiting, constipation, failure to pass meconium, and failure to thrive [12–15]. Aganglionosis is the most common cause of large-bowel obstruction in the young infant [16, 17], and therefore colonic or appendiceal perforation, especially in the young infant, should raise the suspicion of Hirschsprung's disease (Fig. 13.7). Most of the perforations reported in the literature were in the proximal colon (68 %), appendix (1 8 %), or distal small bowel (6 %). In utero perforation producing meconium peritonitis has also been described [15, 18]. The mechanism of perforation appears to be directly related to increased intraluminal pressure from distal obstruction.

Long segment or total colonic aganglionosis accounted for 61 % of documented cases of Hirschsprung's disease that presented with bowel perforation. Appendiceal and ileal perforation were particularly associated with long-segment disease.

Perforation in these cases is in aganglionic bowel, and blind colostomy at the site of perforation or in the transverse or sigmoid colon is an inappropriate treatment.

13.2.4 Meconium Ileus

Meconium abnormalities are at the origin of a series of neonatal intestinal obstructions, characterized by a wide spectrum of severity, from the benign meconium plug syndrome to the complicated meconium peritonitis and perforation. These relatively frequent and benign conditions need prompt recognition to exclude other forms of neonatal intestinal obstruction; among them meconium ileus is frequently associated to severe prematurity and low birth weight. It results from combination of highly viscid meconium in the colon or terminal ileum and poor intestinal motility, resulting in mechanical bowel obstruction.

Clinical signs of delayed meconium passage included gastric residual volumes, abdominal distension, and bilious residua. Perforated cases may be confused with NEC which is excluded by clinical history, no signs of sepsis, lab signs missing, abdominal signs missing, and typical radiological signs missing.

Management of meconium obstruction syndrome included plain radiography that reveals evidence of a mechanical obstruction and enema. Plain abdominal film shows distended small-bowel loops without air fluid levels or pneumatosis. These findings are enough to make diagnosis and exclude other forms of intestinal obstruction, mainly NEC.

Once the obstruction occurred, the risk of perforation becomes higher and is estimated around 30 %.

A softening enema with low osmotic pressure ionic X-ray contrast medium, is the first option whenever overt perforation was not present. The contrast medium leads to a propulsive hyperactive gastrointestinal motility and is diagnostic and therapeutic; however, it is not recommended for hemodynamically unstable patients [19, 20].

Success rate is estimated around 80 % and is strictly time dependent [21, 22]. Where enema has to be performed, fluoroscopy is essential to document contrast medium passing ileocecal valve and mixing with intestinal content, to get an effective clinical result.

13.2.5 Imperforate Anus

Anorectal malformations (ARM) are common anomalies observed in neonates. The reported incidence ranges between 1:3,300 and 1:5,000 live births. They vary in severity from mild anal stenosis to complete caudal regression. These disorders usually require surgical intervention in the neonatal period and postoperative follow-up to obtain and maintain fecal and urinary continence. Diagnostic and therapeutic delays in the management of ARM may lead to complications such as sepsis, aspiration, abdominal distension, colonic perforation, respiratory embarrassment, electrolyte imbalance, and even death.

Colonic perforation due to ARM may not be avoided completely; however, early diagnosis is essential in assuring better outcomes with surgical management. Spontaneous perforation of the colon is estimated to occur in 2 % of neonates with ARM, and the incidence rises to 9.5 % when the diagnosis is delayed [23, 24].

13.2.6 Small Left Colon Syndrome

Intestinal perforation can occur as a complication of the neonatal small left colon syndrome, a condition producing signs and symptoms of low colonic obstruction.

Radiographic examination of the abdomen shows multiple dilated small-bowel loops and sometimes visualization of dilated ascending and transverse portions of the colon.

This syndrome is a benign condition in which contrast enema examination is curative by stimulating meconium evacuation. Contrast enema study demonstrates a characteristic pattern of a small left colon to the level of the splenic flexure where a sharp transition zone exists with the proximal colon being dilated. This study should be done immediately in newborns who develop clinical findings of colon obstruction or fail to pass significant meconium within 24–48 h. This aggressive approach hopefully should reduce the incidence of intestinal perforation as a complication of the neonatal small left colon syndrome. Repeat contrast enema examinations may occasionally be necessary to relieve the obstructive signs in these babies.

13.2.7 Intussusception

Intussusception occurs when a portion of the digestive tract becomes telescoped into the adjacent bowel segment. It generally occurs in children between 6 months and 2 years of age. The vast majority are ileocolic [25–27].

Intussusceptions are the second most common cause of acute intestinal obstructions in children. Once they are diagnosed, they should be treated as early as possible. Though their exact causes are not known in most of the cases, swollen Payer's patches, enlarged lymph nodes, polyps, Meckel's diverticulum, and duplication cysts have been suggested as few of the common etiological factors [28, 29].

The classic triad of intermittent abdominal pain or irritable crying, a palpable mass, and red currant jelly stools is reported to have a positive predictive value of 93 % for intussusceptions [30, 31].

Ultrasonography is a very useful investigation that can be used for the diagnosis. The absence of blood flow in the lesion on color Doppler study correlates significantly with the high incidence of the complications and irreducibility [28, 29, 32].

On the ultrasound image the intussusceptions is a complex structure due to the amount of mesentery [33]. The intussusceptions (the receiving loop) contain the folded intussuscepted (the donor loop), which has two components: the entering limb and returning limbs. Ultrasound obtained at the apex shows a hyperechoic outer ring separated from a hypoechoic center by a thin hyper echoic ring, which likely represents the opposed serous surface of the intussuscepted. Ultrasound obtained near the apex shows multiple concentric rings with a hypoechoic ring surrounding a hyperechoic ring, which surrounds another hypoechoic ring. US scan obtained at the base shows the central limb of the intussusception eccentrically surrounded by the hyperechoic mesentery that show the crescent in doughnut sign.

Contrast medium or gas enemas have been widely used to reduce uncomplicated intussusceptions, but 10–30 % of patients eventually require surgery (Fig. 13.8). Surgery is definitely indicated when patients present with signs of perforation, shock, or peritonitis, when other attempts at reduction fail, or when a pathologic lead point is suspected [34, 35].

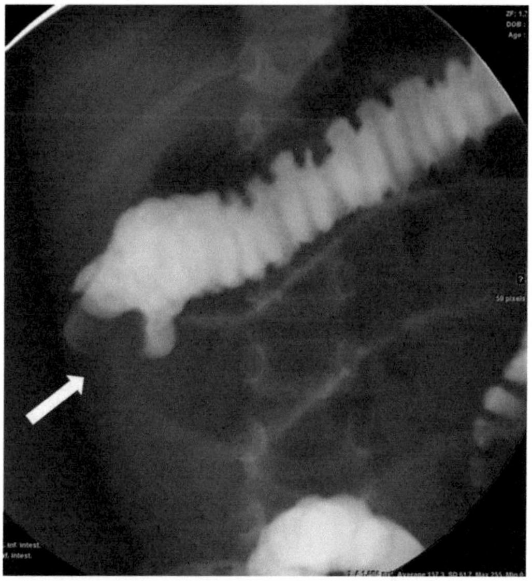

Fig. 13.8 Intussusception: contrast enema shows the "coiled spring" (*arrow*) appearance of bowel at the site of the obstruction

13.2.8 Malrotation/Volvulus

Malrotation/volvulus is a congenital abnormal position of the bowel within the peritoneal cavity and usually involves both the small and the large bowel [36].

Malrotation is accompanied by abnormal bowel fixation by mesenteric bands or absence of fixation of portions of the bowel, leading to increased risks of bowel obstruction, acute or chronic volvulus, and bowel necrosis. Malrotation occurs in approximately 1 in 500 births [37] and is usually diagnosed in newborns and young infants.

The classic clinical manifestation of malrotation in newborns is bilious vomiting with or without abdominal distention associated with either duodenal obstructive bands or midgut volvulus [38]. Midgut volvulus is a life-threatening condition in which the small-bowel or proximal colon twists around the superior mesenteric artery

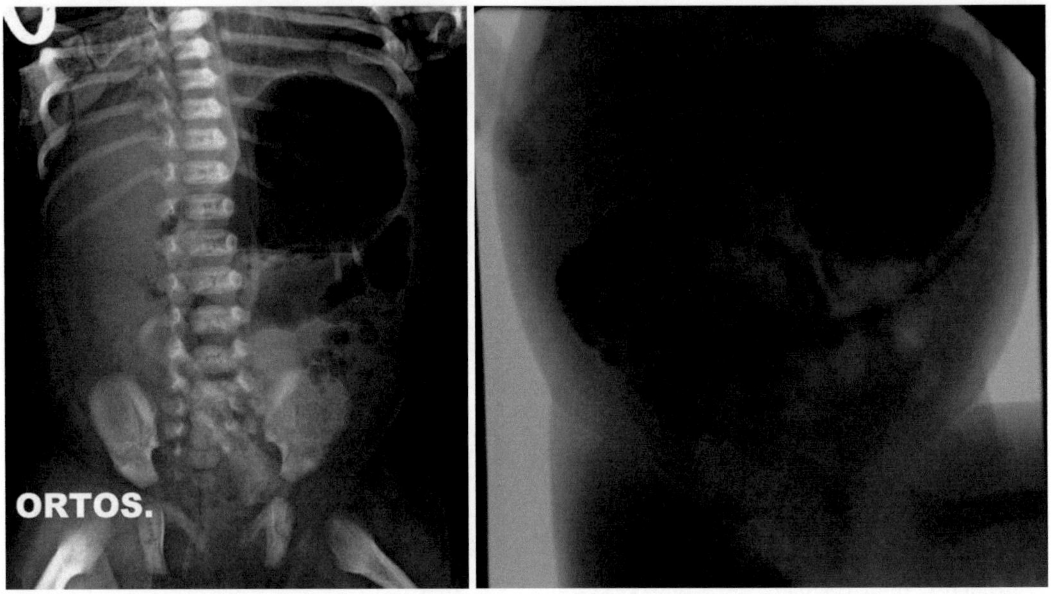

Fig. 13.9 Malrotation in Ladd's bands: evidence of gastric distention on radiography; fluoroscopic examination with contrast medium shows right-sided duodenal-jejunal junction

(SMA) and it commonly presents during the first year of life [39]. The diagnosis of midgut volvulus in infants is facilitated by direct sonographic visualization of the twisted bowel loop. Normally, the superior mesenteric vein is on the right side of the artery. In malrotation, we evaluated on ultrasound image the "whirlpool sign" on the axial scan, formed by the mesenteric vein that is on the left side of the artery. The diagnosis is made with an upper gastrointestinal contrast study (UGI) that demonstrates the right-sided position of the duodenal-jejunal junction or evidence of a midgut volvulus (Fig. 13.9). Treatment requires surgical laparotomy and detorsion or lysis of Ladd's bands (Ladd procedure).

13.2.9 Appendicitis

Appendicitis is the most common condition requiring an emergency abdominal operation in childhood [40]. Despite the relatively high incidence of this common emergency, it remains a difficult diagnosis for clinicians. Early diagnosis of appendicitis in infant and children can prevent perforation and postoperative complications and can decrease costs by shortening hospitalization. Ultrasound is considered to be the imaging test of choice in children. Experienced ultrasonographers can achieve sensitivities of 85–90 % and specificities of 95–100 % in acute appendicitis. On longitudinal images, the inflamed, non-perforated appendix appears as a fluid-filled, uncompressible, blind-ending tubular structure. The maximal appendix diameter, from outside wall to outside wall, is greater than 6 mm. On the axial image, we evaluated a "target sign" characterized by a fluid-filled center and surrounded by an echogenic mucosa and submucosa and hypoechoic muscularis. US features of perforation include loss of the echogenic submucosal layer and presence of a loculated periappendicular or pelvic fluid collection or abscess.

In early inflammation, color flow may be absent or limited to the appendicular tip. Color Doppler findings of appendicular perforation include hyperemia in the periappendicular soft tissues or within a well-defined abscess.

Sometimes, when peritonitis with paralytic ileus is suspected, plain film is useful, and one of the earliest radiographic sign of perforation on radiographic film is dilated transverse colon sign associated with emptiness of the ascending colon.

It is believed to result from a combination of paralytic ileus of the transverse colon and spasm of the ascending colon.

This point can be used to differentiate normal transverse colon gas accumulations from those seen in perforated appendicitis. In the normal individual, the ascending colon usually contains gas and/or fecal material.

13.2.10 Inflammatory Bowel Disease

During the course of the disease, most patients with inflammatory bowel disease (IBD) may eventually develop a stricturing or a perforating complication, and a significant number of patients with both Crohn's disease and ulcerative colitis will undergo surgery.

A young age at onset or pediatric presentation is an important risk factor for developing complicated disease behavior and even disease extension [41, 42].

The radiation-free ultrasound performed with adequate technique and experience by the sonographer should be used as initial imaging method to describe the extension and grading of the inflammation and to appreciate extraintestinal findings (lymph node enlargement, abscesses).

Plain radiography is reserved for acute diseases like obstruction or perforation. Findings are nonspecific and can include large-bowel dilation and small-bowel distension. In the acute abdomen, the toxic megacolon or obstruction can be suspected. These cases have to be followed in order to detect possible bowel perforation. Contrast enema can be helpful for the evaluation of the extension of the disease; moreover, it is helpful to rule out or prove stenosis. Upper gastrointestinal series with small-bowel barium follow-through has been the cornerstone of small-bowel imaging in the past [43].

The more sensitive enteroclysma was considered the gold standard but both methods suffer from one further major disadvantage: its very limited information regarding the extraluminal mesenteric extension of the disease.

Computed tomography (CT) as a cross-sectional imaging method overcomes this and may be helpful in the acute situation, for planning surgery, especially in the evaluation of stricture or obstruction. The major disadvantage of CT is the large amount of radiation exposure [44].

Thus, especially in children, techniques using ionizing radiation should be avoided if possible [45]. MR enterography has definitely advantages including the detection and assessment of disease activity of the entire gut and the ability to evaluate extraluminal disease and is therefore becoming the standard assessment of the small bowel in many centers. However, there is no consensus about the technique, and there is no approved standard protocol for the evaluation of IBD using MRI.

13.2.11 Ingestion of Foreign Objects

Children have a natural tendency to explore objects with their mouths; this can result in the swallowing of foreign objects. Many cases of ingestion of foreign bodies are noted in children between 6 months and 3 years of age [46].

Although the ingested foreign bodies are common and alerting problems of childhood, most of them pass the alimentary tract without any sequel. However, some foreign bodies cause obstruction or perforation of the gastrointestinal tract, requiring surgical intervention. Sharp materials such as fish bones, chicken bones, and needles in contrast may cause complications up to 35 % of the cases, such as peritonitis, abscess formation, inflammatory mass formation, obstruction, fistulae, and hemorrhage [47, 48].

Perforation occurs in less than 1 % of ingestion of a foreign body. The most common sites of intestinal foreign body perforation are the ileocecal and rectosigmoid regions.

Non-radioopaque foreign bodies are especially difficult to detect on plain radiographs of the abdomen. When foreign object swallowing is suspected, an immediate radiographic evaluation is recommended. This evaluation would include a

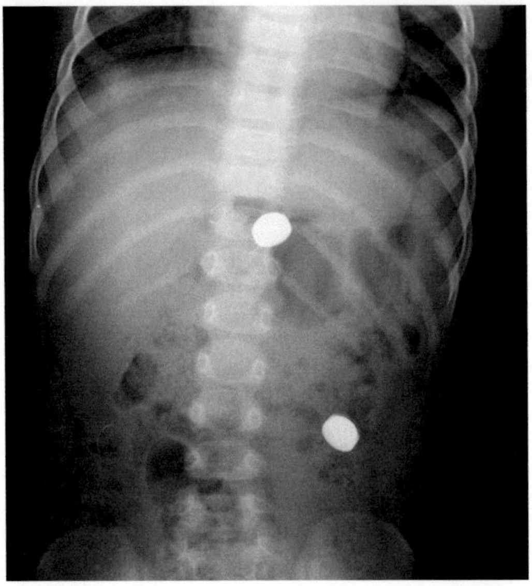

Fig. 13.10 Foreign bodies: button batteries ingestion

frontal radiograph of the abdomen and pelvis, and a lateral radiograph of the neck follow-up with daily radiographs for the documentation of the passage is stated to be appropriate [49].

A particularly ominous scenario is the ingestion of multiple magnetic objects which, when located in different loops of bowel, can attract each other and cause pressure necrosis of the bowel wall and subsequent perforation.

Button battery (BB) ingestion is a common complaint in toddlers. Increased use of lithium BB that are 20 mm in diameter has brought new challenges since they appear more dangerous than earlier types of batteries. Due to their electrochemical composition, impacted BB in the esophagus may cause an extensive damage. Signs of BB should be carefully checked on the anteroposterior (AP) (double rim) and lateral X-ray. Battery ingestion-related injury results from direct pressure necrosis, local electrical currents, and alkali leakage. Signs and symptoms of ingested battery are related to impaction duration, size of battery, battery content, and peristaltic waves of the esophagus (Fig. 13.10).

To prevent morbidity and mortality, in case of an unwitnessed ingestion, coin-like foreign bodies should be assumed BB until proven otherwise.

References

1. Coppolino F, Gatta G, Di Grezia G et al (2013) Gastrointestinal perforation: ultrasonographic diagnosis. Crit Ultrasound J 5(Suppl 1):S4
2. Roh JJ, Thompson JS, Harned RK et al (1983) Value of pneumoperitoneum in the diagnosis of visceral perforation. Am J Surg 146(6):830–833
3. Hefny AF, Abu-Zidan FM (2011) Sonographic diagnosis of intraperitoneal free air. J Emerg Trauma Shock 4(4):511–513
4. Cohen MD (1990) Choosing contrast media for pediatric gastrointestinal examinations. Crit Rev Diagn Imaging 30(4):317–340
5. Zerin JM (1992) Contrast studies of the gastrointestinal tract in the neonate. Semin Pediatr Surg 1(4):284–295
6. Chen SC, Wang HP, Chen WJ et al (2002) Selective use ultrasonography for the detection of pneumoperitoneum. Acad Emerg Med 5(6):643–645
7. Rowe MI, Reblock KK, Kurkchubasche AG et al (1994) Necrotizing enterocolitis in the extremely low birth weight infant. J Pediatr Surg 29:987–991
8. Bălănescu RN, Topor L, Drăgan GC (2013) Clinical and surgical aspects in necrotizing enterocolitis. Chirurgia (Bucur) 108(2):184–188
9. Noerr B (2003) Current controversies in the understanding of necrotizing enterocolitis. Part 1. Adv Neonatal Care 3(3):107–120
10. Tam AL, Camberos A, Applebaum H (2002) Surgical decision making in necrotizing enterocolitis and focal intestinal perforation: predictive value of radiological findings. J Pediatr Surg 37(12):1688–1691
11. Henry MCW, Moss RL (2010) Necrotizing enterocolitis. In: Ashcraft KW, Holcomb GJ, Ostlie DJ (eds) Ashcraft's pediatric surgery. Saunders Elsevier, Philadelphia
12. Sieber WK (1978) Hirschsprung's disease. Curr Probl Surg 15(6):1–93
13. Wylie GG (1957) Course and management of Hirschsprung's disease. Lancet 272:847–855
14. Swenson O, Sherman JO, Fisher JH (1973) Diagnosis of congenital megacolon: an analysis of 501 patients. J Pediatr Surg 8(5):587–594
15. Newman B, Nussbaum A, Kirkpatrick JA Jr (1987) Bowel perforation in Hirschsprung's disease. AJR Am J Roentgenol 148(6):1195–1197
16. Wyllie R (2007) Intestinal atresia, stenosis and malrotation. In: Kliegmann RM, Behrman RE, Jenson HB et al (eds) Nelson textbook of pediatrics. Saunders Elsevier, Philadelphia
17. Karimi A, Gorter RR, Sleeboom C et al (2011) Issues in the management of simple and complex meconium ileus. Pediatr Surg Int 27(9):963–968
18. Sieber WK, Girdany BR (1957) Management of symptomatic aganglionic megacolon in early infancy. AMA Arch Surg 75(3):388–395
19. Raith W, Resch B, Pichler G et al (2013) Delayed meconium passage in small vs. appropriate for gestational age preterm infants: management and short-term outcome. Iran J Pediatr 23(1):8–12

20. Koshinaga T, Inoue M, Ohashi K et al (2011) Therapeutic strategies of meconium obstruction of the small bowel in very-low-birthweight neonates. Pediatr Int 53(3):338–344
21. Nakaoka T, Shiokawa C, Nishihara M et al (2009) Iopamidol enema treatment for meconium obstruction of prematurity in extremely low-birth weight infants: a safe and effective method. Pediatr Surg Int 25:273–276
22. Paradiso VF, Briganti V, Oriolo L et al (2011) Meconium obstruction in absence of cystic fibrosis in low birth weight infants: an emerging challenge from increasing survival. Ital J Pediatr 37:55
23. Turowski C, Dingemann J, Gillick J (2010) Delayed diagnosis of imperforate anus: an unacceptable morbidity. Pediatr Surg Int 26:1083–1086
24. Tong WD, Ludwig KA (2013) Neonatal colon perforation due to anorectal malformations: can it be avoided? World J Gastroenterol 19(25):3915–3917
25. Pracros JP, Tran-Minh VA, Morin de Finfe CH, Basset T et al (1987) Acute intestinal intussusception in children. Contribution of ultrasonography (145 cases). Ann Radiol (Paris) 5(7):525–530
26. Arnaud O, Weil D, Boscq M et al (1986) Acute intestinal intussusception in infants and children and abdominal ultrasonography. J Radiol 5(2):135–136
27. Fonio P, Coppolino F, Russo A et al (2013) Ultrasonography (US) in the assessment of pediatric non traumatic gastrointestinal emergencies. Crit Ultrasound J 5(Suppl 1):S12
28. Krishnakumar Hameed S, Maheshwari U (2006) Ultrasound guided hydrostatic reduction in the management of intussusception. Indian J Pediatr 73(3): 217–220
29. Digant SM, Rucha S, Eke D (2012) Ultrasound guided reduction of an ileocolic intussusception by a hydrostatic method by using normal saline enema in paediatric patients: a study of 30 cases. J Clin Diagn Res 6(10):1722–1725
30. D'Agostino J (2002) Common abdominal emergencies in children. Emerg Med Clin North Am 20:139–153
31. Chang YJ, Hsia SH, Chao HC (2013) Emergency medicine physicians performed ultrasound for pediatric intussusceptions. Biomed J 36(4):175–178
32. Khong PL, Peh WC, Lam CH et al (2000) Ultrasound-guided hydrostatic reduction of childhood intussusception: technique and demonstration. Radiographics 20:1818
33. Del Pozo G, Albillos JC (1999) Intussusception in children-current concept in diagnosis and enema reduction. Radiographics 19:299–319
34. Ksia A, Mosbahi S, Brahim MB et al (2013) Recurrent intussusception in children and infants. Afr J Paediatr Surg 10:299–301
35. Hsu WL, Lee HC, Yeung CY et al (2012) Recurrent intussusception: when should surgical intervention be performed? Pediatr Neonatol 53:300–303
36. Applegate KE, Anderson JM, Klatte EC (2006) Intestinal malrotation in children: a problem-solving approach to the upper gastrointestinal series. Radiographics 26(5): 1485–1500
37. Brandt ML, Pokorny WJ, McGill CW et al (1985) Late presentations of midgut malrotation in children. Am J Surg 150:767–771
38. Howell CG, Vozza F, Shaw S et al (1982) Malrotation, malnutrition, and ischemic bowel disease. J Pediatr Surg 17:469–473
39. West KW, Rescorla FJ, Grosfeld JL et al (1989) Pneumatosis intestinalis in children beyond the neonatal period. J Pediatr Surg 24:818–822
40. Chang YJ, Chao HC, Kong MS et al (2010) Misdiagnosed acute appendicitis in children in the emergency department. Chang Gung Med J 33(5):551–557
41. Vernier-Massouille G, Balde M, Salleron J et al (2008) Natural history of pediatric Crohn's disease: a population-based cohort study. Gastroenterology 135: 1106–1113
42. Gower-Rousseau C, Dauchet L, Vernier-Massouille G et al (2009) The natural history of pediatric ulcerative colitis: a population-based cohort study. Am J Gastroenterol 104:2080–2088
43. Mentzel HJ, Reinsch S, Kurzai M et al (2010) Role of small bowel follow-through in diagnosing inflammation of the terminal ileum in pediatric patients. J Pediatr Gastroenterol Nutr 51:433–436
44. Gaca AM, Jaffe TA, Delaney S et al (2008) Radiation doses from small-bowel follow-through and abdomen/pelvis MDCT in pediatric Crohn disease. Pediatr Radiol 38(3):285–291
45. Brenner DJ (2008) Should computed tomography be the modality of choice for imaging Crohn's disease in children? The radiation risk perspective. Gut 57(11): 1489–1490
46. ASGE Standards of Practice Committee, Ikenberry SO, Jue TL et al (2011) Management of ingested foreign bodies and food impactions. Gastrointest Endosc 73(6):1085–1091
47. Yalçin S, Karnak I, Ciftci AO et al (1999) Sewing-pin perforation of the appendix into the bladder. Pediatr Surg Int 15(1):66–67
48. Karacay S, Topçu K, Sözübir S et al (2013) A rare complication of an ingested foreign body: gallbladder perforation. Case Rep Gastrointest Med 2013: 672572
49. Kunizaki M, Kusano H, Azuma K et al (2009) Cholecystitis caused by a fish bone. Am J Surg 198(2): e20–e22

Imaging of Gastrointestinal Tract Perforation in the Elderly Patient

14

Alfonso Reginelli, Anna Russo, Duilia Maresca, Fabrizio Urraro, Giuseppina Fabozzi, Francesco Stanzione, Alfredo D'Andrea, Ciro Martiniello, and Luca Brunese

14.1 Introduction

Gastrointestinal perforation is a medical emergency that requires immediate medical care. The condition is life-threatening. Chances of recovery improve with an early diagnosis and treatment [1].

Gastrointestinal perforation (GP) occurs when a hole forms all the way through the stomach, small intestine, and large intestine. It might be caused by a number of different diseases, including foreign bodies, colon cancer, diverticulitis, ischaemia, Degos' syndrome, and inflammatory bowel disease. The contents of these organs are then able to spill over into the abdominal cavity. A hole in gastrointestinal system can lead to peritonitis.

Intestinal perforation is an emergency medical situation presented as an acute abdomen, and it is only rarely diagnosed clinically. CT is often the initial modality used to assess patients with acute abdomen, the radiologist may be the first to suggest such a diagnosis [2–6]. CT provides superb anatomical detail and diagnostic specificity by directly imaging of the intestinal wall, detecting secondary signs of bowel disease within the surrounding mesentery and depicting even small amounts of extraluminal air or oral contrast leakage into the peritoneal cavity [5, 6].

Computed tomography allows to identify the site of gastrointestinal perforations and to determine the most predictive signs in this diagnosis. Typically, simple standing chest radiography, including the diaphragm, is the first imaging test that is done in order to identify the presence of extraluminal gas, although, sometimes, it is difficult to establish the diagnosis because the symptoms are non-specific and pneumoperitoneum is only observed on 30–59 % of simple radiographs [7–9]. Recent studies reveal poor sensitivity of plain radiography for the detection of free air, especially in patients with jejuno-ileal or colonic perforation. Several studies have demonstrated that computed tomography (CT) is the best technique for detecting free intraperitoneal air and for the diagnosis of GI perforation.

A. Reginelli (✉) • F. Urraro
Department of Internal and Experimental Medicine, Magrassi-Lanzara, Institute of Radiology, Second University of Naples, Piazza Miraglia, Naples 80100, Italy
e-mail: reginelli@tin.it; furraro@libero.it

A. Russo • D. Maresca • G. Fabozzi • A. D'Andrea C. Martiniello
Department of Radiology, S. G. Moscati Hospital, Via Gramsci, Aversa 81134, Italy
e-mail: annarusso81@yahoo.it; piafabozzi@yahoo.it; dino3doc@libero.it; ciromartiniello@tin.it

F. Stanzione
General, and Emergency Surgery, Metabolic Care, Clinic Pineta Grande, Castel Volturno, Caserta, Italy
e-mail: fstanzione@yahoo.it

L. Brunese
Department of Medicine and Health Sciences, University of Molise, Contrada Tappino, Campobasso, Italy
e-mail: lucabrunese@libero.it

L. Romano, A. Pinto (eds.), *Imaging of Alimentary Tract Perforation*,
DOI 10.1007/978-3-319-08192-2_14, © Springer International Publishing Switzerland 2015

Typical signs to be assessed on CT are:

1. Extravasation of oral contrast
2. Intestinal wall focal defects
3. Free air in the supramesocolic compartment
4. Free air in the inframesocolic compartment
5. Free air in supra- and inframesocolic compartments
6. Gas bubbles adjacent to the intestinal wall
7. Localised extraluminal fluid
8. Segmental wall thickening (>3 mm)
9. Perivisceral fat stranding 'dirty fat sign'
10. Focal collection of extraluminal faecal matter 'dirty mass'
11. Abscesses
12. Sagittal and coronal MPR to view the focal wall defect

Signs 1, 2, and 11 were considered direct signs, meaning that they are signs that indicate where there is a discontinuity in the GI. The remainder were indirect signs of the location of the GI perforation: some indicate the distribution of the extraluminal gas (signs 3, 4, 5, and 6,) and others indicate inflammatory changes (signs 8, 9, and 10) that help estimate the affected GI segment.

CT protocol for evaluating the acute abdomen includes the administration of intravenous contrast or both oral contrasts. The use of a multislice helical scanner with both axial images and multiplanar reformations allows for high-quality visualisation of the entire abdomen [4, 6]. Water-soluble contrast agents do not provoke an inflammatory reaction when leaking into the peritoneal cavity, as they are rapidly absorbed [5]. Assessment of bone and lung window settings, in addition to the routine abdominal window setting, serves as a useful complementary tool for detecting intra- or extraluminal radio-opaque foreign bodies and free intra-abdominal air [10].

Diagnostically, extraluminal oral contrast is a specific sign of gastrointestinal tract (GIT) perforations (more clearly seen on a lung window setting). CT is the most reliable imaging modality for detecting even small amounts of free air [3–6]. Additional CT signs, which may also indicate the site of the perforation, include discontinuity of the bowel wall on an enhanced scan and focal thickening of the bowel wall adjacent to extraluminal gas bubbles, streaky density within the mesentery 'dirty fat' sign, and focal collection of extraluminal faecal matter 'dirty mass' were considered indirect finding of perforation [3, 5, 11] (Fig. 14.1).

The overall accuracy in diagnosing the site of the perforation is 80 % [6]. Yeung et al. [3] also found that the presence of air in both sides of the falciform ligament may differentiate more certainly proximal from distal GIT perforation.

14.2 Foreign Bodies

Generally, the ingestion of foreign bodies occurs involuntarily while eating; meat boluses are the most common foreign bodies ingested in Western countries and fish bones in oriental countries [12–14]. However, in 1 % of cases, it causes complications such as acute abdomen due to intestinal perforation [13]. In some cases, it can cause severe complications and even death; in the USA, 1,500 people die annually from foreign body ingestion [15].

Bowel perforation by a foreign body is less common, as the majority of foreign bodies uneventfully pass to the faeces and only 1 % of them (the sharper and more elongated objects) will perforate the gastrointestinal tract, usually at the level of the ileum [4, 16]. The complications of foreign bodies ingestion with perforation include the formation of localised abdominal abscesses, colorectal, colovesical and enterovascular fistulas, inflammatory masses or omental pseudotumors, pyemia, and endocarditis [4, 17].

In the early patients this condition is more frequent because of persistent two predisposing risk factors for foreign body ingestion: comorbid condition and the use of dentures, because they reduce the sensitivity of the palate [13, 14].

The intestinal tract, where perforations by foreign bodies are most frequent, includes the ileocecal and rectosigmoid regions, because the intestinal lumen narrows and the digestive tract is angulated in these sites. Sites where impaction is most likely include zones with adhesions, areas containing a diverticular process, or surgical

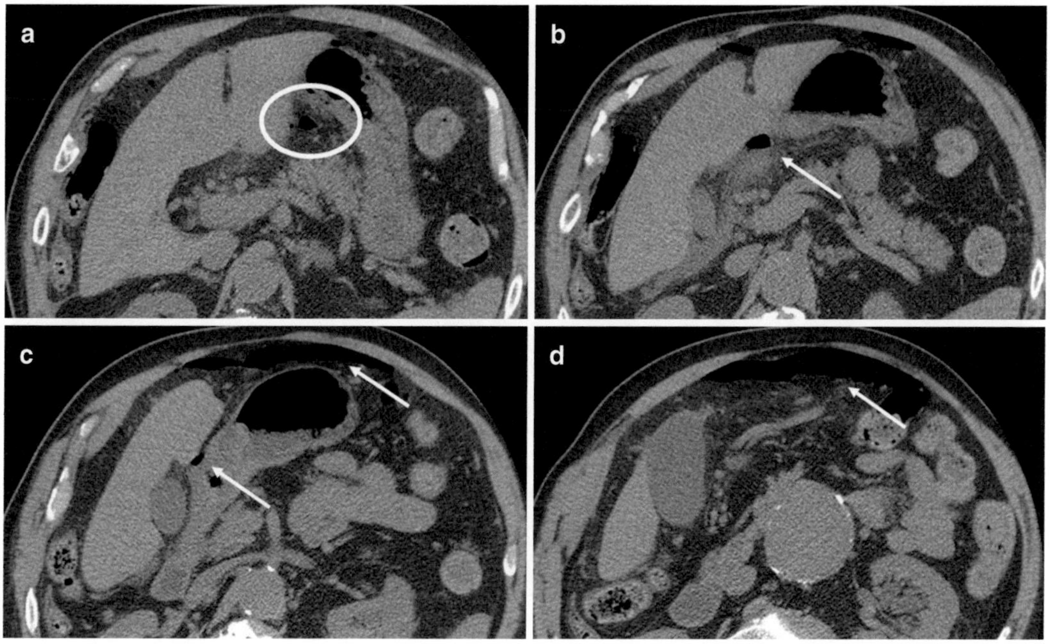

Fig. 14.1 Abdominal CT scan. CT image shows even small amounts of free air (**a–d**). Additional CT shows the site of the perforation (**a**, *white circle*), focal thickening of the bowel wall adjacent to extraluminal gas bubbles (**c**, *white arrows*) and streaky density within the mesentery (**d**, *white arrow*) 'dirty fat' sign (**b**, *white arrow*)

anastomoses [13, 14]. Treatment consists of surgery (from primary suture to rectosigmoid resection with colostomy, removal of the foreign body, and abdominal cavity lavage) and antibiotics.

The patient presented at the emergency department with diffuse abdominal pain with peritoneal irritation and vomiting of 24 h duration. Laboratory tests showed generally leukocytosis and increased C-reactive protein. The supine plain abdominal radiograph demonstrated signs of small-bowel obstruction but do not always shows a radio-opaque foreign body or pneumoperitoneum. This finding is not surprising because, for example, fish bones have variable radio-opacity depending on the fish species; in general, the foreign bodies are minimally radio-opaque and can rarely be detected on plain films, especially if they are masse by coexistent inflammatory tissue, fluid, or abscesses [18]. Moreover, signs of pneumoperitoneum are not usually observed in plain films because impaction of the foreign body into the intestinal wall is gradual, allowing the perforation site to seal with omentum or adjacent loops and limiting the amount of gas or fluid in the peritoneal cavity [18]. The use of US makes it possible to identify foreign bodies, even non-radio-opaque bodies such as fish bones and toothpicks, based on their high reflectivity and variable posterior shadowing [4, 19]. MDCT is currently considered the method of choice for the evaluation of patients with acute abdominal pain and the depiction of foreign bodies due to MDCT's ability to generate high-resolution, thin-collimation, multiplanar reconstructions, which allow the GI tract to be examined in all projections.

Abdominal CT showed generally a foreign body in the small bowel, with pneumoperitoneum and fluid within the abdominal cavity (Fig. 14.2).

14.3 Colorectal Cancer

Colorectal cancer (CRC) is the most common cancer and is also an increasing trend [20, 21]. Computed tomography (CT) has played an

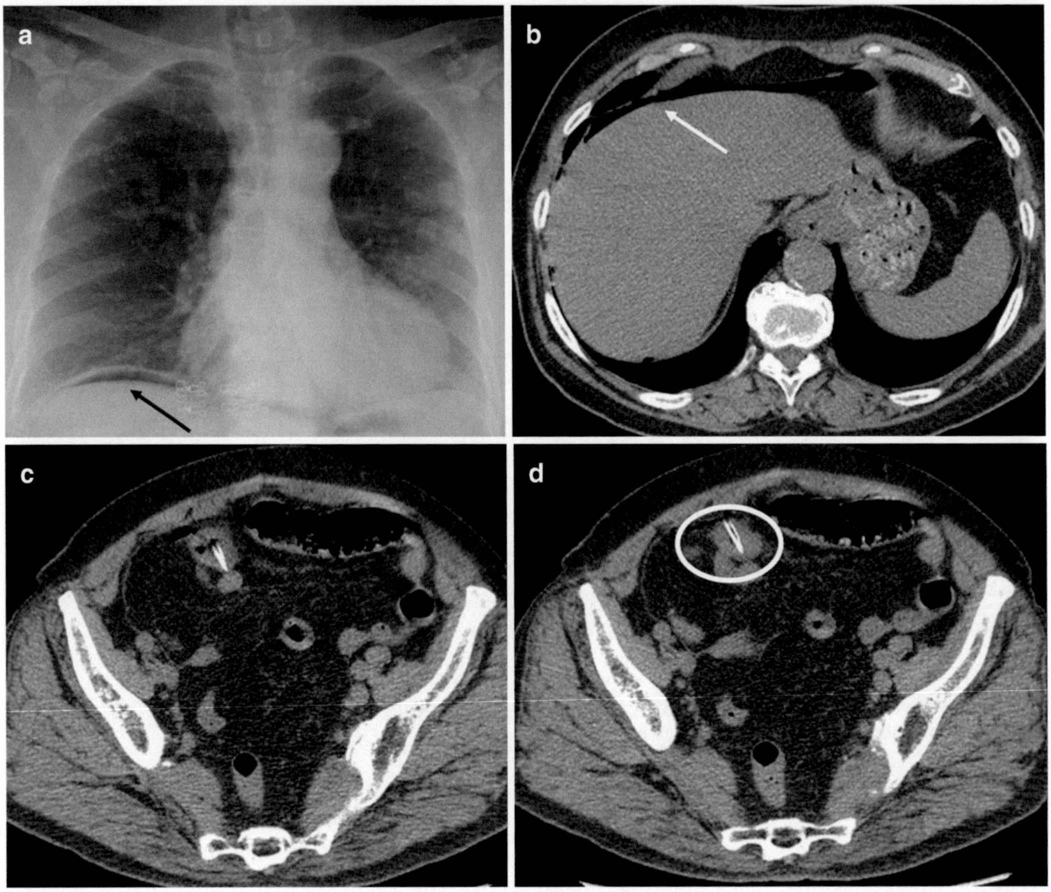

Fig. 14.2 Plain films sign shows gas in the peritoneal cavity (**a**, *black arrows*). Abdominal CT confirms pneumoperitoneum (**b**, *white arrow*) and shows a foreign body in the small bowel with gas and fluid within the abdominal cavity (**c**, **d**, *white circle*)

important role in the preoperative staging and postoperative surveillance of colon cancer. The recent advances in CT technology provide greater accuracy for the preoperative staging of colorectal cancer. The findings associated with adenocarcinoma of the colorectum generally include asymmetric bowel wall thickening with contrast enhancement or the presence of a soft-tissue mass that frequently leads to luminal narrowing or obstruction.

Common presenting symptoms of CRC include abdominal pain, change in bowel habits, rectal bleeding, anaemia, and weight loss [22]. A less frequent presentation is perforation and abscess formation, which is usually intraperitoneal, but may occasionally be located in extraperitoneal spaces. With contained perforation and abscess formation, the clinical picture can closely resemble complicated diverticulitis, whether on clinical examination or on radiological imaging such as computed tomography (CT) scans. Patients typically present fever, abdominal pain and leukocytosis, and CT scans show a pericolic or intra-abdominal abscess.

Bowel obstruction is the most commonly observed complication of colon cancer. Left-sided colon malignancies are more prone to obstruct the colon lumen than are the right-sided malignancies. This is because the diameter of the left colon is smaller than that of the right colon. CT is a sensitive imaging modality for detecting bowel obstruction, and the multiplanar reconstruction images can provide additional information on the transition point in problematic cases [1].

Identifying the transitional zones and an obstructing lesion on CT, and these usually appear as irregular circumferential thickening of the colon, is important to differentiate this entity from other benign conditions such as adynamic ileus, colonic pseudoobstruction, and stercoral colitis, and all these maladies can present with colonic dilatation.

Perforation in association with a colonic tumour is uncommon as a primary presentation, with incidences ranging from 2.6 % [4] to 10 % [23]. Perforation of the colon can be diagnosed by CT with the demonstration of a focal defect in the colon wall that may be accompanied by a fluid-density abscess, free air, or stranding of the pericolic fat. Abscess formation occurs in 0.3–0.4 % of colonic carcinomas and it is the second most common complication of perforated lesions.

Abscesses commonly remain localised in the paracolic region or may develop into a pelvic abscess, but they can also track along various tissue planes and have been reported to present as a flank abscess, psoas abscess, or even a subcutaneous abscess on the trunk [24]. The location of perforation associated with colonic cancers is most commonly at the tumour site and is due to locally invasive disease causing a breach of integrity of the colonic wall. Perforations can also occur proximally to an obstructing primary lesion, for example, a perforated caecum secondary to a closed loop obstruction with a competent ileocecal valve in an obstructed carcinoma of the sigmoid or descending colon [25, 26]. The location of the tumour is also a factor in the likelihood of perforation and abscess formation. In the right and transverse colon, perforations present twice as commonly as peritonitis compared to abscesses. On the other hand, abscess formation is more common than free perforation in the left colon, and the sigmoid and rectosigmoid are the most frequent locations [23, 27]. It is well documented that perforated colonic carcinoma has a lower 5-year survival rate, in comparison to the uncomplicated colonic cancer undergoing elective resection [28]. It is important that the diagnosis of perforated colonic carcinoma is considered as a differential diagnosis whenever a patient presents with an intra-abdominal abscess with the presumptive diagnosis of perforated diverticular disease. All patients who present with complicated 'diverticular disease' and intra-abdominal abscess especially those that do not respond to conservative treatment should be offered surgery with resection of the involved colon and removal of the abscess for histological evaluation (Fig. 14.3).

14.4 Diverticulitis

Diverticular disease has become more prevalent in Western countries [29, 30]. About 10–25 % of individuals with diverticulosis will develop symptomatic diverticulitis, and of these, 15 % will develop significant complications, such as perforation [31]. Although the absolute prevalence of perforated diverticulitis complicated by generalised peritonitis is low, its importance lies in the significant postoperative mortality, ranging from 4 to 26 % regardless of the surgical strategy selected [31, 32]. Optimal treatment strategies are based on disease severity as classified by Hinchey [33]. The usual management of diverticulitis is based on patients symptomatology as well as CT scan results. Simple diverticulitis can be treated with bowel rest and intravenous antibiotics. Complicated diverticulitis is classified using the Hinchey classification, and management strategies depend on the classification. Hinchey III and IV diverticulitis are indications for laparotomy, washout, and resection of the affected colon.

Today, a conservative treatment with antibiotics (and abscess drainage) is advocated for Hinchey 1 and 2 [34]. Patients presenting with perforated diverticulitis with generalised peritonitis (Hinchey 3 and 4) should undergo emergency surgical treatment. Laparoscopic peritoneal lavage without resection of the affected bowel segment in patients with purulent peritonitis (Hinchey 3) appears to diminish the morbidity and improve outcome, whereas acute resection should be performer in patients with gross faecal peritonitis (Hinchey stage 4). The combination of free air and intra-abdominal fluid seen on the CT scan correlated well with

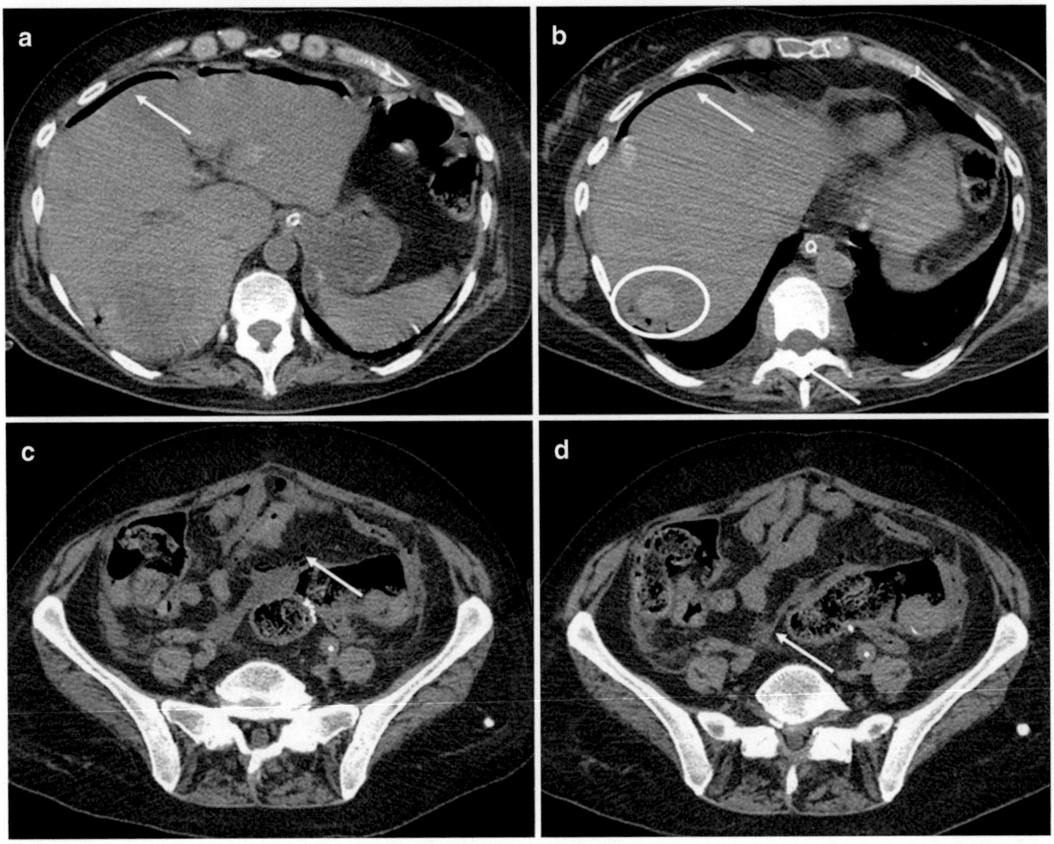

Fig. 14.3 Abdominal CT shows pneumoperitoneum (**a**, **b**, *white arrows*) with liver focal lesion (**b**, *white circle*). Axial CT scan shows irregular thickening of descending colon (**c**, *arrow*) and pericolic fat stranding (**d**, *arrow*). Caudal to colon wall thickening, there are colon wall defect with adjacent peritoneal free fluid and gas (**c**, *arrow*). Free perforation was surgically confirmed

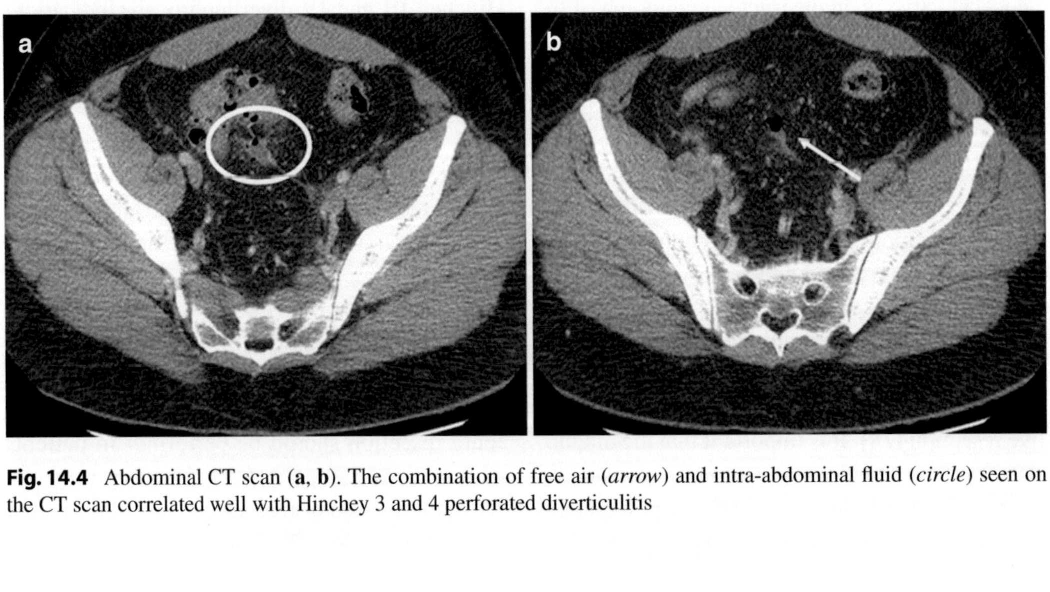

Fig. 14.4 Abdominal CT scan (**a**, **b**). The combination of free air (*arrow*) and intra-abdominal fluid (*circle*) seen on the CT scan correlated well with Hinchey 3 and 4 perforated diverticulitis

Hinchey 3 and 4 perforated diverticulitis, and these are the main findings the radiologists used to for the CT based diagnosis of Hinchey 3 or 4 (Fig. 14.4). Preoperative differentiation between Hinchey stage 3 and 4 is not very important, as both need emergency surgical treatment. Nevertheless, it could be useful in deciding on the surgical approach. In case of purulent peritonitis (Hinchey 3), laparoscopic peritoneal lavage and drainage without resection of the affected bowel segment has shown excellent results. In case of faecal peritonitis, laparotomy is recommended for resection of the affected bowel segment.

The preoperative differentiation between Hinchey 3 and Hinchey 4 is not possible with CT scanning. Today, computed tomography is the modality of choice in the assessment and management of diverticulitis with its high sensitivity and specificity [35, 36]. With CT-guided percutaneous abscess drainage (PCD), it has also become an important therapeutic modality. In recent years, CT scanning has become the imaging modality of choice to determine the extent of the disease and surgeons tend to rely more frequently on the CT findings to decide upon further treatment [37].

14.5 Ischaemia

The two most common aetiologies that cause vascular impairment of the SB wall leading to perforation are direct vascular occlusion and strangulated SB obstruction [38]. Various vasculitides, characterised by inflammation and necrosis of small systemic blood vessels, including the visceral vessels of the GIT, have been reported rarely as a cause of ischaemic intestinal perforation [39]. Prompt diagnosis and treatment is required for a strangulated bowel. The CT findings suggestive of strangulation include intestinal wall thickening, mural hypoperfusion, blurring of the mesenteric vessels with localised mesenteric fluid, and free peritoneal fluid (Fig. 14.5).

More specific findings of bowel infarction are lack of bowel wall enhancement, pneumatosis intestinalis, gas in the portal vein, or pneumoperitoneum [38–40].

Moreover, elderly patient often have underlying pathologies, such as chronic cardiovascular and pulmonary disease, diabetes, malignancies, diverticula, abdominal aortic aneurism, peptic ulcer disease, and biliary tract disease.

They usually take multiple medications, and they often are unable to explain their symptoms

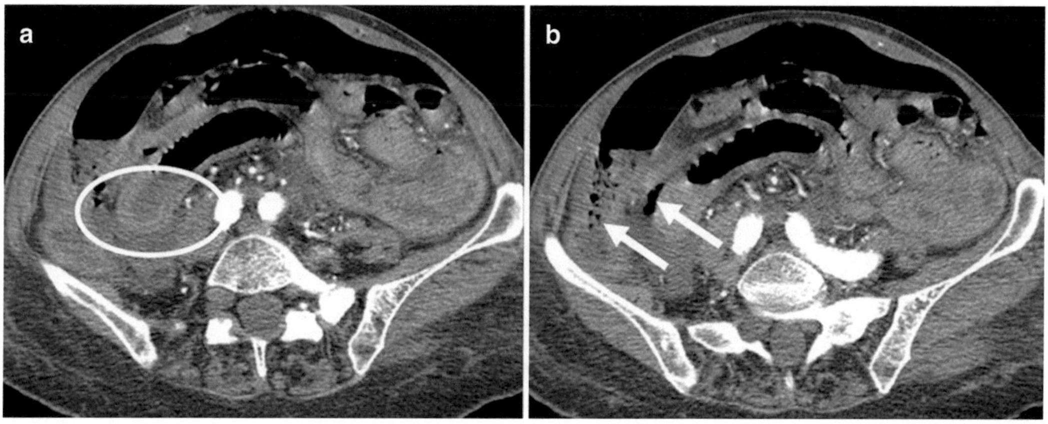

Fig. 14.5 CT scan detects a target appearance of the ischaemic bowel with an inner hyperdense ring due to mucosal hypervascularity, a middle hypodense edematous submucosa, and a normal or slightly thickened muscularis propria. If the vascular impairment persists, CT findings are represented by mural thickening of the involved segments, peritoneal fluid, and mesenteric engorgement (**a**, *circle*). In late-stage venous thrombosis, absence of mural enhancement and the presence of fluid and gas may be evident in the sub-peritoneal or peritoneal space (**b**, *arrows*)

clearly because of an impaired sensorium. Although SBO and mesenteric ischaemia are well-known and common conditions, the diagnosis and the choice of the correct treatment still pose challenges for those working in emergency clinical settings. Clinicians must take into account atypical presentations and the many clinical differentials. Once they have established the diagnosis, they need to decide whether, how, and when to intervene.

Mesenteric ischaemia leading to bowel infarction is a relatively common catastrophic occurrence in the elderly. In this condition the diagnosis may be difficult, but time is of the essence for survival, because the prognosis is poor, and the treatment is almost inconsequential if performed too late. Acute mesenteric ischaemia is a syndrome in which inadequate blood flow through the mesenteric circulation causes ischaemia and eventual gangrene of the bowel wall. The aetiology could be arterial or venous; the arterial disease can be subdivided into nonocclusive and occlusive ischaemia. Diagnostic imaging plays the main role in detecting the degree and severity of intestinal ischaemia and in assessing for evidence of infarction.

14.6 Degos' Syndrome

Kohlmeier described malignant atrophic papulosis in his article 'Multiple Hautrekrosen bei Thromboangiitis obliterans' in 1941 [41]; this same disease entity was described by Degos in 1942. Degos' syndrome is an occlusive small-vessel vasculopathy which causes tissue infarct [42], but its aetiology is unknown and it affects all ages. Degos' syndrome has a benign cutaneous form and a fatal systemic form [43]. Skin lesions may manifest as erythematous papules which heal to leave scars with white atrophic centres. Light microscopy findings of skin lesions may demonstrate wedge-shaped zones of necrosis extending from the epidermis to the reticular dermis, thickened vessel walls, and thromboses [44]. Gastrointestinal lesions may show identical histological findings, and complications such as bowel perforation and peritonitis are often fatal within 2–3 years. Medical treatments such as antiplatelet drugs have been given, but there is not definite effective treatment. The gastrointestinal tract is affected in 50 % of patients with systemic Degos' syndrome. Other systems such as the central nervous system and renal system can also be affected, as demonstrated by the cases described by McFarland et al. and Schade et al. Both the patients described by Kohlmeier and Degos in 1941 and 1942 died from bowel perforation Kim et al. described a case of Degos' syndrome with gastrointestinal involvement in a 59-year-old woman, with a history of multiple skin lesions and small-bowel perforation treated by surgery [45]. The patient developed generalised abdominal pain, and explorative laparotomy revealed multifocal ischaemic changes in the small bowel with perforations. A case of Degos' syndrome described by González Valverde et al. presented with acute abdominal pain due to intestinal perforation and multiple serosal maculae on the intestine; Degos' syndrome was not diagnosed until a few erythematous skin lesions were discovered. The CT findings in a 40-year-old woman with Degos' syndrome were described by Amaravadi et al. They included extensive ascites, nodular thickening of the omentum, small-bowel wall thickening, gross pneumoperitoneum with small-bowel perforations, and intraluminal haemorrhage into a loop of infarcted jejunum. The serial CT images can demonstrate the sites of perforation, peritoneal enhancement, and nodular omentum, of which the features are not specific for Degos' syndrome. The nodular omentum may resemble other conditions such as peritoneal carcinomatosis. The patent mesenteric vessels and absence of atherosclerosis excluded that there was mesenteric artery and vein occlusion.

Tiny pockets of pneumatosis intestinalis were noted in the ileum and ascending colon during the first and third admissions. The pneumatosis was a bubble-like configuration, but without associated portovenous gas. Pneumatosis intestinalis was previously regarded as a sign of transmural necrosis, but it can also be due to different non-ischaemic causes such as chronic obstructive pulmonary disease, connective tissue diseases or infectious enterocolitis, none of which are necessarily associated with unfavourable outcomes. Pneumatosis intestinalis was previously regarded as a sign of transmural necrosis, but it can also be due to different non-ischaemic causes such as chronic obstructive pulmonary disease, connective tissue diseases, or infectious enterocolitis, none of which are necessarily associated with unfavourable outcomes. Kernagis et al. suggested that isolated pneumatosis without portovenous gas and other signs of ischaemia is more likely to have partial mural ischaemia. Wiesner et al. concluded that bubble-like pneumatosis may be related to only partial mura bowel ischaemia. Nonetheless, Degos' syndrome is a vasculopathy that can cause tissue necrosis, and bowel ischaemia cannot be excluded in the presence of pneumatosis.

14.7 Crohn's Disease

Free perforation is a rare complication of Crohn's disease. It occurs during an acute exacerbation of chronic disease, particularly in presence of distal obstruction. The incidence of this complication may become less common and steroid therapy was not a precipitating factor. Primary resection of the perforated and distal obstructed bowel is likely to give the best results [46].

SB perforation may occur in a patient with known CD or may rarely be the first presentation of previously unknown inflammatory bowel disease. Free perforation, although rare, is a life-threatening complication reported in up to 3 % of cases [47, 48].

The perforation occurs during an acute exacerbation of Crohn's disease and was always associated with distal obstruction due to a chronic stenosing lesion.

A low-grade granulomatous process with transmural inflammatory reaction is characteristic of Crohn's disease. It causes affected intestinal loops to become attached to adjacent structures, providing a pathological basis for the more common complications of abscess and fistula formation. While perforation may occur during an active phase of the disease, it does not appear to occur in patients with 'acute ileitis' as was suggested by Crohn (1965) [49]. No perforations have been reported in the series of acute ileitis reported by Atwell and colleagues (1965) [50], Schofield (1965) [51].

CT helps to detect both the perforation and the unsuspected CD as its cause, often presenting with typical findings of active CD.

References

1. Zissin R, Osadchy A, Gayer G (2009) Abdominal CT findings in small bowel perforation. Br J Radiol 82(974):162–171
2. Maniatis V, Chryssikopoulos H, Roussakis A, Kalamara C, Kavadias S, Papadopoulos A et al (2000) Perforation of the alimentary tract: evaluation with computed tomography. Abdom Imaging 25:373–379
3. Yeung KW, Chang MS, Hsiao CP, Huang JF (2004) CT evaluation of gastrointestinal tract perforation. Clin Imaging 28:329–333
4. Coulier B, Tancredi MH, Ramboux A (2004) Spiral CT and multidetector-row CT diagnosis of perforation of the small intestine caused by ingested foreign bodies. Eur Radiol 14:1918–1925
5. Rubesin SE, Levine MS (2003) Radiologic diagnosis of gastrointestinal perforation. Radiol Clin North Am 41:1095–1115
6. Hainaux B, Agneessens E, Bertinotti R, De Maertelaer V, Rubesova E, Capelluto E et al (2006) Accuracy of MDCT in predicting site of gastrointestinal tract perforation. AJR Am J Roentgenol 187:1179–1183
7. Cadenas Rodríguez L, Martí de Gracia M, Saturio Galán N, Pérez Dueñas V, Salvatierra Arrieta L, Garzón Moll G (2013) Use of multidetector computed tomography for locating the site of gastrointestinal tract perforations. Cir Esp 91(5):316–323
8. Lozon AA, Duff JH (1976) Acute perforation of the colon. Can J Surg 19:48–51
9. Levine MS, Scheiner JD, Rubesin SE, Laufer I, Herlinger H (1991) Diagnosis of pneumoperitoneum on supine abdominal radiographs. AJR Am J Roentgenol 156:731–735
10. Zissin R, Konikoff F, Gayer G (2006) CT findings of iatrogenic complications following gastrointestinal endoluminal procedures. Semin Ultrasound CT MR 27:126–138
11. Pinto A, Scaglione M, Pinto F, Romano L, Grassi R, Rotondo A (2000) Helical computed tomography diagnosis of gastrointestinal perforation in the elderly patient. Emerg Radiol 7:259–262
12. Rodríguez-Hermosa JI, Cañete N, Artigau E, Gironès J, Planellas P, Codina-Cazador A (2009) Small bowel perforation by an unusual foreign body. Rev Esp Enferm Dig 101(9):639–641
13. Rodríguez-Hermosa JI, Codina-Cazador A, Sirvent JM, Martín A, Gironès J, Garsot E (2008) Surgically

treated perforations of the gastrointestinal tract caused by ingested foreign bodies. Colorectal Dis 10: 701–707
14. Goh BK, Chow PK, Quah HM, Ong HS, Eu KW, Ooi LL et al (2006) Perforation of the gastrointestinal tract secondary to ingestion of foreign bodies. World J Surg 30:372–377
15. Rodríguez-Hermosa JI, Ruiz-Feliú B, Roig-García J, Albiol-Quer M, Planellas-Giné P, Codina-Cazador A (2009) Lethal intestinal perforation after foreign body ingestion in a superobese patient. Obes Surg 19:1183–1185
16. Drakonaki E, Chatzioannou M, Spiridakis K, Panagiotakis G (2011) Acute abdomen caused by a small bowel perforation due to a clinically unsuspected fish bone. Diagn Interv Radiol 17(2):160–162
17. Goh BK, Tan YM, Lin SE et al (2004) CT in the preoperative diagnosis of fish bone perforation of the gastrointestinal tract. AJR Am J Roentgenol 187: 710–714
18. Ell SR, Sprigg A (1991) The radio-opacity of fish bone species variation. Clin Radiol 44:104–107
19. Rioux M, Langis P (1994) Sonographic detection of clinically unsuspected swallowed toothpicks and their gastrointestinal complications. J Clin Ultrasound 22:483–490
20. Yeo ES, Ng KH, Eu KW (2011) Perforated colorectal cancer: an important differential diagnosis in all presumed diverticular abscesses. Ann Acad Med Singapore 40(8):375–378
21. Wong MTC, Eu KW (2007) Rise of colorectal cancer in Singapore: an epidemiological review. ANZ J Surg 77:446–449
22. Speights VO, Johnson MW, Stoltenberg PH, Rappaport ES, Helbert B, Riggs M (1991) Colorectal cancer: current trends in initial clinical manifestations. South Med J 84:575–578
23. Welch JP, Donaldson GA (1974) Perforative carcinoma of the colon and rectum. Ann Surg 180:734–740
24. Kobayashi H, Sakurai Y, Shoji M, Nakamura Y, Suganuma M, Imazu H et al (2001) Psoas abscess and cellulitis of the right gluteal region resulting from carcinoma of the cecum. J Gastroenterol 36:623–628
25. Biondo S, Kreisler E, Millan M, Fraccalvieri D, Golda T, Marti Rague J et al (2008) Differences in patient postoperative and long-term outcomes between obstructive and perforated colonic cancer. Am J Surg 195:427–432
26. Kim SW, Shin HC, Kim IY, Kim YT, Kim CJ (2010) CT findings of colonic complications associated with colon cancer. Korean J Radiol 11(2):211–221
27. Shucksmith HS (1963) Subcutaneous abscess as the first evidence of carcinoma of the colon. Br J Surg 50:514–515
28. Devitt JE, Roth-Moyo LA, Brown FN (1970) Perforation complicating adenocarcinoma of colon and rectum. Can J Surg 13:9–12
29. Gielens MP, Mulder IM, van der Harst E, Gosselink MP, Kraal KJ, Teng HT, Lange JF, Vermeulen J (2012) Preoperative staging of perforated diverticulitis by computed tomography scanning. Tech Coloproctol 16(5):363–368, Jun 30
30. Painter NS, Burkitt DP (1975) Diverticular disease of the colon, a 20th century problem. Clin Gastroenterol 1:3–21
31. Parks TG (1969) Natural history of diverticular disease of the colon. A review of 521 cases. Br Med J 5684:639–642
32. Vermeulen J, Akkersdijk GP, Gosselink MP et al (2007) Outcome after emergency surgery for acute perforated diverticulitis in 200 cases. Dig Surg 5:361–366
33. Morris CR, Harvey IM, Stebbings WS, Hart AR (2008) Incidence of perforated diverticulitis and risk factors for death in a UK population. Br J Surg 7:876–881
34. Hinchey EJ, Schaal PG, Richards GK (1978) Treatment of perforated diverticular disease of the colon. Adv Surg 12:85–109
35. Soumian S, Thomas S, Mohan PP, Khan N, Khan Z, Raju T (2008) Management of Hinchey II diverticulitis. World J Gastroenterol 47:7163–7169
36. Singh JP, Steward MJ, Booth TC, Mukhtar H, Murray D (2010) Evolution of imaging for abdominal perforation. Ann R Coll Surg Engl 3:182–188
37. Ambrosetti P, Becker C, Terrier F (2002) Colonic diverticulitis: impact of imaging on surgical management—a prospective study of 542 patients. Eur Radiol 5:1145–1149
38. Destigter KK, Keating DP (2009) Imaging update: acute colonic diverticulitis. Clin Colon Rectal Surg 3:147–155
39. Rha SE, Ha HK, Lee SH, Kim JH, Kim JK, Kim JH et al (2000) CT and MR imaging findings of bowel ischaemia from various primary causes. Radiographics 20:29–42
40. Furukawa A, Yamasaki M, Takahashi M, Nitta N, Tanaka T, Kanasaki S et al (2003) CT diagnosis of small bowel obstruction: scanning technique, interpretation and role in the diagnosis. Semin Ultrasound CT MR 24:336–352
41. Zissin R, Osadchy A, Klein E, Konikoff F (2006) Consecutive instances of gallstone ileus due to obstruction first at the ileum and then at the duodenum complicating a gallbladder carcinoma: a case report. Emerg Radiol 12:108–110
42. Yeung JT, Ma JK, Yung AW (2013) Degos' syndrome complicated by bowel perforation: focus on radiological findings. Hong Kong Med J 19(2):174–177
43. Scheinfeld NS. Degos disease. Medscape website: http://emedicine.medscape.com/article/1087180-overview. Accessed Dec 2010
44. Scheinfeld N (2007) Malignant atrophic papulosis. Clin Exp Dermatol 32:483–487
45. Kim DW, Kang SB, Lee KH, Choe GY, Park SY, Nicholay M (2004) Degos' disease (malignant atrophic papulosis) as a fatal cause of acute abdomen: report of a case. Surg Today 38:866–870

46. Steinberg David M, Trevor Cooke W, Alexander-Williams J (1973) Free perforation in Crohn's disease. Gut 14:187–190
47. Berg DF, Bahadursingh AM, Kaminski DL, Longo WE (2002) Acute surgical emergencies in inflammatory bowel disease. Am J Surg 184:45–51
48. Zissin R, Hertz M, Osadchy A, Novis MB, Gayer G (2005) Computed tomographic findings of abdominal complications of Crohn's disease – pictorial essay. Can Assoc Radiol J 56:25–35
49. Crohn BB (1965) The pathology of acute regional ileitis. Am J Dig Dis 10:565–72
50. Atwell JD, Duthie HL, Goligher JC (1965) The outcome of Crohn's disease. Br J Surg 52(12):966–72
51. Schofield PF (1965) The natural history and treatment of crohn's disease. Ann R Coll Surg Engl 36:258–79

15 Imaging of Gastrointestinal Tract Perforation in the Oncologic Patients

Luigia Romano, Sonia Fulciniti, Massimo Silva, Riccardo Granata, and Giuseppe Ruggiero

15.1 Introduction

Gastrointestinal tract cancer can occur with many complications. Perforation, obstruction, bleeding, and invasion of the adjacent organs and structures are the main complications associated with gastrointestinal tumors [1].

One of the most severe complications has been represented by perforation.

Perforation is one of the gastrointestinal tract tumor complications with the worse prognostic factors because it is frequently associated with a severe septic status. It has been reported to occur in 3–10 % of colorectal carcinoma, and it is an emergency condition that requires immediate surgical management [2].

Perforation may occur because of the tumor's lack of desmoplastic response and rapid growth with insufficient blood supply, or it could depend on rapid necrosis due to chemotherapy.

It is generally due to two main conditions that are frequently associated and are represented by tumor necrosis and ischemia. The necrotic degeneration determined by the rapid tumoral growth under a limited blood supply can determine the tumoral perforation. Furthermore, the vascular occlusion by tumor cells and the increasing endoluminal hollow viscus pressure contribute to intestinal cancer perforation. Rarely the perforation occurs distantly from the primary tumor; in this case, it could depend on the mucin production by the tumor associated with the obstructive condition with a high pressure of the intestinal lumen.

The gastrointestinal perforation has two poor prognostic factors represented by the development of a severe septic status and the spillage of cancer cells inside the peritoneal cavity with a high rate of metastatic site diffusion.

In case of a perforated rectal tumor, CT can demonstrate the involvement of soft surrounding tissues represented by subcutaneous cellulitis and myositis associated with gas dissection

L. Romano (✉)
Department of Radiology, "A. Cardarelli" Hospital, Via Manzoni n° 213, Naples 80123, Italy
e-mail: luigia.romano@fastwebnet.it

S. Fulciniti
Department of Radiology, "A. Cardarelli" Hospital, Via Cupa Costa Brancaccio, n°12, Naples 80131, Italy
e-mail: soniafulciniti@libero.it

M. Silva
Department of Radiology, "A. Cardarelli" Hospital, Via Diaz, n° 108, Portici (Naples) 80025, Italy
e-mail: massimosilva@alice.it

R. Granata
Second University of Naples-Italy, Via Quattro Giornate n°15, Giugliano in Campania-Naples 80014, Italy
e-mail: gruggiero1@sirm.org

G. Ruggiero
Department of Radiology, "A. Cardarelli" Hospital, Via Sigmund Freud n°63, Naples 80131, Italy
e-mail: riccardogranata@hotmail.com

L. Romano, A. Pinto (eds.), *Imaging of Alimentary Tract Perforation*,
DOI 10.1007/978-3-319-08192-2_15, © Springer International Publishing Switzerland 2015

composed of multiple air bubbles. Deep fluid collections may coexist in the pelvic and retroperitoneal infected spaces.

The fluid collections are generally distributed in the perirectal and perineal planes, ischiorectal fossa, scrotum, thighs, buttocks, abdominal wall, and retroperitoneum. This kind of rectal cancer perforation associated with adjacent soft tissue gas dissection is called Fourier gangrene.

In patients affected by cancer treated with monoclonal antibody-tyrosine kinase inhibitors, a perforation of gastrointestinal tract can occur as a complication of the chemotherapeutic protocol.

Monoclonal antibodies are tyrosine kinase inhibitors targeting the vascular endothelial growth factor (VEGF) receptor and are used widely in the treatment of various neoplasms, demonstrating an improved selected antitumoral efficacy [3].

Particularly bevacizumab has been utilized for the treatment of advanced colorectal cancer, and it is under investigation for the treatment of other kinds of neoplasms. Unfortunately these new agents have severe collateral effects as gastrointestinal perforation, gastrointestinal fistula, and arterial thrombosis.

VEGF inhibition can damage the capillary bed of the intestinal wall, thus reducing the threshold for the development of microperforation, pneumatosis intestinalis, or frank perforation. Up to the stage of the development of pneumatosis intestinalis, the patient can be managed successfully by stopping anti-angiogenic therapy associated with fasting and parenteral nutrition. In case of perforation the patient has to be treated surgically to prevent sever peritonitis and septic status.

15.2 Computed Tomography

Computed tomography (CT) is increasingly being used as a screening modality for patients with symptoms of acute abdomen and has become the preferred small bowel imaging modality for assessing intestinal disorders.

Early symptoms of gastrointestinal tumor perforation are often nonspecific and could be misinterpreted as other frequent abdominal emergency conditions such as obstruction, intestinal ischemia, and peritonitis.

Patients with abdominal pain and an acute presentation of the gastrointestinal cancer undergo contrast medium emergency CT of the abdomen. In fact for acutely ill patients, CT is often the only study required, providing crucial information for accurate diagnosis of gastrointestinal tract neoplasms and associated complications [4].

15.3 MDCT Protocol Design Consideration

The MDCT protocol described is designed for a 64-row scanner, and images are acquired at 0.625 collimation, with reconstruction axial slice of 2.5 mm., pitch of 0.984, and gantry rotation time of 0.5 s.

The abdominal volumetric scan begins at the level of the diaphragmatic dome and ends at the pubic symphysis.

For gastrointestinal tract evaluation, the use of thin sections, high-volume, rapid-bolus scanning technique with state-of-the-art CT technology is important in differentiating intestinal and abdominal findings.

Preliminary unenhanced abdominal CT is obtained to detect free air bubbles into the peritoneal cavity or in fluid collections, hemoperitoneum, and preexisting hyperattenuating material in the bowel wall and lumen such as suture materials, blood clots, or retained contrast material (c.m).

Intravenous administration of contrast medium is mandatory for discovering gastrointestinal cancer.

Intravenous injection of a volume of 100–120 ml of iodine contrast material is generally necessary for evaluating enhancement alteration of the bowel wall and mesenteric fold.

For better viewing the enhancement alteration of the gastrointestinal wall, contrast agents with higher concentration of iodine (400 mg./ml) and high injection rates (at least 3–4 ml/s.) are preferred and are followed by a 30–50 ml saline chaser, also injected at a rate of 3–4 ml/s.

After the abdominal pre-contrast scan, the automated bolus tracking is used to time the beginning of the c.m. acquisition during the arterial phase. The bolus tracking requires precise placement of the region-of-interest (ROI) cursor in the abdominal aorta lumen. The image acquisition is triggered at an attenuation threshold of 150 UH.

The c.m. arterial phase is mandatory to detect arterial supply and arterial enhancement of hypervascularized gastrointestinal stromal tumors (GISTs) and their distant metastasis. It is also mandatory for evaluating ischemic changes of the intestinal wall that could be associated with cancer.

The scan delay for the next portal-venous phase is 70 s. The portal phase acquisition gives maximum bowel wall and primary tumor attenuation and distant metastasis attenuation, and it is useful in evaluating other intestinal cancer-associated findings, as mesenteric fold spreading, presence of a fistula through adjacent hollow viscus wall, and venous mesenteric drainage neoplastic obstruction. It is useful also for evaluating the CT findings associated with tumor perforation, as generalized peritonitis and septic fluid collections.

In selected cases, oral administration or enema of iodine contrast material (c.m.) could be useful, especially for demonstrating cancer fistulization.

Sagittal and coronal MIP reformatted images are useful for localizing the pathological segment of the bowel within the abdomen and evaluating the map of the distribution of air bubbles, abdominal cavity and peritoneal fold inflammation, and fluid collections.

15.4 CT Findings of Primary Gastrointestinal Cancer

CT is unable to determine whether a neoplasm is localized to the mucosa or infiltrates the muscularis layer. CT staging of the primary tumor is based on the evaluation of an irregular thickness or mass of the gastrointestinal wall, with a dishomogeneous post-contrast medium wall attenuation, with the presence or absence of the neoplastic

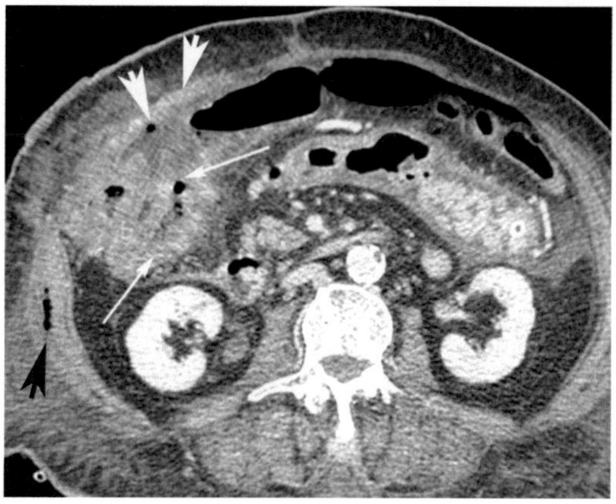

Fig. 15.1 Axial post-contrast medium CT scan shows the ascending colon thickening (*white arrows*) and surrounded by a pericolic fat inflammation associated with dense fluid and air bubbles (*white arrow heads*). Fluid film and air bubbles spread also into the abdominal wall (*black arrow head*)

diffusion to adjacent fat planes, structures, organs, lymph nodes, and distant regions.

A variety of radiological findings that depend on the development of peritoneal and mesenteric fold inflammation and fluid collection associated with gastrointestinal tumor perforation sometimes can hide the underlying primary cancer and can be misinterpreted as an infectious disease [5] (Fig. 15.1).

15.5 Stomach Cancer

The most frequent CT finding of stomach cancer is represented by a focal or diffuse gastric wall thickening, with a dishomogeneous post-contrast medium wall attenuation, particularly of the adenocarcinoma type (Fig. 15.2). Other CT signs are outer and inner lobulated irregular margins, ulceration, and narrowing of the lumen with obstruction and secondary proximal gastrectasia. The areas of dishomogeneous post-contrast enhancement are due to tumoral tissue inhomogeneity for edema, necrosis, or hemorrhage [6].

The tumor could invade surrounding organs and structures as the diaphragmatic muscle, pancreas, spleen, left lobe of the liver, transverse mesocolon, and small and greater omentum.

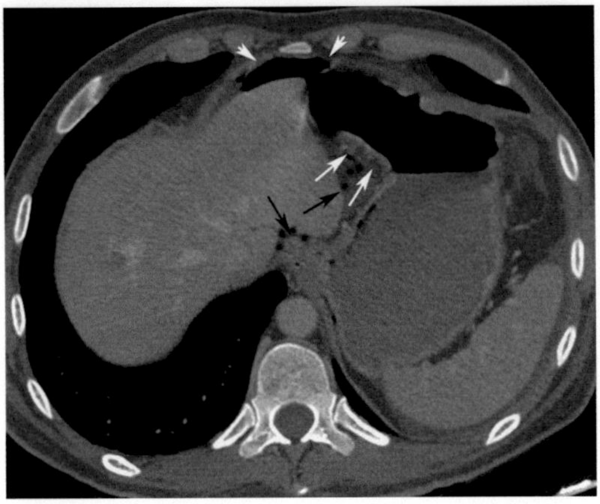

Fig. 15.2 Axial post-contrast medium CT scan shows pneumoperitoneum (*white arrow heads*) and a focal gastric wall thickening, with a dishomogeneous post-contrast medium wall attenuation (*white arrows*), representing a stomach cancer. The perforation of the lesion has been demonstrated by adjacent multiple air bubble spread within the small omentum (*black arrows*)

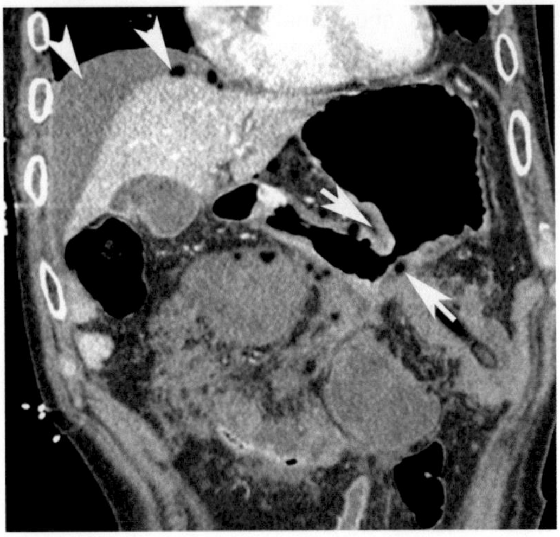

Fig. 15.3 Coronal post-contrast medium CT scan shows the narrowing of the stomach body lumen (*white arrows*) with secondary proximal gastrectasia. There is an open peritoneal perforation, with fluid and free air bubbles diffused around the gastric walls, inside the small omentum, and in the right subphrenic space (*white arrow heads*)

When the greater omentum is diffusely infiltrated, an "omental cake" may be recognized at CT scan as an extensive dishomogeneous thickened soft tissue mass, separating the colon and the small bowel from the anterior abdominal wall.

Metastasis could be evidenced at the liver, adrenal glands, lymph nodes, ovaries, and peritoneal cavity.

Gastric lymphoma can occur as a part of a generalized lymphomatous process or, in 10 % of cases, could be represented by an isolated primary gastric localization [7].

The lymphomatous process generally spreads submucosally, determining an irregular diffuse inhomogeneous and hypodense smooth thickening of the gastric wall greater than 1 cm. involving more than half of the circumference of the stomach. The inner and outer margins of the lymphoma are frequently waved; the perigastric flat planes are generally obliterated by the tumor invasion. Associated diffuse bulky lymphadenopathies indicate a disseminated disease.

The perforation of gastric carcinoma and lymphoma is a rare condition with an incidence of 0.4–0.6 % [8].

It generally occurs in elderly patients with a locally ulcerated advanced tumor. The use of thin high-resolution axial CT slices can demonstrate in some cases a direct discontinuity of the gastric neoplasm. In open peritoneal perforation, an amount of fluid and free air bubbles is diffused principally around the gastric walls, in the subphrenic left space, and inside the umbilical fissure of the liver and the small omentum (Fig. 15.3).

15.6 Small Intestinal Cancer

Tumors of the small intestine are uncommon, accounting for no more than 6 % of all gastrointestinal apparatus neoplasms, and are frequently represented by annular, aneurysmally dilated or ulcerated mass, associated with thickening or retractive desmoplastic reaction of the adjacent mesenteric fold. An endoluminal mass with a dishomogeneous post-contrast medium wall attenuation can be visualized. The evidence of ulceration is indicative of adenocarcinoma. Other CT signs are ulceration, necrotic areas, inner undulated margins, irregular outer profiles, and narrowing and obstruction of the lumen (Fig. 15.4). The perforation occurs in sites of the small intestine

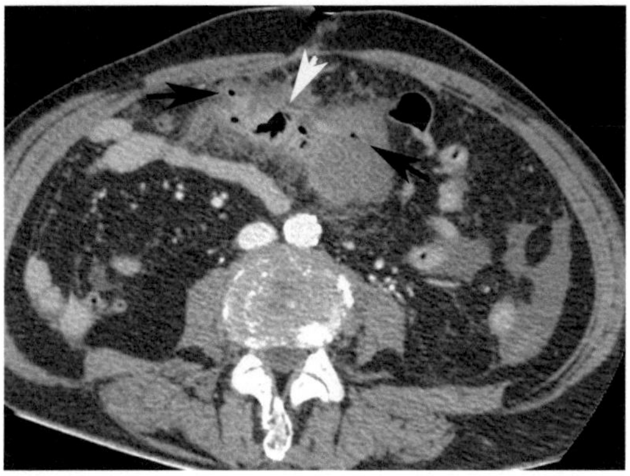

Fig. 15.4 Axial post-contrast medium CT scan shows a small bowel ulcerated mass (*white arrow head*), associated with narrowing of the lumen and retractive desmoplastic reaction with irregular outer profiles of the adjacent mesenteric fold in which there are multiple air bubbles (*black arrows*)

where an intramural infiltration by neoplastic cells has developed and has been followed by tumor necrosis. Perforation of a bowel metastasis can occur also after chemotherapy due to the cellular necrotic effect produced by the drug [9].

15.7 Small Intestinal Lymphoma

Small intestinal involvement of a lymphoma is one of the crucial points in the course of the pathology. The perforation or fistulization of this kind of localization can occur at any site including the duodenum, jejunum, and ileum [10] (Fig. 15.5).

Free intestinal perforation may occur both spontaneously and after chemotherapy, and it is due to tumor necrosis (Fig. 15.6). The diagnosis is often delayed because this kind of pathology has been frequently treated with cortisone that can reduce significantly abdominal acute symptoms.

If the perforation involves a small intestinal lymphoma, it is possible that in the peritoneal cavity there will be the presence only of free fluid without air. The peritoneal fluid can be evidenced by ultrasonography, but the site of the intestinal lymphoma could be better visualized by computed tomography.

The bowel wall can get ruptured due to the mechanical action of the bowel that resulted in

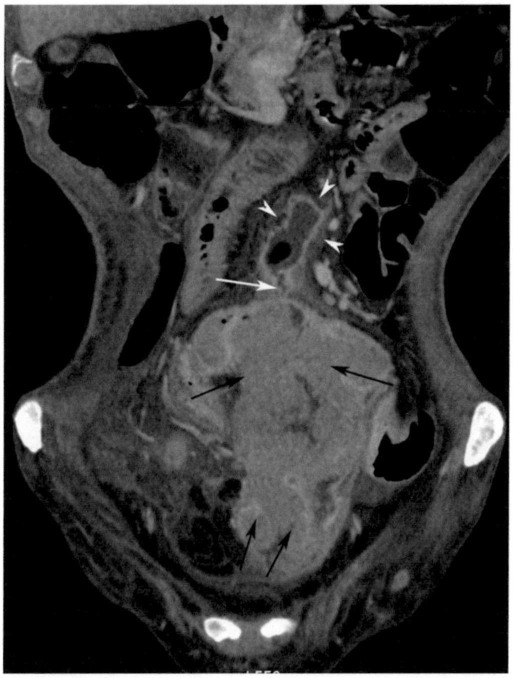

Fig. 15.5 Coronal post-contrast medium CT scan shows a very large dishomogeneous ileal mass (*black arrows*), associated with a thin fistula (*white arrow*) communicating with a mesenterial abscess (*white arrow heads*)

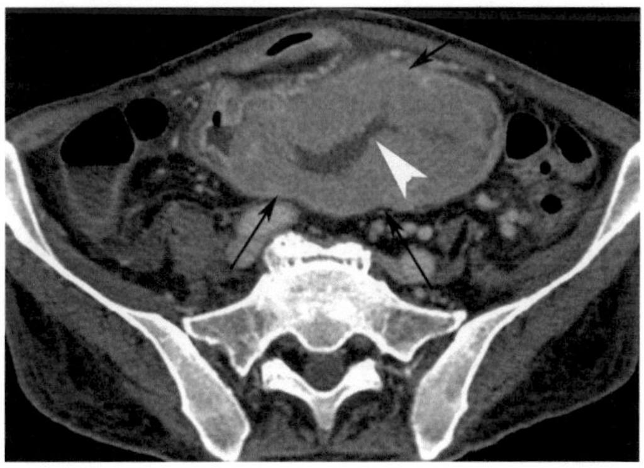

Fig. 15.6 Axial post-contrast medium CT scan shows a very large small intestinal mass (*black arrows*), in which there is a necrotic area (*white arrow head*)

mucosal ulceration, the depth of which increased gradually with the depth and degree of lymphoma cell infiltration, until eventually with the increase in intraluminal pressure (Fig. 15.7a, b).

If the lymphoma is located in the mesenteric fold, it can invade and obstruct the adjacent bowel loops leading to their perforation in the abdominal

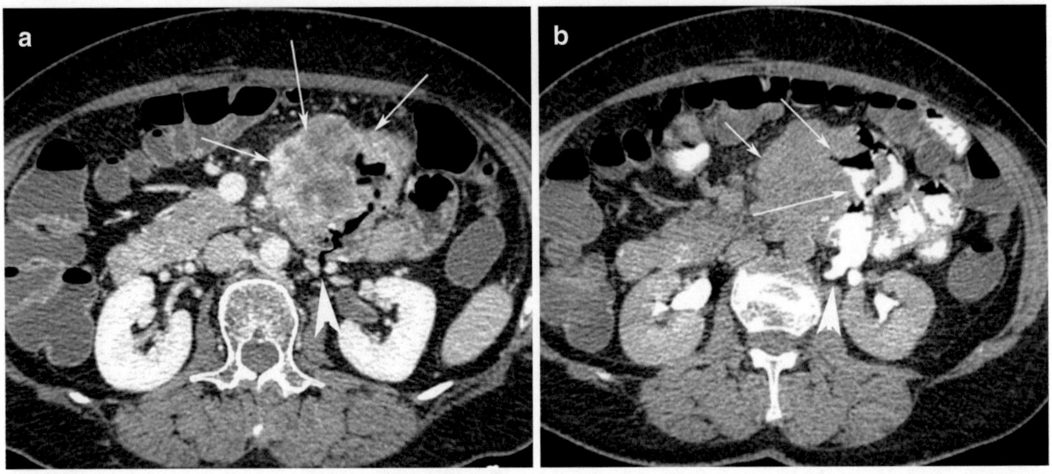

Fig. 15.7 (**a**) Axial post-contrast medium CT scan shows a very large dishomogeneous mass *(white arrows* in **a** and *small arrow* in **b**) of the abdominal left flank, involving an ileal loop and the adjacent mesenteric fold in which there is an ulcerated area associated with a long posterior fistula (*white arrow head*) communicating with the retroperitoneal space. (**b**) After oral administration of contrast medium, the intestinal fistula is clearly demonstrated (two *white arrows*), with extravasation of c.m. into the left anterior pararenal space (*white arrow head*)

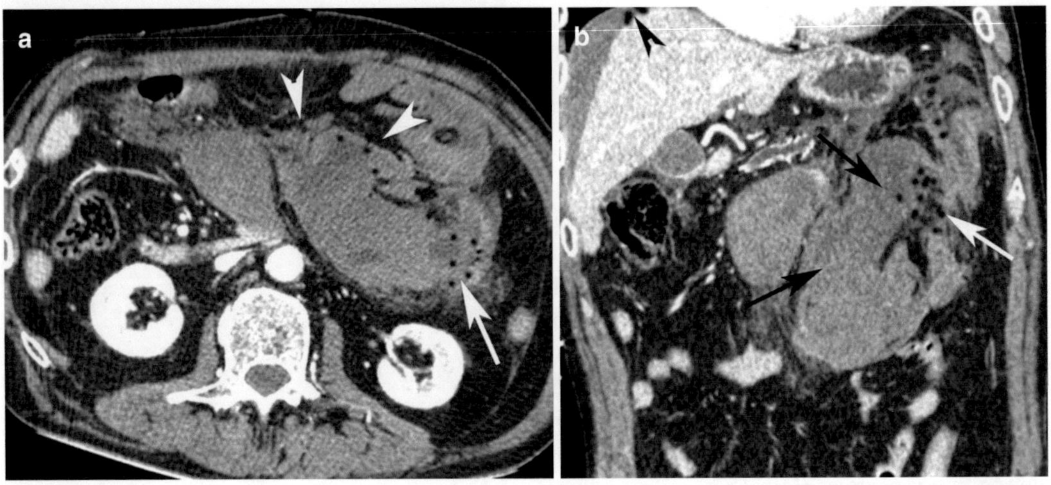

Fig. 15.8 (**a**) Axial post-contrast medium CT scan shows a large lymphoma located into the mesenteric fold (*white arrow heads*) that invades and obstructs the adjacent bowel loops (*white arrow*). (**b**) Coronal reconstruction CT image shows the involved bowel loops (*black arrows*) and their perforation with air bubbles into the adjacent mesenteric fold (*white arrow*) and into the abdominal cavity (*black arrow head*)

cavity (Fig. 15.8a, b) or to their fistulization in an adjacent structure, as the excretory renal system or psoas muscle [11] (Fig. 15.9a, b).

The steroid treatment itself can induce ulceration, tumor necrosis, and perforation of the intestinal bowel loop lymphoma.

15.8 Small Intestinal Metastasis

Solitary or multiple metastases spread in the small intestinal wall is much less common, although small bowel involvement in the late stage of abdominal carcinomatosis is frequently observed.

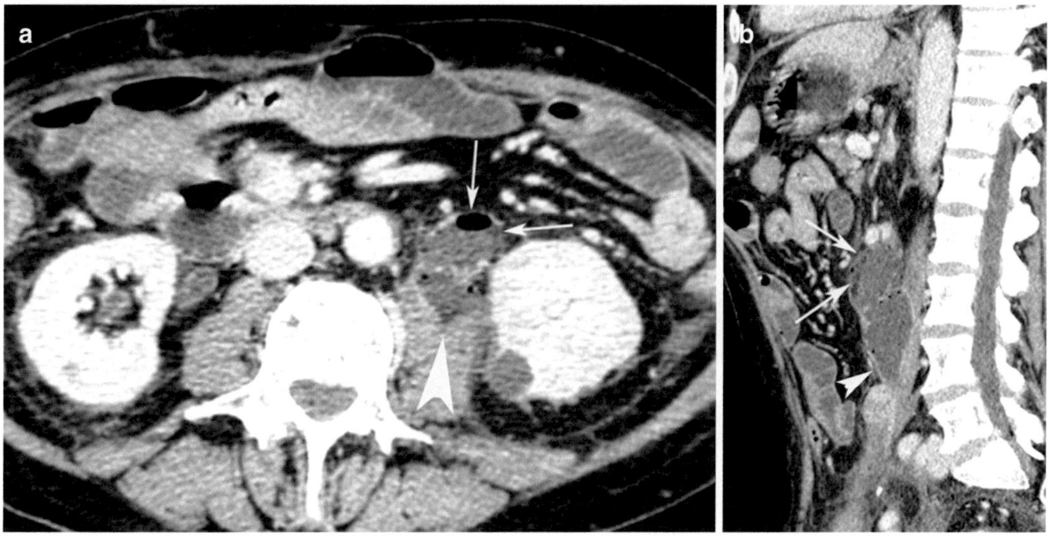

Fig. 15.9 (**a**) Axial post-contrast medium CT scan shows an obstructed small intestinal loop (*white arrows*) perforated into the psoas muscle fascia (*white arrow head*). (**b**) Sagittal reconstruction CT image better shows the perforated bowel loop (*white arrows*) with the development of a muscle abscess (*white arrow head*)

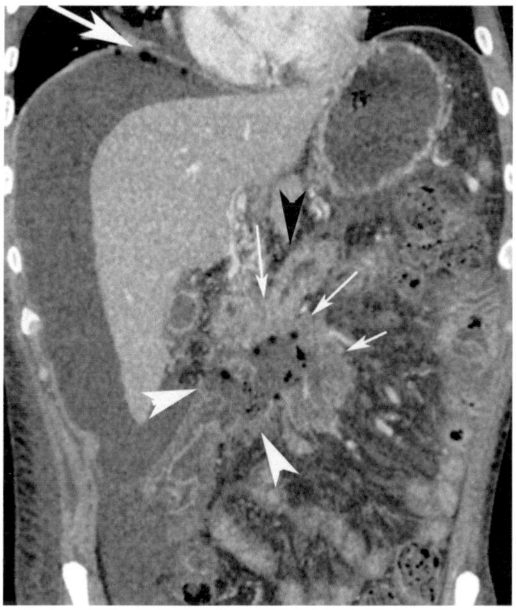

Fig. 15.10 Post-contrast medium CT coronal reconstruction shows a large mesenterial mass (*thin white arrows*) with a large necrotic area and irregular borders (*white arrow heads*) involving the duodenum (*black arrow head*). The necrotic mass perforation has been demonstrated by the presence of air and fluid into the peritoneal cavity (*white arrow*)

When metastatic lesions of the small intestine cause symptoms, the usual presentation is that of either complete or incomplete bowel obstruction, intestinal bleeding due to ulceration and erosion, and more rarely intestinal perforation [12].

Perforation of a bowel metastasis can occur also after chemotherapy due to the cellular necrotic effect produced by the drug [9] (Fig. 15.10).

The most frequent histologic types that can determine hematogenous metastasis into the intestinal wall are oat cell, epidermoid, giant cell carcinomas, and melanomas. The primary tumor generally has an abdominal or pelvic cancer origin as colon, uterine, and ovarian cancer or extra-abdominal origin as pulmonary cancer, breast cancer, and melanoma [13].

15.9 Colorectal Cancer

The ascending and descending colon tumors can be readily assessed because of their fixed retroperitoneal locations. Tumors localized in the flexures and transverse colon are less

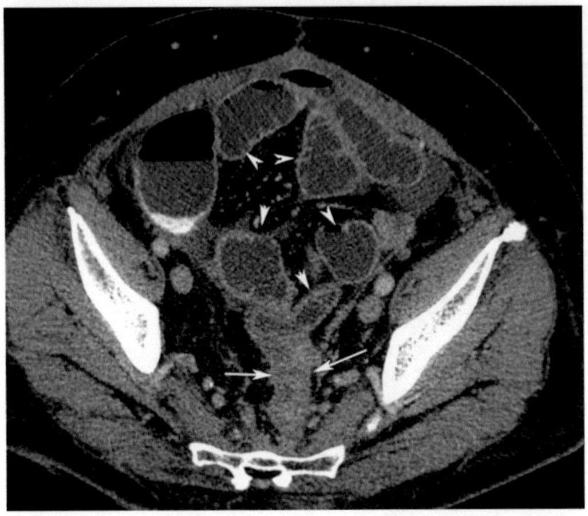

Fig. 15.11 Post contrast medium axial reconstruction shows a focal thickening of the sigmoid colon wall with a dishomogeneous post-contrast medium wall attenuation narrowing the intestinal lumen (*white arrows*), with mechanical obstruction of the proximal intestinal loops (*white arrow heads*)

frequently well evidenced by CT, for their position, retained fecal material, incomplete distension of the wall, peristaltic activity, and respiratory excursions.

The most frequent CT finding of colon cancer is represented by a focal thickening of the wall greater than 6 mm with a dishomogeneous post-contrast medium wall attenuation, frequently narrowing the intestinal lumen (Fig. 15.11).

Particularly in the adenocarcinoma type, an endoluminal polypoid mass with a dishomogeneous post-contrast medium wall attenuation can be visualized. Other CT signs are ulceration, necrotic areas, inner undulated margins, irregular outer profiles, stenosis, and obstruction of the lumen (Fig. 15.12a, b).

The rectum and rectosigmoid tract are easily evaluated by CT because of the fixed position in the pelvic cavity.

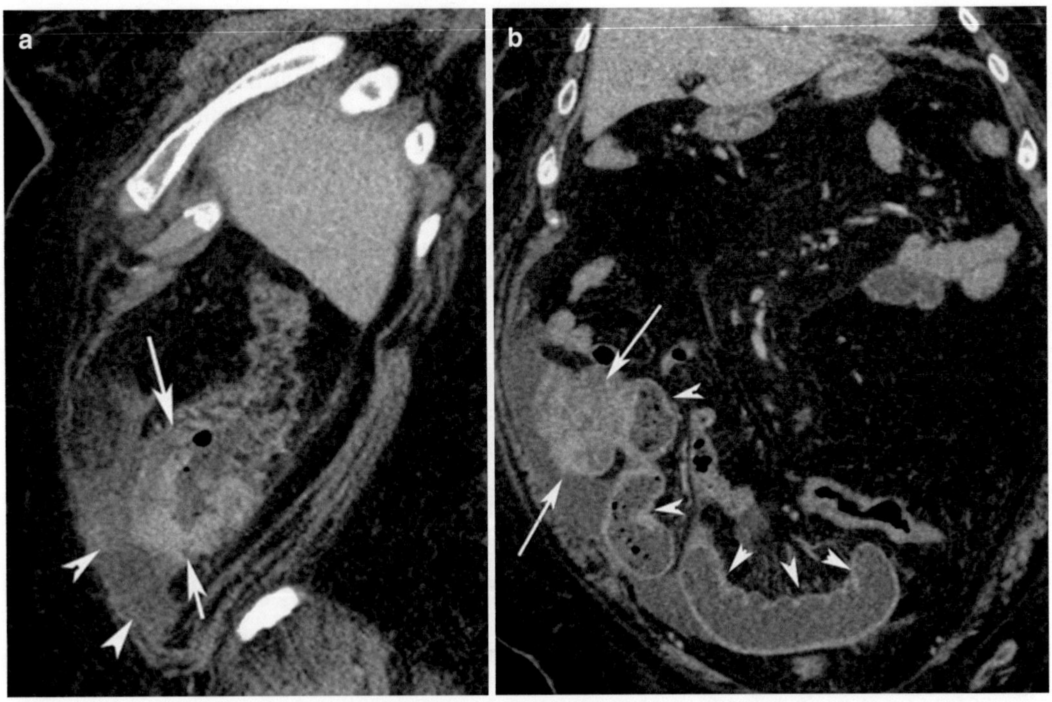

Fig. 15.12 (**a**) Sagittal reconstruction post-contrast medium CT image shows a neoplastic mass of the cecum pouch with inner undulated margins and irregular outer profiles (*white arrows*, **a** and **b**), surrounded by peritoneal fluid (*white arrow heads*). (**b**) Coronal reconstruction post-contrast medium CT image shows a mechanical obstruction of the proximal ileal loops (*white arrow heads*) with the lumen filled with fluid and air bubbles

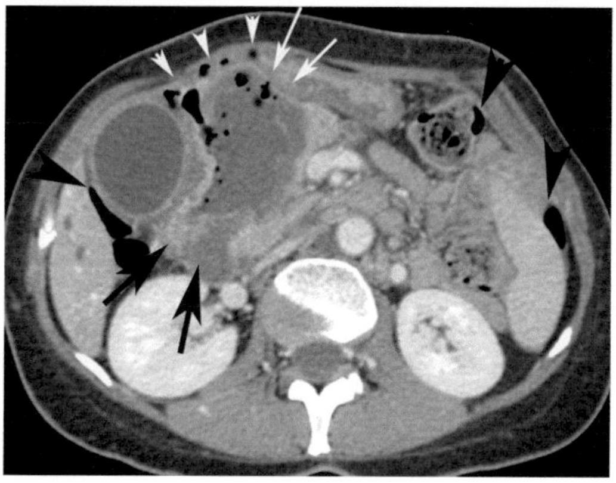

Fig. 15.13 Axial post-contrast media CT scan shows a focal thickening of the wall of the right flexure of the colon with a dishomogeneous post-contrast medium wall attenuation narrowing the intestinal lumen (*black arrows*). The neoplastic stenosis has been complicated both with a covered perforation due to the development of a pericolic abscess (*white arrows*) and open perforation with free air bubbles around the abscess wall (*white arrow heads*) and into the peritoneal cavity (*black arrow heads*)

Extracolon tumor spread is suggested by loss tissue fat planes between the large intestine and the surrounding structures as the seminal vesicles, prostate, bladder, uterus, ovaries, ureters, and muscles as the iliac, levator ani, obturator internus, piriformis, and coccygeal. Rectum and rectosigmoid tumor can invade bones as the sacrum and coccyx.

In selected cases it is possible to evidence a discontinuity of the colorectal cancer wall, with associated findings of open perforation or covered perforation (Fig. 15.13). In open perforation, an amount of dense fluid and free air bubbles is located principally in the subphrenic spaces, around the liver and the gastric walls, along the mesenteric folds, and in the peritoneal recesses of the pelvic cavity.

The cover perforation with the development of an abscess has been demonstrated by a low-density unilocular or multilocular collection with air-fluid level or air bubbles (Fig. 15.14a, b),

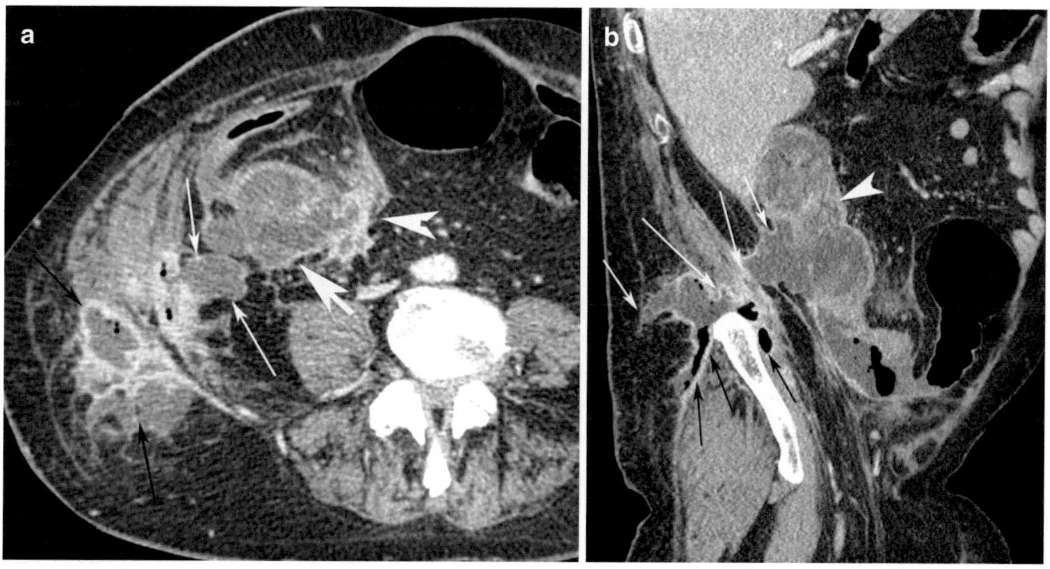

Fig. 15.14 (**a**) Axial post-contrast medium CT scan shows the cover perforation of the ascending colon cancer (*white arrow head*) with the development of an abscess, demonstrated by a low-density multilocular collection with air bubbles (*white arrows*), associated with inflamed surrounding fat tissue. The multiloculated abscess has been complicated with an abdominal wall fistula and development of a subcutaneous fat abscess (*black arrows*). (**b**) Sagittal reconstruction CT image shows the paracolic internal (*white arrow head*) and subcutaneous external abscesses (*white arrows*). The infection has spread also inside the muscle fasciae (*black arrows*)

associated with an increased peripheral density of the infiltrated or inflamed surrounding fat tissue. It is generally associated with a limited amount of free peritoneal fluid mainly localized in the vesical-rectal pouch.

Associated metastasis could be evidenced at the liver, adrenal glands, local lymph nodes, and peritoneal cavity. Additional findings are frequently represented by omental cake diffused distant lymph nodes.

15.10 CT Findings of Associated Intestinal Obstruction

Abnormal accumulation of gas and fluid in the distended intestinal tract occurs in the mechanical obstruction of both the small and large bowels affected by cancer (Figs. 15.11 and 15.12a, b). The distended intestinal loops contain air-fluid levels and are located proximal to the site of the neoplastic obstruction. During the acute phase of the mechanical obstruction, peristalsis become hyperactive with thickened plicae mucosae as the intestine attempts to work against the site of occlusion. When the obstruction lasts for a long time and is persistent, the intestine becomes atonic and plicae mucosae disappear.

At the level of the small intestine, the occlusion can determine an accumulation of small droplets of gas within the recesses between the valvulae conniventes, producing a series of small air bubbles referred to as the "string of pearls."

If the site of neoplastic mechanical obstruction is the colon, a competent ileocecal valve prevents the reflux of gas and fluid in the lumen of the small intestine, resulting in a "closing loop" obstruction of the colon. The wall of the cecum, being thinner and weaker than the wall of the remainder portions of the colon, distends more rapidly and to a greater degree. Therefore the rupture of the obstructed colon most likely occurs at the cecum level.

If the ileocecal valve is incompetent, allowing gas and fluid to reflux into the lumen of the small intestine, the tear of the cecum is not probable.

The high pressure in the intestinal lumen caused by occlusion can lead to a hypoperfusion of the intestinal wall with consequent ischemia and infarction [14].

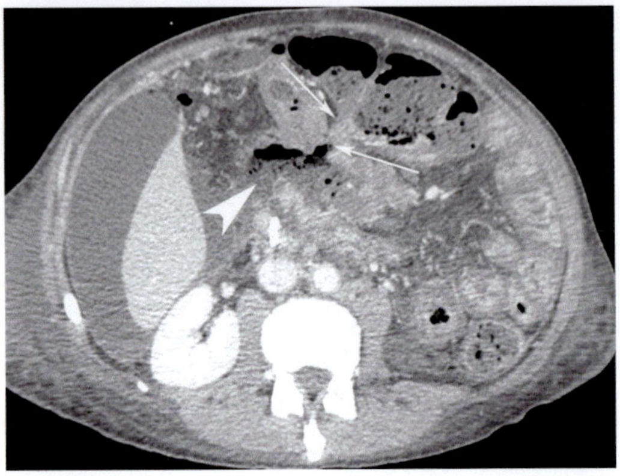

Fig. 15.15 Axial post-contrast medium CT scan shows a metastatic tissue that involves the transverse colon and adjacent ileal bowel loop (*white arrows*) with intestinal perforation and spread of air bubbles and enteric fluid into the mesenteric fold (*white arrow head*)

15.11 Primary Tumors and Metastasis of Small Bowel Perforation

Primary tumors and metastasis of the small bowel intestine can determine various complications as obstruction, bleeding, malabsorption, and perforation.

Mural replacement by metastatic tissue occurs after hematogenous or lymphatic spread of cancer cells. The spontaneous necrosis or the induced necrosis by chemotherapy can lead to metastasis perforation (Fig. 15.15). Also the increased luminal pressure due to the obstructed bowel loop or the embolization procedure performed for occluding the arterial supply to stop the severe bleeding of a metastasis can lead to the perforation [15].

15.12 Gastrointestinal Stromal Tumor (GIST) Perforation

Gastrointestinal stromal tumors (GISTs) are the most common mesenchymal tumors of the gastrointestinal tract and are 2.5 % of all gastrointestinal tumors [16]. The stomach is the most common site accounting for 50–70 % of GISTs, the small intestine for 25–30 %, and the colon-rectum for 5 % [17]. They are well-circumscribed masses that range in size from several millimeters to 30 cm and do not have a true capsula. They are frequently inhomogeneous with hyperdense areas that depend on a significant arterial blood supply, with focal areas of hemorrhage, necrosis, calcifications, cystic degeneration, and cavitations that can communicate with the intestinal lumen, the abdominal cavity, or both. Extension into the adjacent small bowel mesentery and encasement of noncontiguous segments of the small intestine, colon, bladder, ureter, and abdominal wall can occur [18].

They involve the muscularis propria of the intestinal wall and have the propensity for outer growth, projecting into the abdominal cavity.

The most common GISTs have an exophytic growth pattern and are shown by a mass located outside the gastrointestinal tract of origin (Fig. 15.16).

Obstruction of the intestine occurs very rarely, whereas the most frequent complication is hemorrhage [19].

GIST spontaneous perforation is a rare condition and can be due to the bleeding of the mass and capsula rupture that lead to a severe hemoperitoneum rather than pneumoperitoneum [20].

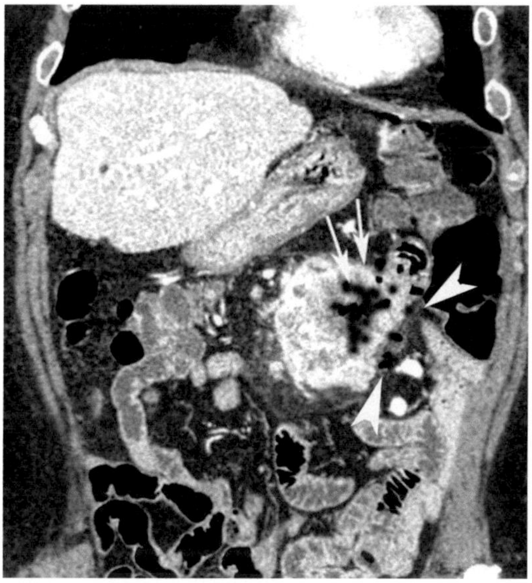

Fig. 15.16 Post-contrast medium CT coronal reconstruction shows a large hypervascularized and perforated gastrointestinal stromal tumor (GIST) involving the wall of a jejunal loop (*white arrows*) with air bubbles spread into the adjacent mesenteric fold (*white arrow heads*)

Extensive necrosis and fistula development may occur determining the growth of a cavity inside the tumoral tissue and bleeding. An air-fluid level can occur in these lesions with the formation of a fistula between an adjacent bowel loop and the primary tumor.

15.13 Colon Cancer Perforation

The perforation of colon neoplasms can occur in 2.5–10 % of cases [21].

Michowitz et al. [22] have proposed the following classification of perforated colon cancer:

1. Free perforation with leakage of the enteric fluid into the abdominal cavity
2. Covered perforation with local abscess development
3. Perforation into adjacent structures or organs or development of a fistula

Perforation of colon cancer has been reported to be a poor prognostic condition because it is evaluated as a sign of advanced disease and associated with two risks. The first is the diagnosis of the cancer itself and the second the septic complication that is joined with the perforation, the tumor dissemination, and consequent high rate of recurrence for the peritoneal seeding [23] (Fig. 15.17).

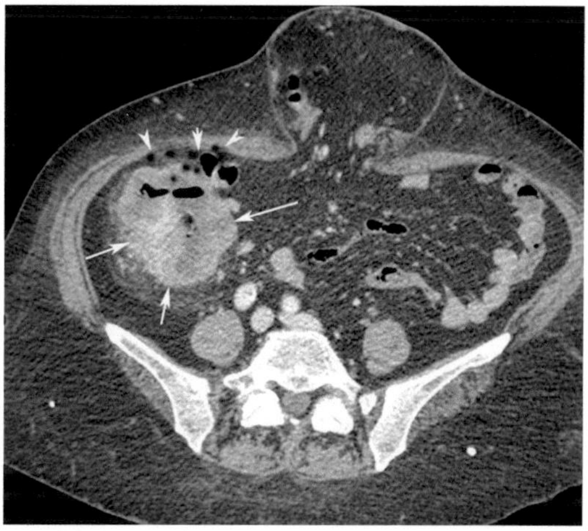

Fig. 15.17 Axial post-contrast medium CT scan shows the irregular thickening and narrowing of the cecum (*white arrows*) surrounded by a pericolic fat inflammation associated with free air bubbles (*white arrow heads*)

Particularly if there is a competent ileocecal valve, the presence of the tumor can lead to an obstruction complicated with a significant dilatation of the lumen producing a closed-loop colon occlusion that can be complicated by the perforation of the intestinal wall.

Perforation and penetration of the intestinal tumor in the pericolic fat can lead to a pericolic abscess that could be the early presentation of the tumor.

Abscess development occurs in 0.3–0.4 % of colonic carcinoma, and it is the second most common complication of perforative lesions [24].

One of the most common presenting conditions of colonic abscess is the development of an anterior abdominal wall frequently determined by a transverse colon fistulized tumor. It is not rare that the tumor can determine an adhesion with a solid organ capsula. Colon flexure carcinoma can involve the liver or the spleen that could become the presenting site of abscesses [25].

Retroperitoneal perforation of ascending and descending colon cancer can involve the fat planes of the retroperitoneum, the posterior wall muscles, and the subcutaneous fat. The most frequent complication of these abscesses is represented by the entero-cutaneus fistula (16.7 %) [26] (Fig. 15.14a, b).

Abscess development occurs in 0.3–4 % of cases of colon cancer and is the second most common presentation of this type of tumor [27].

Tumor growth can contribute to abscess development due to the presence of bacteria in the bowel content. Suppuration of the intestinal content can lead also to more rare infectious collections as muscle, anterior abdominal wall, retroperitoneal, perirenal, and periappendicular abscesses [28].

The application of a drainage catheter into the fluid collection, when it is achievable by CT or ultrasound guide, is the best preliminary treatment for reducing patient toxemia. The next diverting colostomy followed by the resection of the affected colon tumor portion can definitely remove the source of the sepsis.

The tumor perforation could depend on the necrotic degeneration of the neoplastic tissue, next colonization of the necrotic fluid by enteric bacteria, and then fistulization of the necrotic and inflamed wall in the peritoneal cavity. It could depend also on the neoplastic occlusion of the lumen, dilatation of the proximal colon, and secondary perforation of the thin distended wall.

As consequence of a perforated colon cancer, an adjacent localized air-fluid collection can occur, associated with pericolic folds and fat inflammation or a peritoneal open spreading with evidence of air bubbles and dense fluid in all peritoneal recesses and pouches [29].

Especially open peritonitis can cause spreading of primary cancer cells into the abdominal cavity with peritoneal seeding. Afterward a peritoneal carcinosis can develop.

The pericolic abscess can occur as a consequence of the perforation or direct tumor invasion of the surrounding structures [30].

The most frequent localization is represented by the pelvic peritoneal cavity and the paracolic recesses. From the first site, the infectious dense fluid can spread into other spaces with the development of new abdominal collections. The diaphragmatic aspiration movement can facilitate the development of a right subphrenic fluid collection.

In rare cases ascending or descending colon tumor can develop a posterior perforation or a fistula in the retroperitoneal iliac cavity. The inflammation can distribute along fascial and muscle planes, especially the iliopsoas muscle, and can spread up to the groin and the inferior limb [31].

In these cases, the diagnosis of primary colon cancer is very difficult.

Another difficult differential diagnosis is represented by the primary colon cancer stranding the adjacent fat tissue and inflammatory conditions as diverticulitis and appendicitis. In some cases colonic perforation can depend also on an underlying pathology as diverticulitis. Sigmoidal diverticulitis could be associated with a chronic inflammatory thickening of the wall of the affected loop, so it is difficult for making a diagnosis of a perforated colon cancer associated with diverticulitis.

Marked asymmetric intestinal wall thickness with loss of stratified contrast attenuation that regard a segmental colon loop could be evaluated as colon cancer, whereas the presence of stratified enhancement is an important sign of benignant inflammatory pathologies [32]. Another finding in favor of colon cancer is represented by a sudden transitional loop from a normal thin wall to a thickened segmental wall, associated with pericolic fat stranding and lymph nodes.

The overlap in the radiological appearances of the perforated colon cancer often complicates the differential diagnosis of a pericolic infiltration with a cover perforation with an inflammatory abscess that could depend on appendicitis or diverticulitis.

15.14 Obstructing Colon Cancer Complicated with Perforation

The effect of obstruction of colorectal carcinoma complicated with perforation influences significantly the outcome. The consequences of the perforation are represented by the tumor cells spread into the peritoneal cavity and the development of abdominal abscesses and/or peritonitis.

The perforation can depend directly on the tumor necrosis or can occur proximally to the cancer site for ischemic or marked dilatation of the proximal bowel loop.

The perforation of the tumor occurs at the immediate localization of the primary cancer, whereas the perforation proximal to the tumor occurs at least 2 cm proximal to the cancer site.

An obstructing colon cancer can increase strongly the endoluminal pressure of the proximal loops. If the ileocecal valve is efficient, there is not any decompression of the dilated lumen, and the consequent severe dilatation of the colon lumen can lead to the collapse of the submucosal vascular plexus, with consequent ischemia and perforation of the wall. This severe complication can lead to a pericolic abscess if the perforation is covered by surrounding mesenteric folds or to open peritoneal perforation complicated with stercoraceous peritonitis [33].

During the ischemic phase, the colon wall proximal to the obstructed loop is thickened due to intramural edema and hyperemia, and this finding is similar to nonspecific colitis [34].

Ischemia that occurs proximally to a colon carcinoma has an incidence of 1–7 % [35].

15.15 Colon Cancer Complicated with Ischemia and Perforation

The main site of ischemic alteration in colon cancer is the segment contiguous with the primary tumor. In a minority of cases, the ischemic site is located in a noncontiguous colon segment (skip zone).

Colon ischemia with transmural edema can appear on CT axial images as a smooth, annular wall thickening with a layered pattern enhancement proximal to a dishomogeneous tissue of irregular thickness of a fungine mass that represents the colon neoplasm [36].

The CT appearance of the ischemic segment is a concentrically thickened wall with a target double halo sign, due to the mucosal congestion and ulceration and submucosal hemorrhage. Obstructive ischemia, mucosal ulceration, submucosal edema, and hemorrhage determine the most frequent CT findings that are represented by colon wall thickening.

Especially ischemic colitis that can develop proximally to a colonic cancer can be complicated with bowel perforation.

The colon is particularly involved in colonic ischemia when the tumor arises in two critical areas: at the junction between the superior and inferior mesenteric artery, proximally the splenic flexure, and between the inferior mesenteric artery and the hypogastric artery, proximally the rectosigmoid segmental tract.

The bowel lumen dilatation for a rectosigmoidal cancer has a significant role in the development of ischemia, because distended bowel lumen may produce local hemodynamic alterations and vascular supply insufficiency [37].

15.16 CT Findings of Associated Peritonitis

Bacterial peritonitis usually results from gastrointestinal tumor perforation complicated with seeding of the peritoneal cavity with multiple enteric bacteria. In its early stage peritonitis is manifested by a thickened peritoneum due to edema associated with exudative free fluid. These findings could be generalized or localized [38].

CT can demonstrate loculated ascites, omental or mesenteric thickness, and ectopic air bubbles that generally surround the perforation site and are distributed in both supramesocolic and inframesocolic compartments.

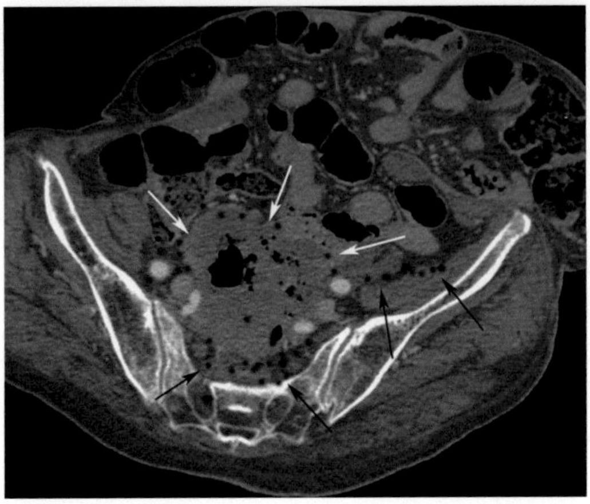

Fig. 15.18 Axial post-contrast medium CT scan shows a perforated rectal cancer (*white arrows*) surrounded by free air bubbles spread into the perirectal and left iliac fat planes (*black arrows*)

15.17 Rectal Cancer Perforation: Fourier Gangrene

Fourier gangrene is defined as a polymicrobial necrotizing fasciitis of the perineal, perirectal, or genital area. Soft tissue gas represents the product of anaerobic bacteria metabolism.

In elderly, debilitating, alcoholic, and diabetic patients, a Fourier gangrene could be a severe complication of rectal tumors. The gangrene is due to the leakage of intestinal content along the perirectal or ischiorectal fossa with the formation of an anaerobic infection (Fig. 15.18).

The pathogenesis of Fourier gangrene is due to soft tissue necrosis based on infectious cellulitis, myositis, and fasciitis associated with subcutaneous vessel thrombosis with endoarteritis and disruption and necrosis of the overlying dermal and epidermal tissue.

Anatomically the perineum is divided into two triangles with an anterior urogenital area and a posterior anorectal area. The two areas are divided by the imaginary line connecting the ischial tuberosities.

The superficial perineal fascia, or Colles fascia, is fixed laterally to the pubic branches and is in relation with the bulbocavernous muscle, where it is fenestrated. The fenestrated fascia may allow the perirectal infection to distribute into the scrotum (Fig. 15.19a, b). The connection of the Colles fascia with Scarpa fascia allows the infection to spread to the buttocks, the thighs, and the abdominal wall (Fig. 15.20).

Furthermore the infection may spread above the urogenital diaphragm into the perivesical space and then into the retroperitoneal space.

The characteristic CT appearance of Fourier gangrene is of soft tissue thickening, fat stranding of the surrounding tissue, and diffuse development of air bubbles.

CT can demonstrate the perirectal infection adjacent to the rectal tumor and the distribution of infectious subcutaneous cellulitis and myositis associated with gas dissection composed of multiple air bubbles. Deep fluid collections may coexist in pelvic and retroperitoneal infected spaces.

The fluid collections are generally distributed in the perirectal and perineal planes, ischiorectal fossa, scrotum, thighs, buttocks, abdominal wall, and retroperitoneum [39].

The testis and epididymis are spared from the infection and are of normal size and structure.

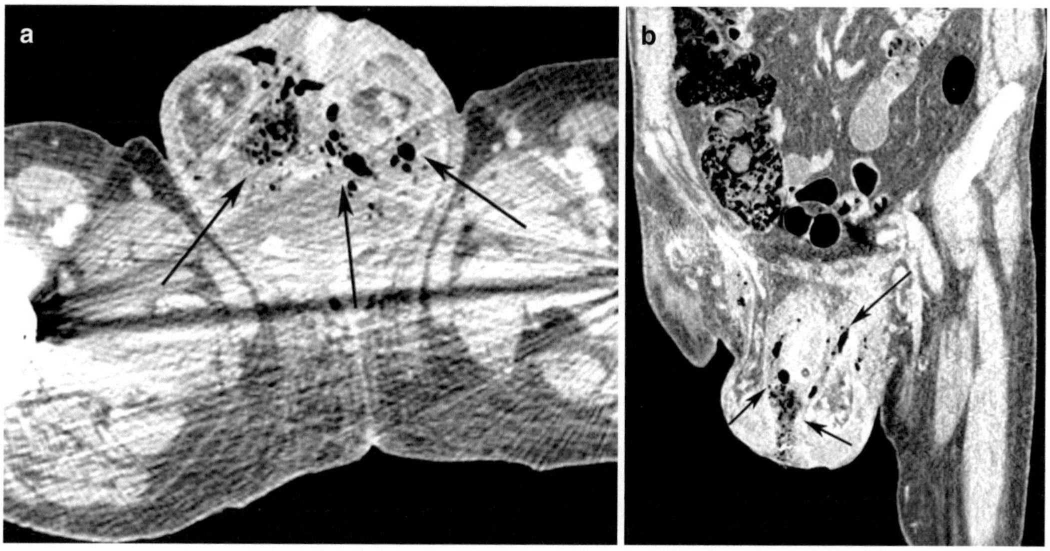

Fig. 15.19 Axial (**a**) and sagittal (**b**) post-contrast medium CT images show Fourier gangrene with multiple air bubbles spread into the scrotum (*black arrows*)

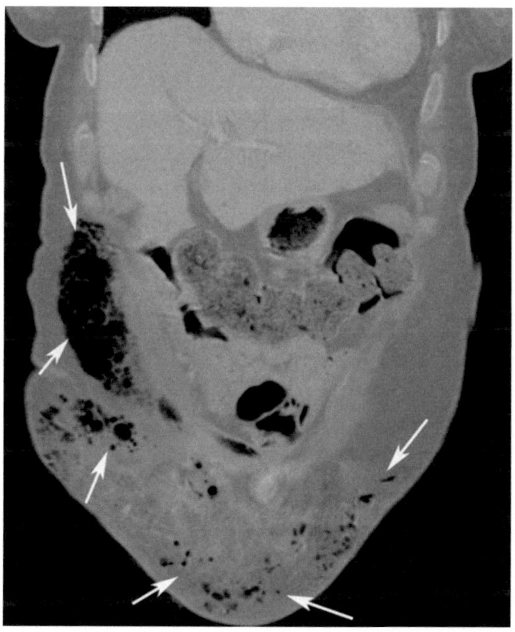

Fig. 15.20 Coronal reconstruction CT scan shows Fourier gangrene with multiple air bubbles spread into the subcutaneous fat of the abdominal wall (*white arrows*)

15.18 Bowel Perforation Associated with Chemotherapy

Monoclonal antibodies are tyrosine kinase inhibitors targeting the vascular endothelial growth factor (VEGF) receptors and are used widely in the treatment of various neoplasms, demonstrating an improved selected antitumoral efficacy [3].

Vascular endothelial growth factor-targeted therapies (VEGF) including bevacizumab, sunitinib, and sorafenib can give intestinal toxicity, especially bowel loop perforation, gastrointestinal fistula, and arterial thrombosis. Time exposure to the drug may induce chronic damage to the intestinal microvasculature due to VEGF inhibitors.

Multifactorial causes could determine these complications, as the compromise of intestinal wall consistency, interruption of intestinal wall determined by the necrosis of superficial micrometastasis, ischemia due to peripheral mesenterial

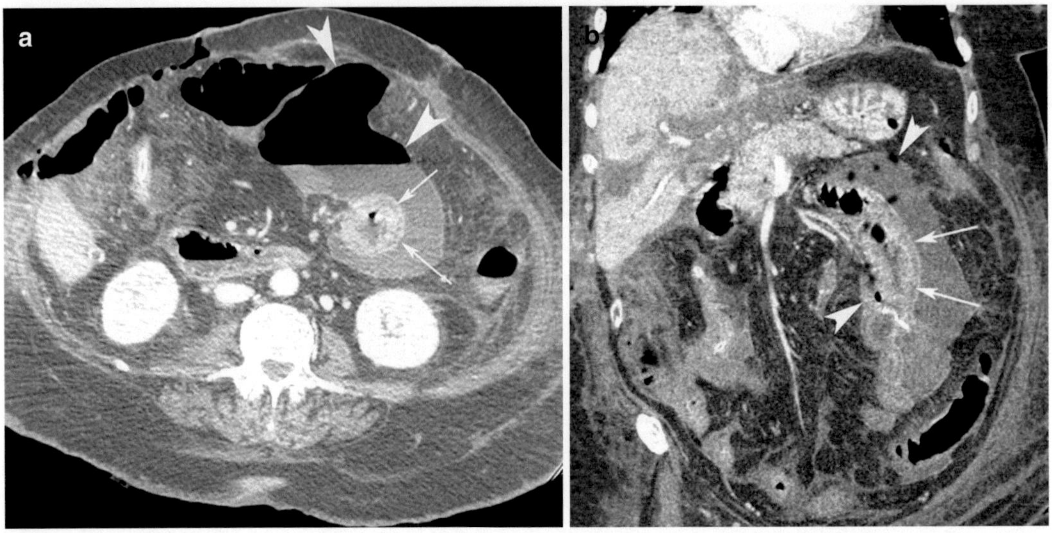

Fig. 15.21 Axial (**a**) and sagittal (**b**) post-contrast medium CT images show an ischemic ileal bowel loop with a thickening of the wall due to edema and submucosal hyperemia (*white arrows*). The ischemia has been complicated with a cover perforation represented by a surrounding large air-fluid collection (*white arrow heads*)

arteries thrombosis, and dehiscence of surgical intestinal sutures [40].

Thromboembolic events could occur in 3 % of cases [41].

The venous and especially arterial vessels are at thrombotic risk, and it is due to the VEGF inhibitors with the progressive loss of the vascular protection by the endothelial cells.

The disruption of the endothelial vascular layer of the arterial wall induces platelet aggregation and then thrombosis of the lumen [42].

Gastrointestinal perforation, determined by a direct effect of the drug on the intestinal wall or by the intestinal necrosis induced by the arterial thrombosis, has been paid particular attention nowadays and has an overall risk of 5.4 % and a specific risk for colorectal cancer of 2.4 %.

One of the reasons of bowel perforation could be represented by the necrosis of the tumor up to the serosal layer predisposing the wall to the development of perforation. Also the thrombosis of intestinal mesenteric vessels and the resulting ischemia can lead to bowel wall perforation.

Other gastrointestinal-related risk factors that can lead to intestinal perforation during VEGF inhibitor treatment have been represented by the site of the intestinal colorectal anastomosis, presence of colon diverticulitis, or bowel obstruction associated with intestinal cancer. Particularly the presence of peritoneal carcinomatosis complicated with intestinal poor canalization is a predisposing factor to bowel wall perforation during VEGF inhibitor treatment, for the increasing lumen pressure with multiple ischemic sites along the wall of the intestinal loop [43].

Particularly bevacizumab has been utilized for the treatment of advanced colorectal cancer, and it is under investigation for the treatment of other kinds of neoplasms.

Bevacizumab is known to be associated with intestinal perforation in 0.5–1.7 % of patients with colon cancer [44].

Bevacizumab could limit the blood flow to the splanchnic vasculature by thrombosis or vasoconstrictions, which can be responsible for poor ulcer healing inducing bowel perforation.

The drug can modify the endothelial cells of the vascular submucosal plexus of the intestinal wall leading to thrombosis, ischemia, and perforation [45] (Fig. 15.21a, b).

Pneumatosis intestinalis is another condition that could be determined by bevacizumab chemotherapy. It is a pathologic condition represented by an infiltration of air bubbles into the wall of the intestinal loops.

Every pathology that could determine chronic bowel hypoxia can develop a pneumatosis intestinalis.

VEGF inhibitors can act through two mechanisms for developing pneumatosis intestinalis. The first is due to the disconnection of cholesterol particles from atheromas with the development of microembolus that can determine a peripheral mesenterial microvascular occlusion and ischemia; the second has been represented by the penetration of air bubbles in the submucosal layer of the intestinal wall [46].

It is characterized by submucosal and subserosal gas microbubbles distributed along the wall of the gastrointestinal tract. The gas-filled microcystic aspect of the gastrointestinal wall can be well recognized by CT.

There are three possible sources of intestinal wall gas represented by bacterial production, intraluminal production, and pulmonary source [47].

The intraluminal gas can go through the ruptured mucosa due to an increasing intraluminal pressure. Also enteric bacteria can cross the injured mucosa and develop gas microbubbles in the bowel wall. Finally pulmonary gas can depend on a barotrauma complicated with alveolar wall injuries. In this case the associated pulmonary interstitial emphysema can spread up to the mesenterial interstitium developing pneumatosis intestinalis [47].

Bevacizumab inhibits the capillary network of small intestinal wall and reduces the microvasculature of the intestinal villi, inhibiting the intestinal mucosa to grow, contributing to microperforation that leads to pneumatosis intestinalis.

Associated risk factors can be linked to the bevacizumab effects as the previous exposure to radiation therapy or a recent intestinal surgery, both of which can affect the intestinal vasculature integrity increasing the risk of bowel perforation [43].

References

1. Kim SW, Kim HC, Yang DM et al (2012) Perforated tumors in the gastrointestinal tract: CT findings and clinical implications. Br J Radiol 85:1307–1313
2. Kelley WE, Brown PW, Lawrence W et al (1981) Penetrating obstructing and perforating carcinomas of the colon and rectum. Arch Surg 116:381–384
3. Abou-Jawde R, Choueiri T, Alemany C et al (2003) An overview of targeted treatments in cancer. Clin Ther 25(8):2121–2137
4. Horton KM, Abrams RA, Fishman EK (2000) Spiral CT of colon cancer: imaging features and role in management. Radiographics 20:419–430
5. Boormans JL, Hesp WL, Tenue TM et al (2006) Carcinoma of the sigmoid presenting as a right inguinal hernia. Hernia 10:93–99
6. Kasakura Y, Ajani JA, Fujii M et al (2002) Management of perforated gastric carcinoma. A report of 16 cases and review of world literature. Am Surg 68:434–440
7. Brady LW, Asbell O (1980) Malignant lymphoma of the gastrointestinal tract. Radiology 137:291–296
8. Roviello F, Rossi S, Marrelli D et al (2006) Perforated gastric carcinoma: a report of 10 cases and review of the literature. World J Surg Oncol 4:19
9. Zissin R, Osadchy A, Gayer G (2008) Abdominal CT findings in small bowel perforation. Br J Radiol 82:162–171
10. Freeman HJ (2003) Free perforation due to intestinal lymphoma in biopsy-defined or suspected celiac disease. J Clin Gastroenterol 37:299–302
11. Wada M, Onda M, Tokunaga A et al (1999) Spontaneous gastrointestinal perforation in patients with lymphoma receiving chemotherapy and steroids. J Nippon Med Sch 66:37–40
12. Catena F, Ansaloni L, Gazzotti F et al (2005) Small bowel tumors in emergency surgery: specificity of clinical presentation. ANZ J Surg 75:997–999
13. Berger A, Cellier C, Daniel C (1999) Small bowel metastasis from primary carcinoma of the lung: clinical findings and outcome. Am J Gastroenterol 94:1884–1887
14. Kim SH, Shin SS, Jeong YY et al (2009) Gastrointestinal tract perforation: MDCT findings according to the perforation sites. Korean J Radiol 10:63–70
15. Shiraishi M, Hirayasu S, Nosato E et al (1998) Perforation due to metastatic tumors of the ileocecal region. World J Surg 22:1065–1068
16. Miettinen M, Majidi M, Lasota J (2002) Pathology and diagnostic criteria of gastrointestinal stromal tumors (GISTs); a review. Eur J Cancer 38(5):39–51
17. Debiec-Rychter M, Wasag B, Stul M et al (2004) Gastrointestinal stromal tumors (GISTS) negative for KIT (CD 117 antigen) immunoreactivity. J Pathol 202:430–438
18. Crosby JA, Catton CN, Davis A et al (2001) Malignant gastrointestinal stromal tumors in the small intestine: a review of 50 cases from a prospective database. Ann Surg Oncol 8:50–59
19. Hohenberger P, Ronellenfisch U, Oladeji O et al (2010) Pattern of recurrence in patients with ruptured primary gastrointestinal stromal tumor. Br J Surg 97:1854–1859

20. Cegarra-Navarro MF, Corral de la Calle MA, Gerela-Baena E et al (2005) Ruptured gastrointestinal stromal tumors: radiologic findings in six cases. Abdom Imaging 30:535–542
21. Hulnik DH, Megibow AJ, Balthazar EJ et al (1987) Perforated colorectal neoplasm: correlation of clinical, contrast enema and CT examinations. Radiology 164:611–615
22. Michowitz M, Avnieli D, Lazarovici I et al (1982) Perforation complicating carcinoma of the colon. J Surg Oncol 19:18–21
23. Setti Carraro PG, Segala M, Orlotti C et al (1998) Outcome of large bowel perforation in patients with colorectal cancer. Dis Colon Rectum 41:1421–1426
24. Chen HS, Shen-Chen SM (2000) Obstruction and perforation in colorectal adenocarcinoma: an analysis of prognosis and current trends. Surgery 127:370–376
25. John PW (1976) Unusual abscess in perforating colorectal cancer. Am J Surg 131:270–274
26. Tsai HL, Hsieh JS, Yu FJ et al (2007) Perforated colonic cancer presenting as intra-abdominal abscess. Int J Colorectal Dis 22:15–19
27. Mandava N, Kumar S, Pizzi WF et al (1996) Perforated colorectal carcinoma. Am J Surg 172:236–238
28. Panwalker AP (1988) Unusual infections associated with colorectal cancer. Rev Infect Dis 10:347–364
29. Biondo S, Kreisler E, Millan M et al (2008) Differences in patients postoperative and long-term outcomes between obstructive and perforated colonic cancer. Am J Surg 195:427–432
30. Okita A, Kubo Y, Tanada M et al (2007) Unusual abscesses associated with colon cancer: report of three cases. Acta Med Okayama 61:107–113
31. Tsukuda K, Ikeda E, Miyake T et al (2005) Abdominal wall and thigh abscess resulting from the penetration of ascending colon cancer. Acta Med Okayama 59:281–283
32. Pereira JM, Sirlin CB, Pinto PS et al (2004) Disproportionate fat stranding: a helpful CT sign in patients with acute abdominal pain. Radiographics 24:703–715
33. Tan KK, Hong CC, Zhang J et al (2010) Surgery for perforated colorectal malignancy in an Asian population: an institution's experience over 5 years. Int J Colorectal Dis 25:989–995
34. Ko GJ, Ha HK, Lee HJ et al (1997) Useful of CT in patients with ischemic colitis proximal to colonic cancer. AJR Am J Roentgenol 168:951–956
35. Rha SE, Ha HK, Lee SH et al (2000) CT and MR imaging findings of bowel ischaemia from various primary causes. Radiographics 20:29–42
36. Xiong L, Chintapalli KN, Dodd GD et al (2004) Frequency and CT patterns of bowel wall thickening proximal to cancer of the colon. AJR Am J Roentgenol 182:905–909
37. Boley SJ, Agruwal GP, Warren AR et al (1969) Pathophysiologic effects of bowel distention on intestinal blood flow. Am J Surg 117:228–233
38. Abdelrazeq AS, Scott N, Thorn C et al (2008) The impact of spontaneous tumor perforation on outcome following colon cancer surgery. Colorectal Dis 10:775–780
39. Wysoki MG, Santora TA, Shah RM et al (1997) Necrotizing fasciitis: CT characteristics. Radiology 203:859–863
40. Han ES, Monk BJ (2007) What is the risk of bowel perforation associated with bevacizumab therapy in ovarian cancer. Gynecol Oncol 105:3–6
41. Scappaticci FA, Skillings JR, Holden SN et al (2007) Arterial thromboembolic events in patients with metastatic carcinoma treated with chemotherapy and bevacizumab. J Natl Cancer Inst 99(16):1232–1239
42. Gonzales-Pacheco FR, Deudero JJ, Castllanos MC et al (2006) Mechanisms of endothelial responses to oxidative aggression: protective role of autologous VEGF and induction of VEGFR2 by H2O2. Am J Physiol Heart Circ Physiol 291(3):H1395–H1401
43. Scappaticci FA, Fehrenbacher L, Cartwright T et al (2005) Surgical wound complications in colorectal cancer patients treated with bevacizumab. J Surg Oncol 91(3):173–180
44. Sugrue M, Kozloff M, Hainsworth J et al (2006) Risk factors for gastrointestinal perforations in patients with metastatic colorectal cancer receiving bevacizumab plus chemotherapy. J Clin Oncol 24:3535
45. Choueiri TK, Schutz FA, Je Y et al (2010) Risk of arterial thromboembolic events with sunitinib and sorafenib; a systematic review and meta analysis of clinical trials. J Clin Oncol 28:2280–2285
46. Hapani S, Chu D, Wu S (2009) Risk of gastrointestinal perforation in patients with cancer treated with bevacizumab; a meta analysis. Lancet Oncol 10:559–568
47. St Peter SD, Abbas MA, Kelly KA (2003) The spectrum of pneumatosis intestinalis. Arch Surg 138:68–75

16 Role of Multidetector Row Computed Tomography in the Diagnosis of Acute Peritonitis Due to Gastrointestinal Perforation

Vittorio Miele and Barbara Sessa

16.1 Introduction

Peritonitis can be defined as an inflammatory process of the peritoneal space caused by numerous sources, generally by an infectious agent as bacteria, fungi and virus or by irritant agents as talc, drugs or foreign bodies [1].

The inflammatory process could be localized with the formation of abscesses or diffuse; on the basis of the pathogenesis, it could be classified as primary, secondary or tertiary peritonitis.

Primary peritonitis is generally caused by an extraperitoneal source, frequently from haematogenous dissemination in patients with cirrhosis or in children who have nephrosis.

Secondary peritonitis is caused by an infection by the resident flora of the gastrointestinal tract resulting from a break of the integrity of the intestinal tract or the urogenital system or solid organs; it could be classified as acute peritonitis by perforation, postoperative peritonitis or post-traumatic peritonitis [2].

Mortality of secondary peritonitis is still 30–50 % despite advances in pharmacological and resuscitation therapy and surgical and imaging technique [1, 3].

V. Miele (✉) • B. Sessa
Cardiovascular and Emergency Radiology Department, S. Camillo Hospital, C.ne Gianicolense 87, Rome 00152, Italy
e-mail: vmiele@sirm.org; barbara.sessa@tiscali.it

16.2 Peritonitis from Gastrointestinal Tract Perforation

From proximal to distal the gastrointestinal tract is composed of the stomach, duodenum, jejunum, ileum, appendix, colon, and peritonealized rectum.

A break of the integrity of the intestinal wall causes intra-abdominal contamination resulting in a secondary peritonitis, localized with abscess formation or diffuse [1].

The type and degree of peritoneal contamination depends on the site and duration of the pathological process and on the physiologic state of the patient, including the time of the last meal, other coexistent diseases and the presence or absence of a bowel obstruction with bacterial overgrowth.

Microbiological contamination depends on the anatomic site of perforation increasing from proximal to distal.

The stomach and duodenum have the lowest number of microorganism per cubic centimetre of luminal contents (less than 10^3 organisms per gram) for the presence of acidic, biliary and pancreatic secretions which produce a hostile local milieu. They are yeast, aerobic bacteria (predominantly *Staphylococci*, *Streptococci* and *Haemophilus* species) and anaerobic bacteria (predominantly *Bacteroides*, *Veillonella* and *Bifidobacterium* species).

Gastric and duodenal perforation produce a highly acute pain due to a rapid chemical peritonitis, often followed by a systemic

L. Romano, A. Pinto (eds.), *Imaging of Alimentary Tract Perforation*,
DOI 10.1007/978-3-319-08192-2_16, © Springer International Publishing Switzerland 2015

inflammatory response syndrome (SIRS) with a rapid clinical deterioration and a progress to an infected peritonitis and sepsis.

The small bowel and colon contain a relatively neutral environment.

The proximal jejunum contains 10^4 organisms per gram of luminal contents to 10^7 organisms per gram in the terminal ileum.

The frequency of aerobes progressively increases along the small bowel with the major percentage of Gram-negative in the terminal ileum.

The highest percentage of microorganism per gram (10^{12}) is present in the colon, with an abrupt change of the microfloral load and composition between the terminal ileum and the colon. In fact in this tract, anaerobes outnumber aerobes by up to 1,000-fold, with a prevalence of *Bacteroides*, *Bifidobacterium*, *Eubacterium*, *Clostridium*, *Lactobacillus* and *Fusobacterium*; also a limited variety of Gram-positive anaerobes are present [4, 5].

Colonic perforations cause a neutral, nonerosive environment and may present with a slower clinical progression, without immediate pain. But they produce a secondary bacterial peritonitis which progressively leads to purulent or faecal peritonitis or localized intra-abdominal abscess formation [5].

16.3 Major Causes of Gastrointestinal Tract Perforation and Related Peritonitis

Common causes of peritonitis include appendicitis, diverticulitis, perforated gastrointestinal ulcer, perforated carcinoma, acute cholecystitis, acute pancreatitis, and abdominal surgery.

Gastrointestinal perforation with lack of gastrointestinal wall integrity causes acute peritonitis for the release of intraluminal contents into the normally sterile peritoneal cavity.

The more frequent causes of gastrointestinal perforation are:

1. Penetrating foreign body.

   It results from the ingestion of sharp, pointed or jagged objects such as chicken bones, fish bones, razor blades and toothpicks [6, 7] and is more frequently localized in the small intestine and colon.

   Other causes are penetrating trauma and endoscopy/iatrogenic perforation for invasive diagnostic and therapeutic medical procedures as upper endoscopy, colonoscopy, interventional radiologic-guided tissue biopsy and fluid drainage, laparoscopy, etc.
2. Extrinsic obstruction, caused by benign or malignant neoplasms or by non-gastrointestinal tumours located adjacent to the compressed segment of bowel.
3. Other causes are surgical adhesions, malrotation, volvulus or herniation. These conditions produce perforation especially when they occur as a closed-loop obstruction; in these cases, there was a progressive increase in venous congestion followed by arterial stasis, necrosis and loss of mural integrity [8, 9].
4. Intrinsic gastrointestinal obstruction, more frequently in cases of appendicitis and diverticulitis, but also from the gastrointestinal tract for intraluminal neoplasms, phytobezoars, ischaemic strictures and Crohn disease.
5. Direct loss of gastrointestinal wall integrity especially for peptic ulcer perforation but also from neoplastic growth or from adjuvant or neoadjuvant therapy [10].
6. Gastrointestinal ischaemia especially in elderly and critically ill patients.
7. Infection from *Clostridium difficile*, *Salmonella typhi*, *Mycobacterium tuberculosis* and cytomegalovirus [11].

16.4 Imaging of Gastrointestinal Perforation and Related Peritonitis

The diagnosis of gastrointestinal perforation is generally based on the identification of extraluminal leakage and consequent inflammatory reaction which is around the perforated site or diffuse (peritonitis).

Plain radiography has been the first imaging step in patients with suspected GI perforation for the detection of free air outside the gut lumen.

The reported sensitivity in the identification of extraluminal air on plain radiography is 50–70 % [12].

CT is the diagnostic modality of choice in diagnosing GI tract perforation [13].

It can depict the presence of a small amount of intra- and extraperitoneal air but also the site of perforation, cause and associated complications such as phlegmon, abscess and peritonitis.

The diagnosis of alimentary tract perforations is based on direct findings as focal bowel wall discontinuity, extraluminal gas and extraluminal enteric contrast (when administrated); indirect signs of GI perforation and related peritonitis include segmental bowel wall thickening, abnormal bowel wall enhancement, perivisceral fat stranding, or fluid and abscess.

It is important for the clinical management and surgical approach of the identification of the site of GI perforation; CT is accurate in detecting the site of perforation in about 85 % of cases [13, 14].

The site of perforation can be evaluated by CT signs as (a) discontinuation of the GI wall, (b) the site of luminal contrast medium leakage, (c) the level of bowel obstruction and (d) abrupt GI wall thickening with or without an associated phlegmon, inflammatory mass or abscess [15].

On the basis of location of extraluminal air, it could be possible to presume the site of perforation: air in the lesser sac is commonly due to posterior perforation of the stomach or duodenum or less commonly from the rupture of the lower oesophagus or transverse colon. When perforation is in the duodenal bulb or stomach, free air is confined in the intrahepatic fissure or the ligamentum teres. Air in the mesenteric folds is generally depicted in the perforation of the colon and small bowel.

Pneumoretroperitoneum is found in the perforation of the extraperitoneal gastrointestinal tracts as the duodenum (descending and horizontal portions), ascending and descending colon and rectum [16].

Also three-fourths of the diverticulum is located in the extraperitoneum, and so perforation of the sigmoid diverticula also can produce a pneumoretroperitoneum.

When gas is located in the retroperitoneum, it generally tends to remain confined in the retroperitoneal space without a free spread in the peritoneal space.

When gas is located bilaterally into the anterior and/or posterior pararenal spaces, it generally originates in the pelvis; gas in the anterior pararenal space is generally produced by duodenal or ascending colon perforations, whereas gas in the left anterior pararenal space indicates descending or sigmoid colon perforations.

Rectal perforation causes bilateral pneumoretroperitoneum [17].

When it is depicted as intraperitoneal and extraperitoneal air, generally the source of perforation is an extraperitoneal structure [17].

16.4.1 Oral Contrast Administration

In case of suspected gastrointestinal perforation, an oral contrast should be administrated during CT exam, consisting in a dilute water soluble iodinated solution.

When an extravasation of ingested contrast material was depicted, it must be considered a specific direct sign of bowel perforation with a high specificity in the diagnosis of the perforation site.

The sensitivity of extravasation of oral contrast material varies from 19 to 42 % [13] due to the rapid sealing of perforation sites and the supine position during the CT exam so that the absence of visible extravasation does not exclude a perforation.

16.5 Perforation of the Stomach/Duodenum

Peptic ulcer disease remains the most common cause of gastroduodenal perforation [14], most commonly from the gastric antrum or duodenal bulb.

Other causes of stomach or duodenum perforation are traumatic injuries, especially in the descending and horizontal portions of the duodenum, mostly by blunt trauma in children and by penetrating trauma in adults, with

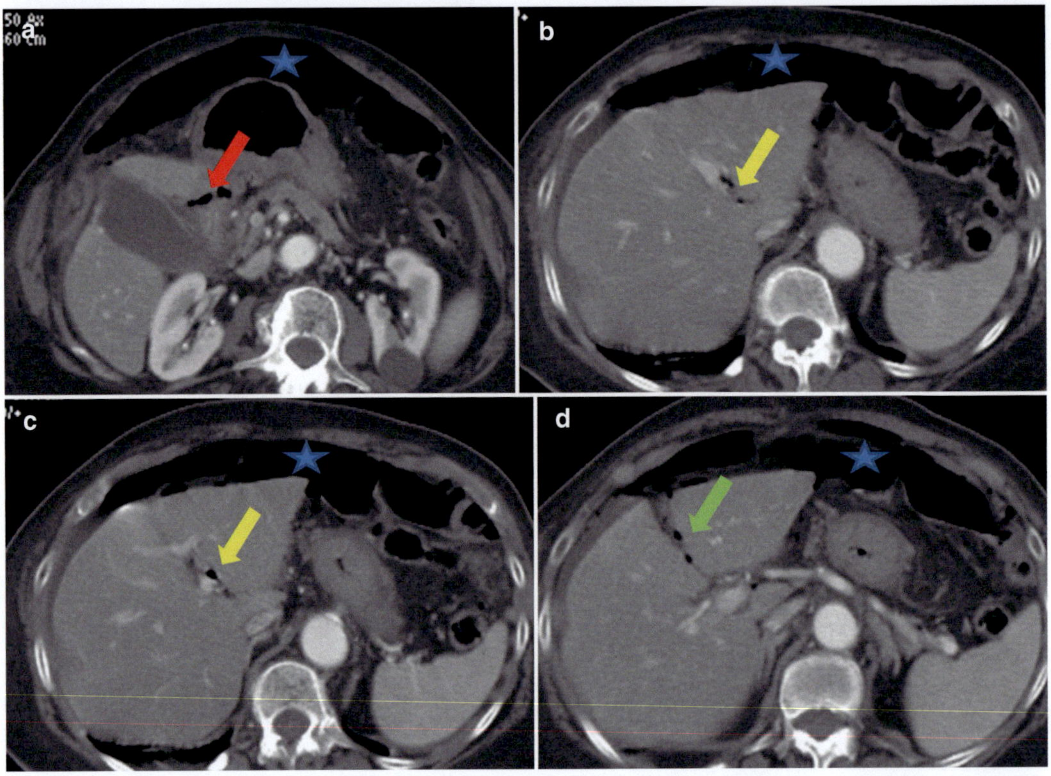

Fig. 16.1 Contrast-enhanced axial scans (**a**-**d**). Ulcer of the anterior bulb of the duodenum (*red arrow*), perforated in the peritoneal cavity. Signs of peritonitis are air in the lesser sac, in the intrahepatic fissure (*green arrow*), periportal free gas (*yellow arrows*) and free air in the peritoneal cavity (*blue star*)

pneumoretroperitoneum in the anterior pararenal space [18]. Rarely malignant tumours at advanced stage can produce a gastric perforation (reported incidence of 0.4–6 %) [19].

Reported perforation rates for diagnostic and therapeutic procedures such as esophagogastroduodenoscopy and endoscopic retrograde cholangiopancreatography are 0.03–0.3 % [20], especially of the oesophagus, followed by the duodenum, jejunum and stomach.

CT direct signs of gastroduodenal perforation are extraluminal air with gas bubbles in close proximity to the discontinuity in the gastrointestinal wall, focal wall defect and leakage of luminal contrast when administrated.

Ulcers of the anterior wall of the stomach and duodenum may perforate directly into the peritoneal cavity, whereas posterior stomach and duodenum wall defect often caused a confined peritonitis. Generally ulcers are located on the anterior bulb of the duodenum and produce, therefore, a peritoneal peritonitis with air especially in the lesser sac and in the intrahepatic fissure of the ligamentum teres (Fig. 16.1).

The most significant sign to distinguish upper from lower GI tract perforation is the periportal free gas for the anatomical relationship between the portal tract and the gastric antrum or duodenal bulb (Fig. 16.1).

A distal duodenal perforation produces extraluminal air in the right anterior pararenal space because of the retroperitoneal position of the duodenum distal to the bulb (Fig. 16.2).

Other CT signs about the perforated wall are wall thickening and wall focal enhancement.

The stomach and duodenum contain acidic, biliary and pancreatic secretions so that gastric and duodenal perforation produce a rapid chemical peritonitis which can be followed by a systemic inflammatory response syndrome (SIRS) with a possible progress to an infected peritonitis and sepsis.

CT signs of peritonitis due to gastrointestinal perforation are increased fat density adjacent to

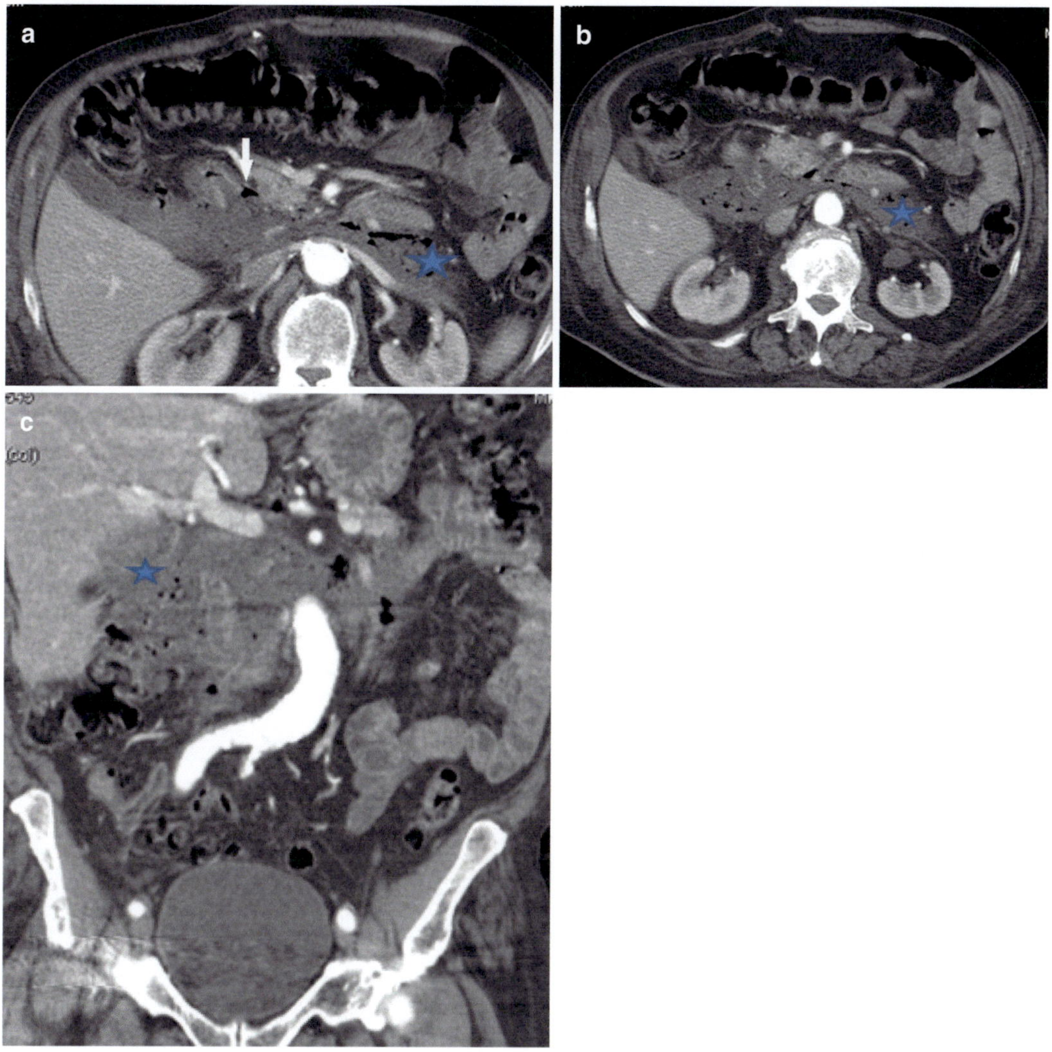

Fig. 16.2 Ulcer in the III portion of the duodenum. (**a**, **b**) Axial scans, (**c**) coronal reconstruction shows a wall defect in the III portion of the duodenum (*white arrow*) with an inflammatory collection in the retroperitoneal space (*blue star*)

the site of wall defect, perigastroduodenal fluid, stranding and gas bubbles in close proximity to the site of perforation and fluid between the duodenum and pancreatic head (Fig. 16.2).

16.6 Small Bowel Perforation

The incidence of small bowel perforation is low, but it can be produced by a variety of causes including ischaemic or bacterial enteritis, Crohn disease, diverticulitis, ingested foreign bodies, bowel obstruction, volvulus and intussusceptions [21].

The amount of extraluminal air in these cases is small or absent, and it is depicted only in 50 % of CT performed in patients with small bowel perforation.

When present free air is depicted in the mesenteric folds.

Indirect signs of small bowel perforation and related peritonitis are an increased attenuation of small bowel mesenteric fat, free fluid in the mesenteric folds or leaking of intestinal contents into the interloop spaces.

Crohn disease is a common small bowel inflammatory condition but can rarely lead to free perforation, from the colon (1.6 %) or small bowel (0.7 %) [22].

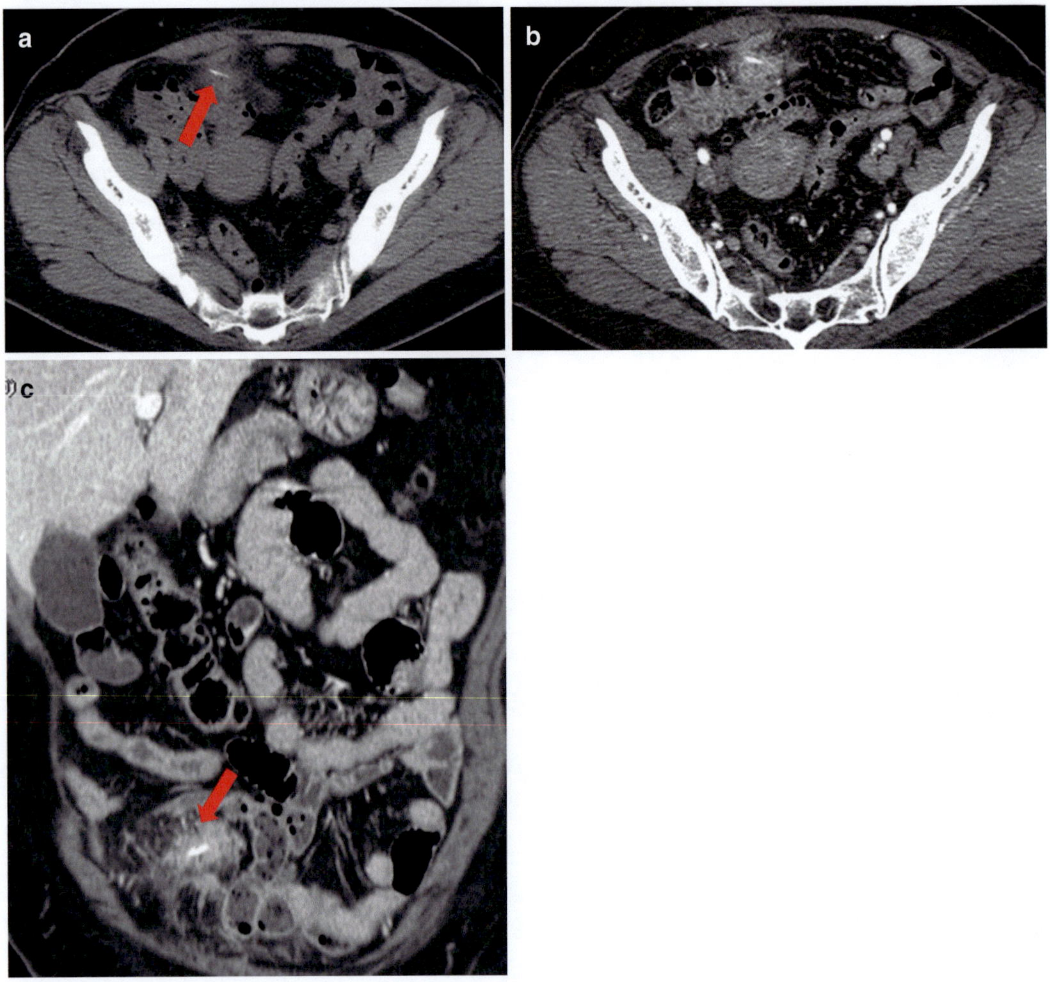

Fig. 16.3 Localized peritonitis. (**a**) Unenhanced axial scan, (**b**) enhanced axial scan and (**c**) coronal MPR reconstruction depicted an extraluminal ingested foreign body, a toothpick (*red arrows*) close to an ileal loop, at the site of perforation. An inflammatory reaction of the mesenteric fat around the foreign body is also present

Small bowel perforation could be a complication of wall ischaemia with transmural necrosis, leading to peritonitis.

Also penetrating abdominal trauma can produce small bowel perforation; in these cases abdominal CT has a sensitivity of 64 % and accuracy of 82 % in detecting the site of perforation even in the absence of the free air but especially with the help of indirect signs as infiltration of the mesentery and/or intraperitoneal fluid [23].

Small bowel perforation can also result from GI lymphoma, GISTs or metastasis.

Fish bones and chicken bones are the most common ingested foreign bodies to cause perforation (Fig. 16.3).

16.7 Appendix Perforation

CT has a high sensitivity and specificity for diagnosing acute appendicitis ranging from 94 to 98 % [24]. Unfortunately detecting appendiceal perforation is not so simple in CT especially in early stage; rupture of the appendix, in fact, can be a localized process, and the amount of extraluminal air is usually small or absent (no more than 1 or 2 ml) because acute appendicitis is typically initiated by luminal obstruction.

CT reaches a sensitivity and specificity of 95 % in the diagnosis of perforated appendicitis when it presents a combination of these five findings: (1) extraluminal air, (2) extraluminal

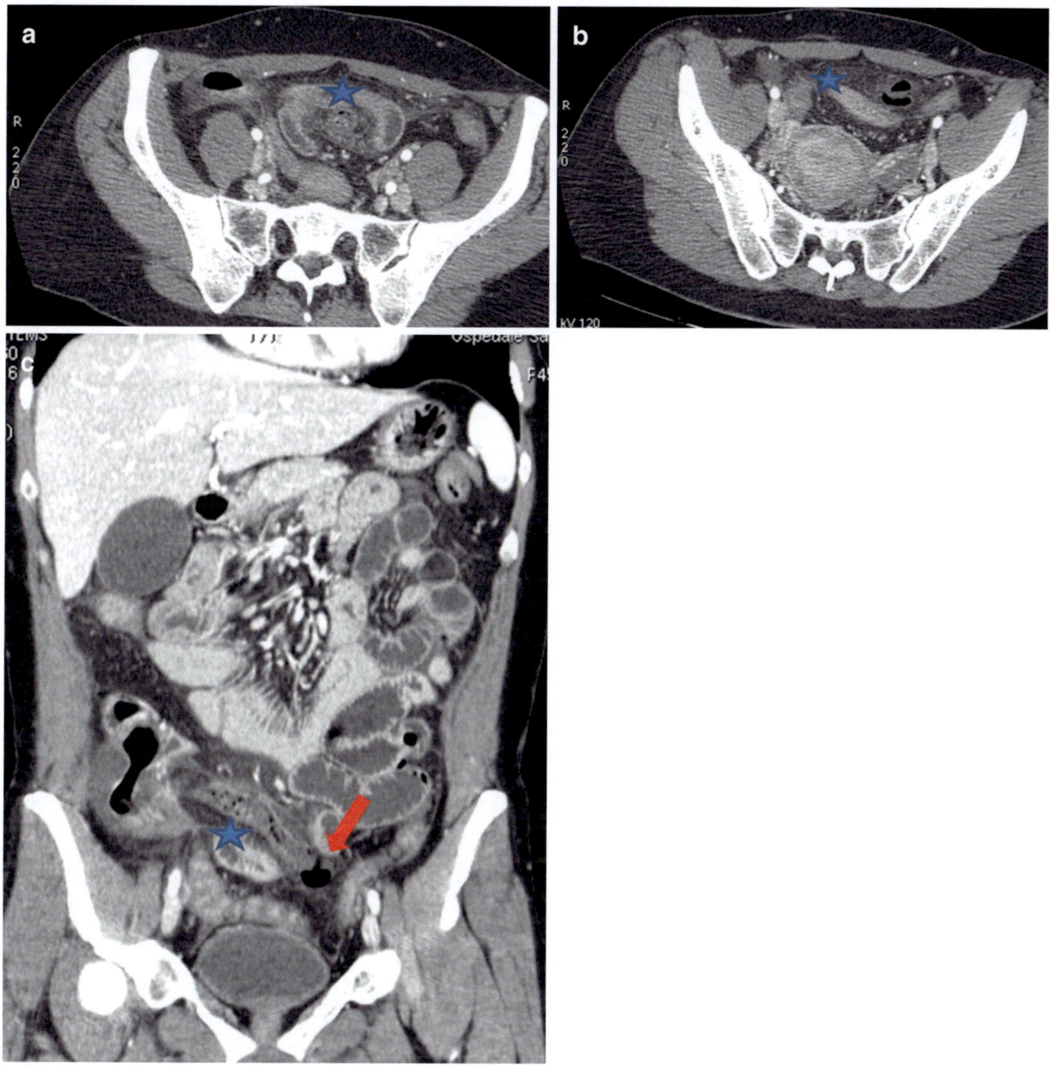

Fig. 16.4 Peritonitis due to mesoceliac perforated appendicitis. (**a**, **b**) Axial scans, (**c**) coronal MPR reconstruction: a long mesoceliac appendicitis (*blue star*) perforated on the top with free air (*red arrow*) and inflammatory reaction of the perivisceral fat

appendicolith, (3) abscess, (4) phlegmon and (5) defect in enhancing the appendiceal wall [24] (Figs. 16.4 and 16.5).

The signs of peritonitis as periappendiceal stranding and fluid can be detected in the perforated but also in non-perforated appendicitis.

16.8 Colon Perforation

Malignant neoplasm and diverticulitis are the major causes of large bowel perforation, followed by trauma, ischaemia, inflammatory lesions and iatrogenic causes.

Inflammatory lesions and penetrating trauma are frequently observed in the right colon, whereas malignant neoplasm, spontaneous perforation, diverticulitis, blunt trauma and ischaemia are generally detected in the left colon [21]; perforation of cecum can occur when the intraluminal pressure of the colon is increased, as in the case of bowel obstruction or in malignant tumour (Fig. 16.6).

Iatrogenic injuries produce perforations especially of the rectum and sigmoid colon.

Perforation of the large bowel may occur in intraperitoneal or extraperitoneal space depending on the perforated portion.

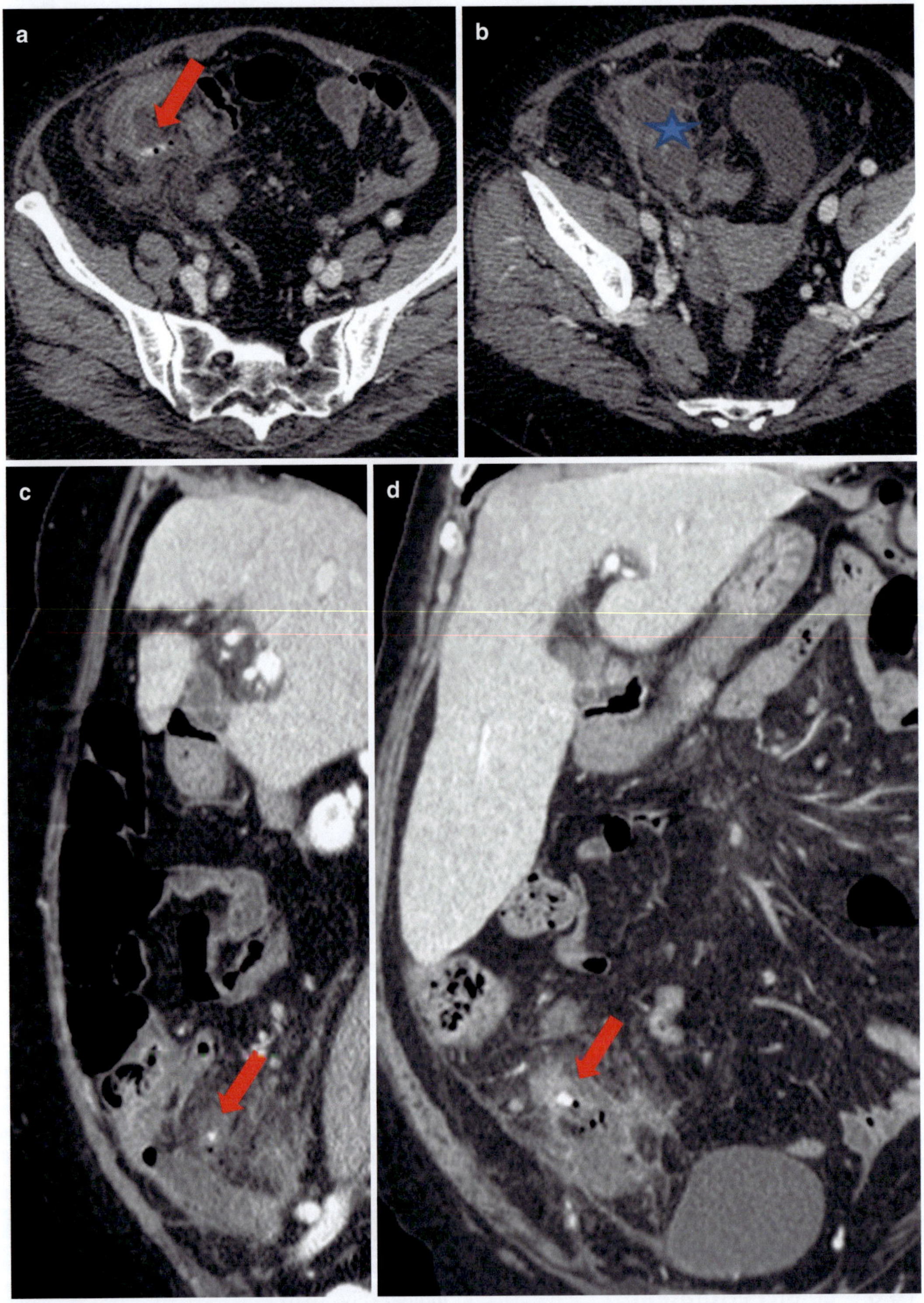

Fig. 16.5 Peritonitis due to gangrenous perforated appendicitis. (**a**, **b**) Axial scans, (**c**) sagittal reconstruction, (**d**) coronal reconstruction detects a gangrenous perforated appendicitis with extraluminal bubbles and extraluminal appendicoliths (*red arrow*); also a perivisceral abscess is present (*blue star*)

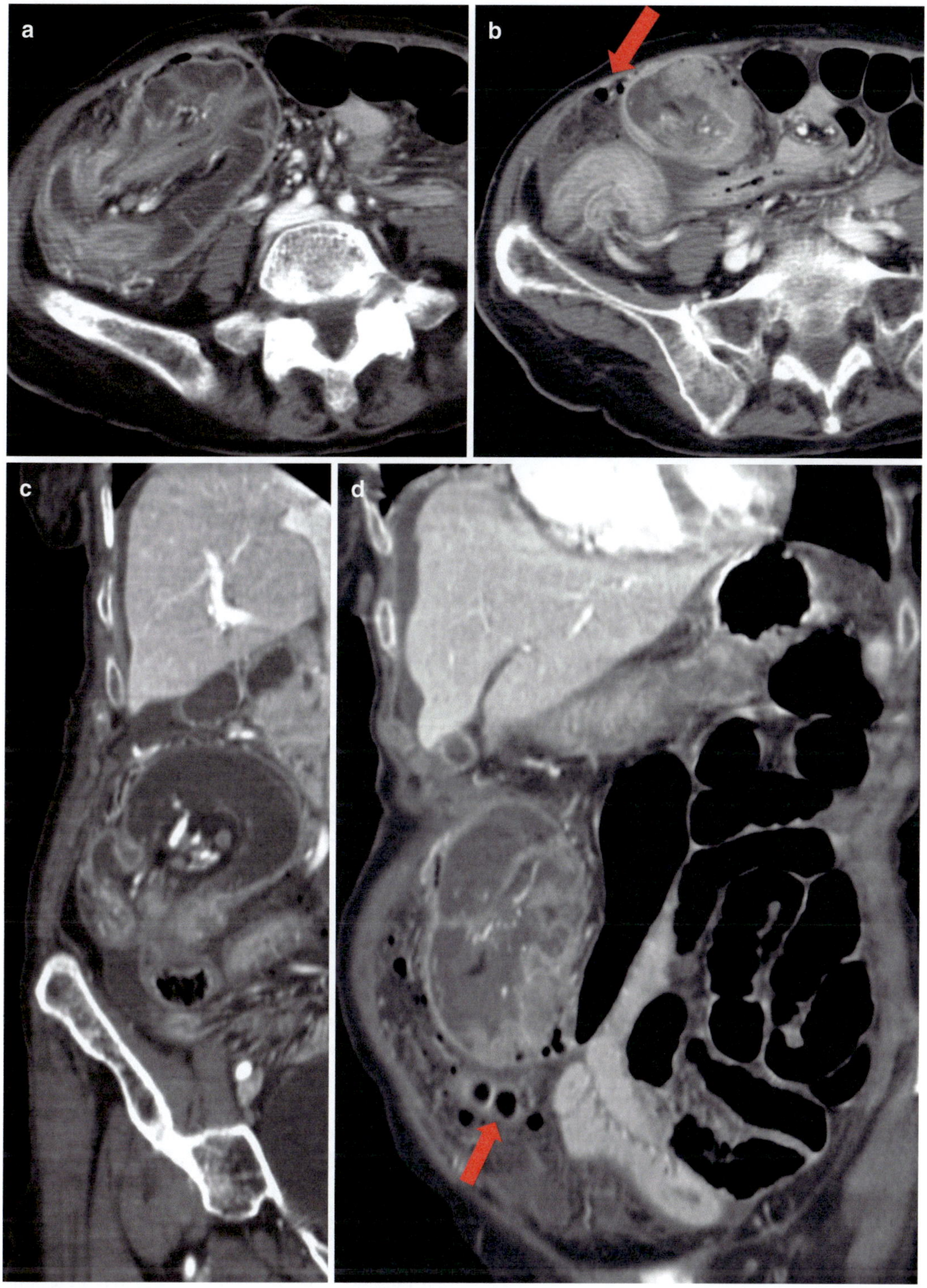

Fig. 16.6 Peritonitis due to perforation of the cecum neoplasm with intussusception. (**a**, **b**) Axial scans, (**c**, **d**) coronal reconstruction shows a pathological cecum wall thickening with an ileum-cecum-colon intussusception and wall perforation with gas bubbles (*red arrow*) and an increased attenuation in mesenteric fat

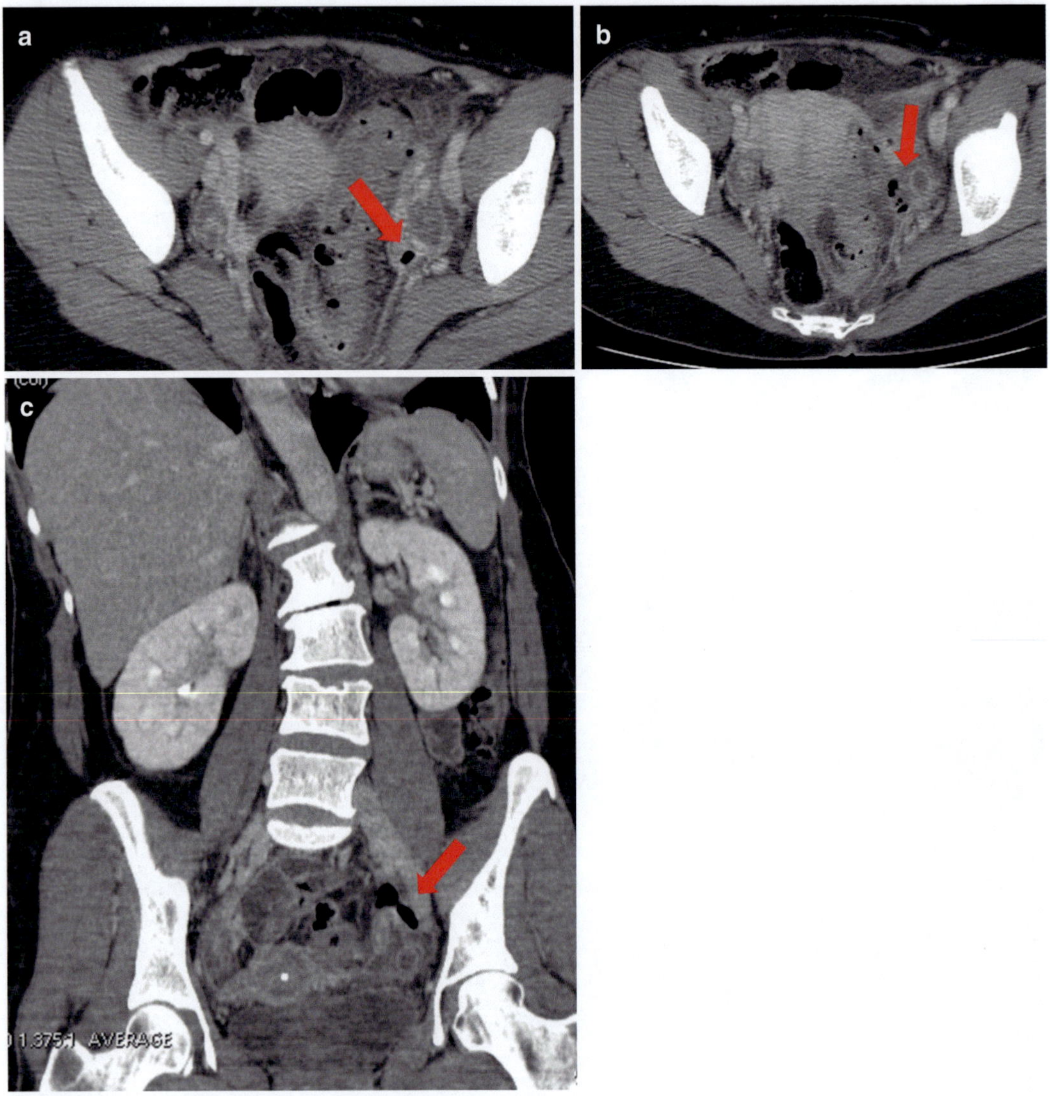

Fig. 16.7 Peritonitis due to perforated sigmoid diverticulitis. (**a**, **b**) Axial scans, (**c**) MPR coronal reconstruction. Perforation of a sigmoid diverticula with an obturatory space abscess containing free bubbles (*red arrows*)

Gas only in the pelvis suggests a colon perforation; diverticula perforation may produce extraperitoneal or intraperitoneal free bubbles (Figs. 16.7 and 16.8) because most colon diverticula are located in the retroperitoneum between the taenia mesocolica and taenia libera and between the taenia mesocolica and taenia omentalis [17].

A large amount of free air is seen in the perforation for complicated large bowel obstruction and iatrogenic procedure; colonoscopic perforation of the posterior walls of the sigmoid, ascending and descending colon causes free gas in the retroperitoneal space, often in the anterior pararenal space.

In case of perforated colorectal neoplasm without large bowel obstruction, the amount of extraluminal air is usually small.

CT findings of colonic perforation and peritonitis are free air, dirty mass, dirty fat sign, extraluminal fluid collection, bowel wall thickening around the perforated site and interruption of colonic wall.

A dirty mass is a focal collection of extraluminal faecal matter containing small air bubbles (Fig. 16.9). The dirty fat sign is a diffuse increase in attenuation of mesenteric fat [25].

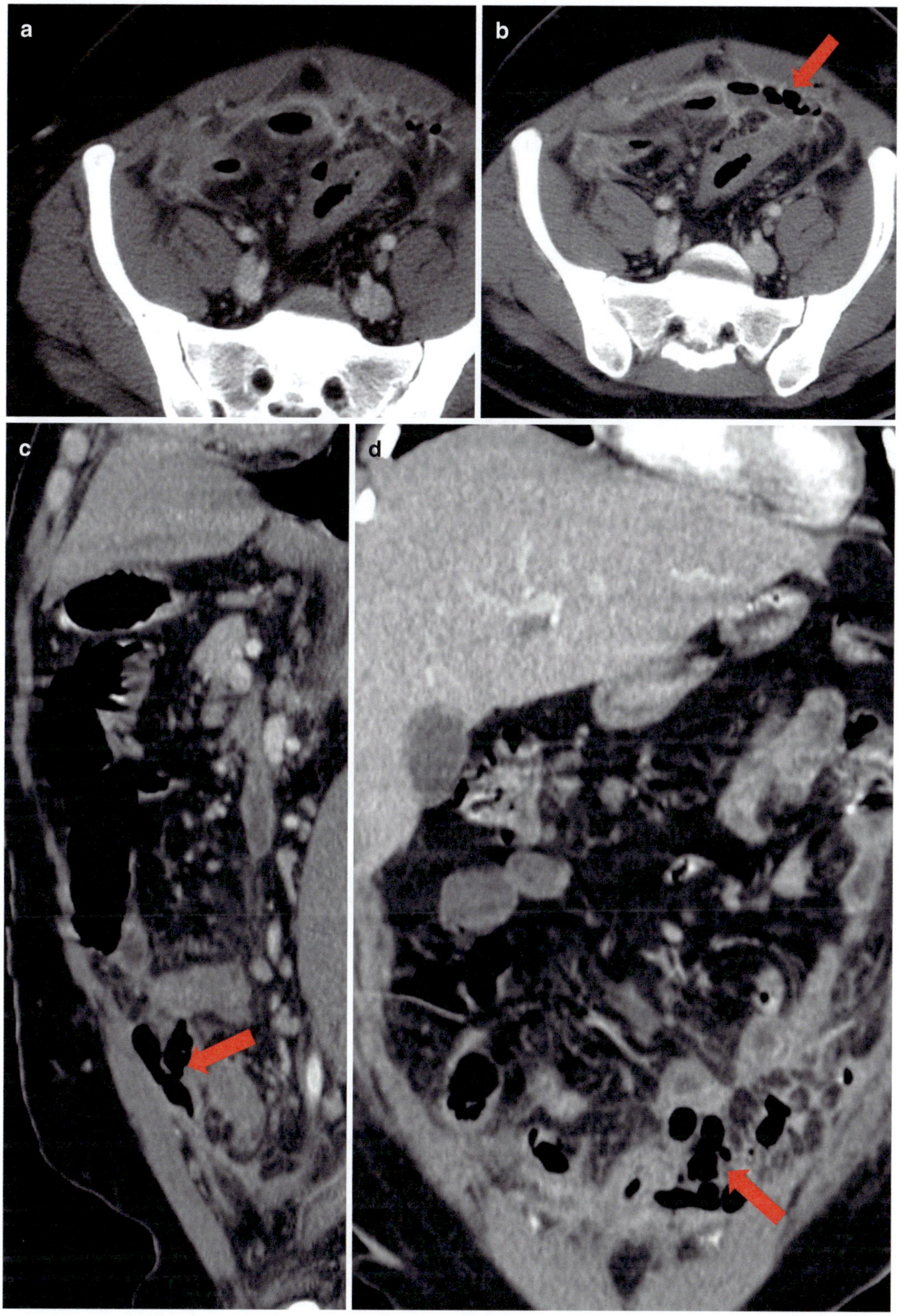

Fig. 16.8 Peritonitis due to perforation of sigmoid diverticula. (**a**, **b**) Axial scans, (**c**) sagittal scan and (**d**) coronal scans show a sigmoid diverticulitis with perivisceral phlegmon and free bubbles (*red arrows*)

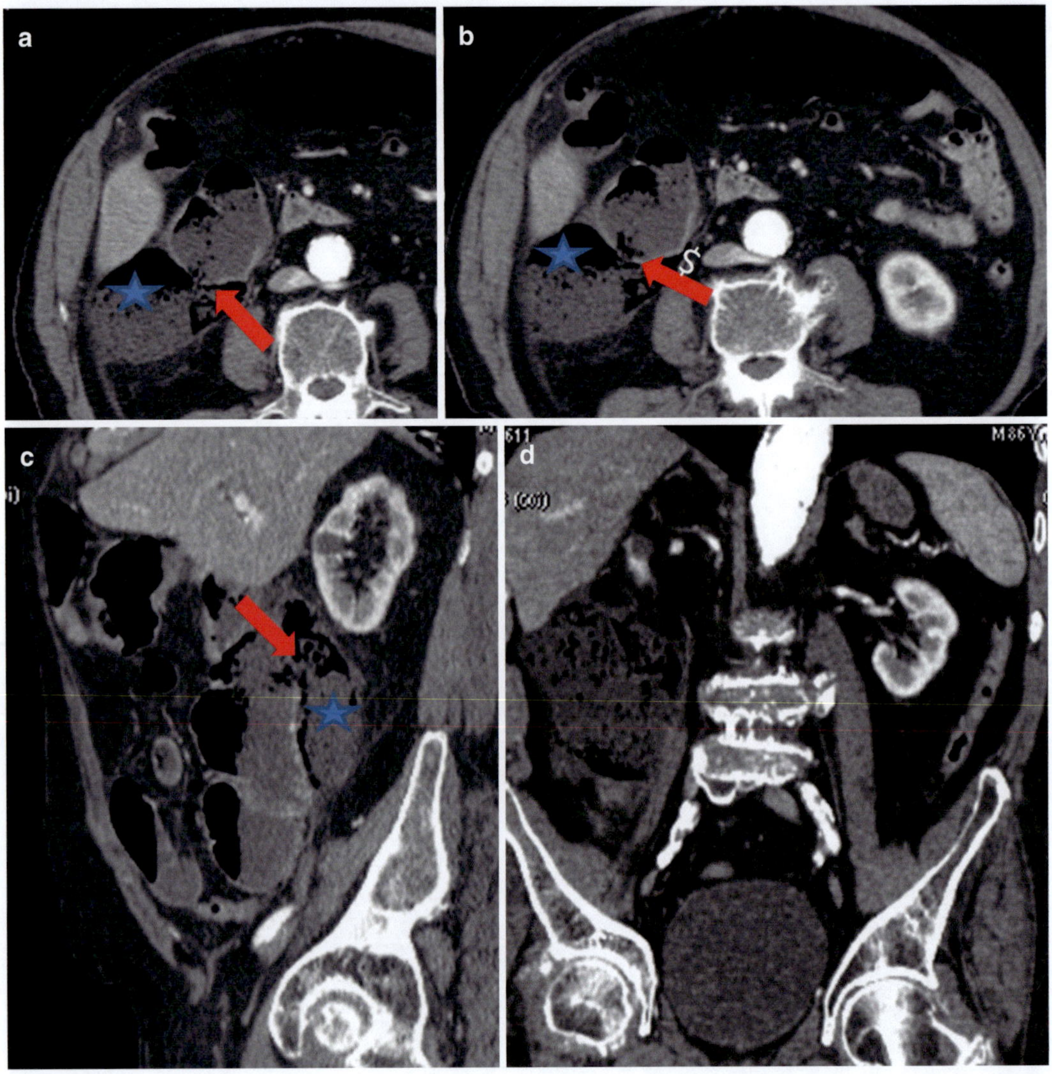

Fig. 16.9 Faecal peritonitis due to perforation of the ascending colon. (**a**, **b**) Axial scans, (**c**) sagittal reconstruction and (**d**) coronal reconstruction. A leakage of the posterior wall of the ascending colon (*red arrow*) produces an extraluminal faecal matter containing small air bubbles (dirty mass) (*blue star*)

Acute colon perforation may produce a faecal peritonitis (diffuse or localized-dirty mass) which is associated with high risk of morbidity and mortality [5].

16.9 Anorectal Perforation

The perforation of the extraperitoneal portion of the rectum and anal canal is most commonly seen following trauma or surgery [26].

References

1. Ordonez CA, Puyana JC (2006) Management of peritonitis in the critically ill patient. Surg Clin North Am 86:1323–1349
2. Pinto A, Romano L (2013) Peritonitis. In: Guglielmi G et al (eds) Geriatric imaging. Springer, Berlin/Heidelberg, pp 741–751
3. Wittman DH, Schein M, Condon RE (1996) Management of secondary peritonitis. Ann Surg 224(1):10–18
4. Guarner F (2006) Enteric flora in health and disease. Digestion 73(Suppl 1):5–12

5. Guarner F, Malageleda JR (2003) Gut flora in health and disease. Lancet 361:512–519
6. Goh BK, Chow PK, Quah HM et al (2006) Penetration of the gastrointestinal tract secondary to ingestion of foreign bodies. World J Surg 30(3):372–377
7. Ozel H, Topaloglu S, Yuksel BC et al (2003) Jejunal perforation in mentally retarded patient due to an ingested chicken bone. Hepatogastroenterology 50(Suppl 2):ccxxxviii–ccxxxix
8. Kimchi NA, Brodie E, Shapiro M et al (2002) Non-traumatic perforation of the small intestine: report of 13 cases and review of the literature. Hepatogastroenterology 49(46):1017–1022
9. Moran BJ (2007) Adhesion-related small bowel obstruction. Colorectal Dis 9(Suppl 2):39–44
10. Kashakura Y, Ajani JA, Fugii M et al (2002) Management of perforated gastric carcinoma: a report of 16 cases and review of world literature. Am Surg 68:434–440
11. Hayetian FD, Read TE, Brozovich M et al (2006) Ileal perforation secondary to Clostridium difficile enteritis. Arch Surg 141:97–99
12. Maniatis V, Chryssikopoulos H, Roussakis A et al (2000) Perforation of the alimentary tract: evaluation with computed tomography. Abdom Imaging 25:373–379
13. Haianaux B, Agneessens E, Bertinotti R et al (2006) Accuracy of MDCT in predicting site of gastrointestinal tract perforation. AJR Am J Roentgenol 187(5): 1179–1183
14. Kim SH, Shin SS, Jeong YY et al (2009) Gastrointestinal tract perforation: MDCT findings according to the perforation sites. Korean J Radiol 10(1):63–70
15. Chen CH, Huang HS, Yang CC et al (2001) The features of perforated peptic ulcers In conventional computed tomography. Hepatogastroenterology 48:1393–1396
16. Shaffer HA (1992) Perforation and obstruction of the gastrointestinal tract. Assessment by conventional radiology. Radiol Clin North Am 30:405–426
17. Meyers MA (2000) The extraperitoneal space: normal and pathologic anatomy. In: Meyers MA (ed) Dynamic Radiology of the abdomen. Springer, New York, pp 333–492
18. Glazer GM, Buy JN, Moss AA et al (1981) Ct detection of duodenal perforation. AJR Am J Roentgenol 137:333–336
19. Kim SW, Kim HC, Yang DM (2012) Perforated tumours in the gastrointestinal tract: CT findings and clinical presentation. Br J Radiol 85:1307–1313
20. Enns R, Eloubeidi MA, Mergener K et al (2002) ERCP-related perforation: risk factors and management. Endoscopy 34(4):293–298
21. Ghahremani GG, Ghahremani GG (1993) Radiologic evaluation of suspected gastrointestinal perforations. Radiol Clin North Am 31:1219–1234
22. Greenstein AJ, Mann D, Sachar DB et al (1985) Free perforation in Crohn's disease: I. A survey of 99 cases. Am J Gastroenterol 80(9):682–689
23. Zissin R, Osadchy A, Gayer G (2009) Abdominal CT findings in small bowel perforation. Br J Radiol 82(974):162–171
24. Horrow MM, White DS, Horrow JC (2003) Differentiation of perforated from non perforated appendicitis at CT. Radiology 227:46–51
25. Saeki M, Hoshikawa Y, Miyazaki O et al (1998) Computed tomographic analysis of colonic perforation: "dirty mass" a new computed tomographic finding. Emerg Radiol 5:140–145
26. Thomas PR (1987) Ano-rectal injury causing extraperitoneal and subcutaneous emphysema. Injury 18:426–427

17 Abdominal Compartment Syndrome and Gastrointestinal Tract Perforation

Ciro Acampora, Rosa Ignarra, and Antonio Pinto

17.1 Introduction

The term abdominal compartment syndrome was primarily used by Kron et al. [1] in the early 1980s to depict the physiologic effects of intra-abdominal hypertension complicating a ruptured aortic aneurysm surgery. However, the majority of our knowledge about this disease has evolved over the past few years [2, 3].

Abdominal compartment syndrome can involve both nonsurgical and surgical patients, either preoperatively or postoperatively. Abdominal compartment syndrome is most commonly diagnosed in patients sustaining abdominal or pelvic trauma or suffering from intra-abdominal hemorrhagic diseases. Less common etiologic factors include retroperitoneal hematoma or edema, bowel obstruction, ascites, and necrotizing pancreatitis [2]. Although the incidence of abdominal compartment syndrome ranged between 5 and 15 % of trauma patients [4], an increased intra-abdominal pressure (18 mmHg) was observed in up to 41 % of surgical patients [5].

Abdominal compartment syndrome occurs when there is an acute rise in the intra-abdominal pressure above physiological limits [6, 7]. The diagnosis of this syndrome is generally rapidly performed at the bedside with the intravesical pressure measurements and is based on clinical findings, with the pulmonary, renal, and cardiovascular systems being most adversely affected by the acute rise in the intra-abdominal pressure [8].

C. Acampora • R. Ignarra • A. Pinto (✉)
Department of Radiology, "A. Cardarelli" Hospital, Via Cardarelli 9, Naples I-80131, Italy
e-mail: itrasente@libero.it; rosa_ignarra@hotmail.com; antopin1968@libero.it

17.2 Definitions

Usually, a compartment syndrome represents a pathological situation with an increased pressure in a confined anatomical space that negatively affects the circulation and threatens the function and viability of the tissues therein [7]. Such a syndrome may occur within any enclosed space that is subject to distension. The typical example is an extremity compartment syndrome following trauma to the major inflow or outflow vessels of the lower limb. Abdominal compartment syndrome occurs when there is an acute increase in the intra-abdominal pressure above physiological limits [7].

In 2004, a consensus conference was convened by the World Society of the Abdominal Compartment Syndrome (WSACS) consisting of European, Australasian, and North American surgical, trauma, and medical critical care specialists. Recognizing the lack of accepted definitions, the WSACS tasked these specialists to create evidence-based definitions for "intra-abdominal hypertension" (IAH) and "abdominal compartment syndrome" (ACS) [9]. The intra-abdominal pressure (IAP) is the steady-state

L. Romano, A. Pinto (eds.), *Imaging of Alimentary Tract Perforation*,
DOI 10.1007/978-3-319-08192-2_17, © Springer International Publishing Switzerland 2015

pressure concealed within the abdominal cavity: the normal IAP is approximately 5–7 mmHg in critically ill adults. The intra-abdominal pressure can be measured using various direct and indirect techniques. Direct measurement requires placement of an intraperitoneal catheter connected to an external pressure transducer or saline manometer. Indirect measurements are more practical in clinical situations: the most common technique used in clinical practice is the measurement of the urinary bladder pressure. After instilling 50–100 mL of liquid into the bladder through an indwelling transurethral catheter and clamping the distal tubing, pressure measurements can be obtained by attaching a manometer or bedside monitor to a needle inserted in the specimen collection port of the catheter. With the patient in supine position, the symphysis pubis is used as the zero point for monitor calibration [10–12]. IAH is defined as a sustained or repeated pathologic elevation of IAP ≥12 mmHg. ACS is defined as a sustained IAP >20 mmHg (with or without an abdominal perfusion pressure <60 mmHg) that is associated with new organ dysfunction/failure.

ACS may be further classified as either primary, secondary, or recurrent based upon the duration and etiology of the patient's IAH [13]. Primary, or "surgical," ACS is characterized by IAH of relatively short duration occurring as a result of an intra-abdominal etiology such as abdominal trauma, ruptured abdominal aortic aneurysm, hemoperitoneum, acute pancreatitis, secondary peritonitis, retroperitoneal hemorrhage, or liver transplantation. Primary ACS is therefore defined as a condition associated with injury or disease in the abdominopelvic region that frequently requires early surgical or interventional radiological intervention. Secondary, or "medical," ACS is characterized by IAH that develops as a result of an extra-abdominal etiology such as sepsis, capillary leak, major burns, or other conditions requiring massive fluid resuscitation. It is most commonly encountered in medical or burn patients [14]. Recurrent ACS represents a redevelopment of ACS symptoms following resolution of an earlier episode of either primary or secondary ACS.

17.3 Etiology and Pathophysiology

Any abnormality that elevates the pressure within the abdominal cavity can result in intra-abdominal hypertension. Spontaneous causes include massive ascites, intra-abdominal abscess, ileus, intestinal obstruction, ruptured aortic aneurysm, tension pneumoperitoneum, acute pancreatitis, pregnancy, chronic ambulatory peritoneal dialysis, and mesenteric venous thrombosis [15–19].

Nevertheless, blunt abdominal trauma with intra-abdominal bleeding from splenic, hepatic, and mesenteric injuries is the most common cause of intra-abdominal hypertension [2, 20]. Postoperative and iatrogenic causes include hemorrhage (intraperitoneal or retroperitoneal), visceral edema, acute gastric dilatation, abdominal closure under tension, abdominal packing, and reduction of large peritoneal or diaphragmatic hernias. Posttraumatic elevations of the intra-abdominal pressure typically occur as a result of hemorrhage or postresuscitation visceral edema [11].

If ACS is allowed to develop, the resultant pathophysiology is extensive and system-wide. As initially described 80 years ago, rising IAP increases the intrathoracic pressure through cephalad deviation of the diaphragm [21].

An increased intrathoracic pressure notably reduces venous return, resulting in reduced cardiac output [22]. IAP is transmitted to the thorax both directly and through cephalad deviation of the diaphragm. This significantly increases the intrathoracic pressure, resulting in extrinsic compression of the pulmonary parenchyma and development of pulmonary dysfunction [23]. IAH-induced atelectasis has been demonstrated to cause an increase in the rate of pulmonary infection [24]. Beyond the heart, lungs, and kidneys, almost every other organ system is impacted in the critically ill patient with IAH, even if these effects are not clinically obvious. Of all the organ systems, the gut appears to be one of the most sensitive to elevations in IAP.

In addition to reducing arterial blood flow, IAP compresses thin-walled mesenteric veins, promoting venous hypertension and intestinal edema. Visceral swelling further increases IAP, initiating a vicious cycle which results in worsening malperfusion, bowel ischemia, decreased intramucosal pH, feeding intolerance, systemic metabolic acidosis, and significantly increased patient mortality [25].

Abdominal compartment syndrome caused by perforated peptic ulcer is rare owing to early diagnosis and management. Delayed recognition of perforated peptic ulcer with pneumoperitoneum, bowel distension, and decreased abdominal wall compliance can make up a vicious circle and lead to ACS [16]. The perforated peptic ulcer results in pneumoperitoneum and bowel distension. The progressive increase of the intra-abdominal pressure with obstruction of lymph and venous return can result in diffuse lymphedema of the abdominal wall. The increasing intra-abdominal pressure with abdominal tamponade compromises the blood circulation with initial presentations of a distended abdomen, edema of the lower legs, and cyanosis with deterioration of function of the intra-abdominal organs. Emergent laparotomy is indicated in this clinical setting [16].

Tension pneumoperitoneum is an unusual event. In trauma intraperitoneal air is observed in elective and emergency surgery and, most commonly, is due to a leak from a gastrointestinal anastomosis or perforation. Tension pneumoperitoneum can be associated with positive-pressure ventilation, pneumothorax, spontaneous gastrointestinal perforation, and other more rare syndromes. In each situation, early recognition and treatment of abdominal hypertension is critical to the care of the patient [17].

17.4 Clinical Diagnosis

Findings suggestive of abdominal compartment syndrome include a tensely distended abdomen; increased peak airway pressure; difficulty in maintaining ventilation, with hypoxia and hypercarbia; increasing creatinine; and oliguria [26]. However, most patients with abdominal compartment syndrome are in intensive care units, and clinical examination is usually not sensitive for diagnosing this entity [27]. The diagnosis of abdominal compartment syndrome is complicated by the fact that these patients have many other explanations for renal or pulmonary failure. Sepsis, acute respiratory distress syndrome, hypovolemic shock, and multiorgan failure syndrome are frequently seen in patients who are also at risk of abdominal compartment syndrome. In some patients, these diverse and potentially lethal conditions may coexist [28].

17.5 Radiologic Findings

Although ACS is diagnosed clinically, a number of computed tomography (CT) features have been described to aid the diagnosis of IAH and ACS. Pickhardt et al. [8] described several CT features associated with ACS in four patients with clinically proven abdominal compartment syndrome, which included compression of the inferior vena cava (Fig. 17.1), round belly sign (Figs. 17.1 and 17.2) (abdominal distension indicated by a tense or rounded morphology on axial CT, with a relative increase in the anteroposterior abdominal diameter compared with the transverse diameter)), renal and other solid abdominal

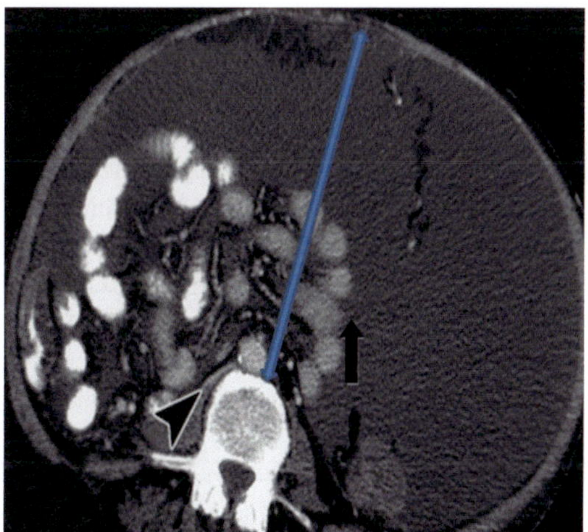

Fig. 17.1 A 51-year-old woman presenting with dyspnea after a liver transplant. Axial CT image shows free intraperitoneal liquid (*black arrow*), the collapsed inferior vena cava (*arrowhead*), and the "round belly sign" (*blue arrow*). The intravesical pressure was 21 mmHg. The occurrence of abdominal compartment syndrome is about 30 % after liver transplantation

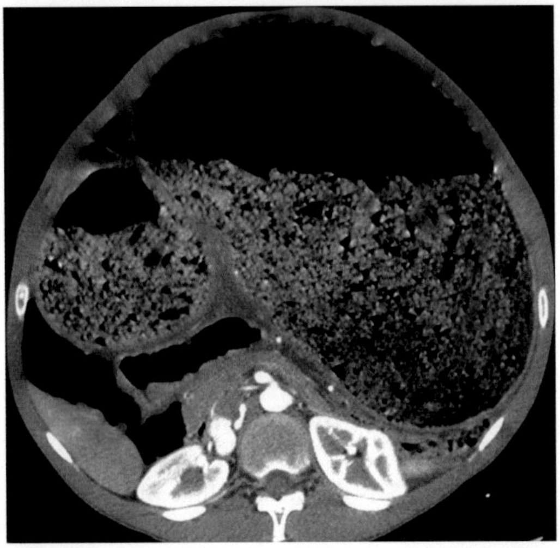

Fig. 17.2 A 19-year-old man with acute abdominal pain. Axial contrast-enhanced CT image shows massive dilatation of colic loops over spread by fecal material (toxic megacolon). The "round belly sign" and bilateral renal displacement and compression are evident. The patient underwent colectomy

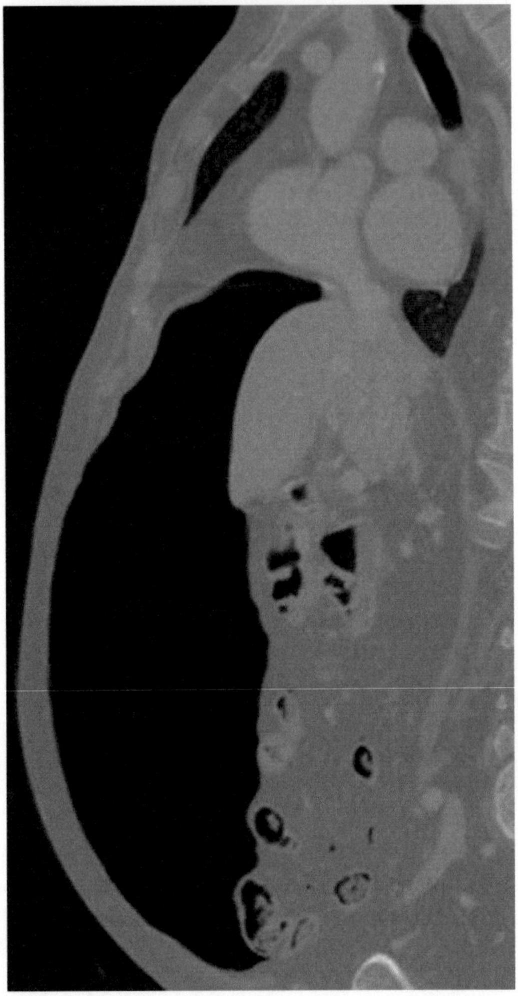

Fig. 17.3 An 84-year-old woman with colonic perforation. Multidetector-row computed tomography (sagittal reconstruction) with intravenous contrast medium showing pneumoperitoneum with compression of the intra-abdominal viscera

visceral compression (Fig. 17.3) or displacement (Fig. 17.2), bowel wall thickening with enhancement (Fig. 17.4), and bilateral inguinal herniation.

Epelman et al. [29] evaluated the preoperative abdominal CT scans of three children with proven ACS to identify signs of elevated IAP. Findings common to these patients included narrowing of the inferior vena cava, direct renal compression or displacement, bowel wall thickening with enhancement, and a rounded appearance of the abdomen. Other investigators described elevation of the diaphragm (Fig. 17.4) in association with IAH [30]. Al-Bahrani et al. [31] evaluated the abdominal CT examination performed in 24 critically ill patients and affirmed that the presence of the round belly sign and the bowel wall thickening with enhancement on CT images of critically ill surgical patients should alert clinicians to the possibility of the presence of IAH and ACS.

It is important to recognize that the CT examination should be viewed as an adjunct toward the recognition of IAH, but not as a substitute to the measurement of the intravesical pressure in at-risk patients. Individual CT signs such as elevated hemidiaphragm, flattened inferior vena cava and renal veins, and increased bowel wall enhancement are neither sensitive nor likely specific for abdominal compartment syndrome. However, when a combination of these findings is present in the appropriate clinical setting or if the signs are seen to worsen on sequential imaging studies, the radiologist should raise the possibility of abdominal compartment syndrome [27, 32]. Identifying patients with IAH and/or ACS at earlier stages could potentially improve the outcome of these patients by early radiological drainage of large fluid collections and/or surgical intervention with abdominal decompression (laparotomy).

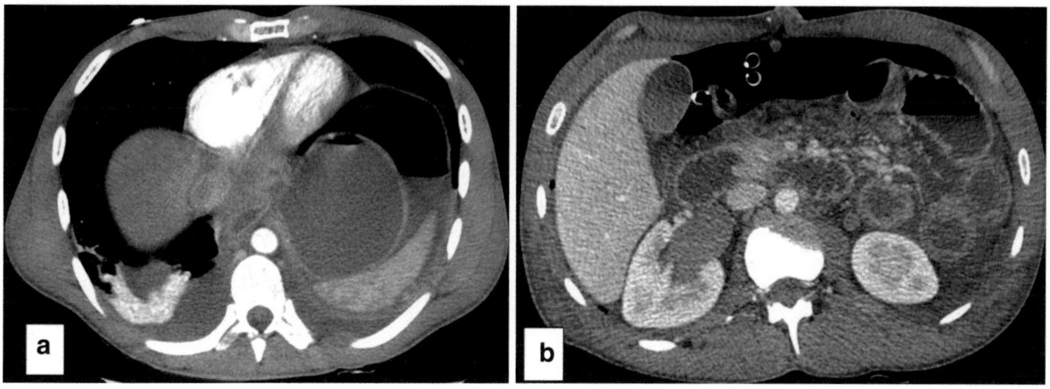

Fig. 17.4 A 19-year-old man (the same patient of Fig. 17.2) with sudden hypotension, tachycardia, and respiratory failure after colectomy due to toxic megacolon. Axial contrast-enhanced CT images show (**a**) an elevated left diaphragm and free intraperitoneal air and liquid and (**b**) bowel wall thickening. The intravesical pressure was 20 mmHg. The patient underwent emergency abdominal laparotomy but died due to severe heart failure

Conclusions

ACS has tremendous relevance in the practice of surgery and the care of critically ill patients because of the effects of elevated pressure within the confined space of the abdomen on multiple organ systems. ACS has been identified to be a cause of significant morbidity and mortality among critically ill surgical, medical, and pediatric patients. With an incidence of IAH that approximates 30–80 % and from 4 to 30 % for ACS depending on the population, this disease entity can no longer be ignored in the critically ill/injured.

The most important factor in the diagnosis of abdominal compartment syndrome is proper suspicion in the appropriate clinical setting. Multidetector row Computed Tomography can provide evidence of an increased intra-abdominal pressure in patients at risk for developing abdominal compartment syndrome.

References

1. Kron IL, Harman PK, Nolan SP (1984) The measurement of intra-abdominal pressure as a criterion for abdominal re-exploration. Ann Surg 199:28–30
2. Saggi BH, Sugerman HJ, Ivatury RR et al (1998) Abdominal compartment syndrome. J Trauma 45:597–609
3. Biffl WL, Moore EE, Burch JM et al (2001) Secondary abdominal compartment syndrome is a highly lethal event. Am J Surg 182:645–648
4. Ertel W, Oberholzer A, Platz A et al (2000) Incidence and clinical pattern of the abdominal compartment syndrome after "damage-control" laparotomy in 311 patients with severe abdominal and/or pelvic trauma. Crit Care Med 28:1747–1753
5. Sugrue M, Jones F, Deane SA et al (1999) Intra-abdominal hypertension is an independent cause of postoperative renal impairment. Arch Surg 134:1082–1085
6. Burch JM, Moore EE, Moore FA et al (1996) The abdominal compartment syndrome. Surg Clin North Am 76:833–842
7. Ball CG, Kirkpatrick AW (2007) Intra-abdominal hypertension and the abdominal compartment syndrome. Scand J Surg 96:197–204
8. Pickhardt PJ, Shimony JS, Heiken JP et al (1999) The abdominal compartment syndrome: CT findings. AJR Am J Roentgenol 173:575–579
9. Malbrain ML, De laet I, Cheatham M (2007) Consensus conference definitions and recommendations on intra-abdominal hypertension (IAH) and the abdominal compartment syndrome (ACS) – the long road to the final publications, how did we get there? Acta Clin Belg Suppl (1):44–59
10. Hammond KL, Margolin DA (2006) Surgical hemorrhage, damage control, and the abdominal compartment syndrome. Clin Colon Rectal Surg 19:188–194
11. Schein M, Wittmann DH, Aprahamian CC et al (1995) The abdominal compartment syndrome: the physiological and clinical consequences of elevated intra-abdominal pressure. J Am Coll Surg 180:745–753
12. Ivatury RR, Diebel L, Porter JM et al (1997) Intra-abdominal hypertension and the abdominal compartment syndrome. Surg Clin North Am 77:783–800

13. Cheatham ML (2009) Abdominal compartment syndrome: pathophysiology and definitions. Scand J Trauma Resusc Emerg Med 17:10
14. Sugrue M (2005) Abdominal compartment syndrome. Curr Opin Crit Care 11:333–338
15. Karkos CD, Harkin DW, Giannakou A et al (2009) Mortality after endovascular repair of ruptured abdominal aortic aneurysms: a systematic review and meta-analysis. Arch Surg 144:770–778
16. Lynn JJ, Weng YM, Weng CS (2008) Perforated peptic ulcer associated with abdominal compartment syndrome. Am J Emerg Med 26:1071.e3–5
17. Alder AC, Hunt JL, Thal ER (2008) Abdominal compartment syndrome associated with tension pneumoperitoneum in an elderly trauma patient. J Trauma 64:211–212
18. Dambrauskas Z, Parseliunas A, Gulbinas A et al (2009) Early recognition of abdominal compartment syndrome in patients with acute pancreatitis. World J Gastroenterol 15:717–721
19. Cil T, Tummon IS, House AA et al (2000) A tale of two syndromes: ovarian hyperstimulation and abdominal compartment. Hum Reprod 15:1058–1060
20. Walker J, Criddle LM (2003) Pathophysiology and management of abdominal compartment syndrome. Am J Crit Care 12:367–371
21. Coombs H (1922) The mechanism of the regulation of intra-abdominal pressure. Am J Physiol 161:159–170
22. Cullen DJ, Coyle JP, Teplick R et al (1989) Cardiovascular, pulmonary, and renal effects of massively increased intra-abdominal pressure in critically ill patients. Crit Care Med 17:118–121
23. Simon RJ, Friedlander MH, Ivatury RR et al (1997) Hemorrhage lowers the threshold for intra-abdominal hypertension-induced pulmonary dysfunction. J Trauma 42:398–403
24. Aprahamian C, Wittmann DH, Bergstein JM et al (1990) Temporary abdominal closure (TAC) for planned relaparotomy (etappenlavage) in trauma. J Trauma 30:719–723
25. Reintam A, Parm P, Kitus R et al (2008) Gastrointestinal failure score in critically ill patients: a prospective observational study. Crit Care 12:R90
26. Ivatury RR, Porter JM, Simon RJ et al (1998) Intra-abdominal hypertension after life-threatening penetrating abdominal trauma: prophylaxis, incidence, and clinical relevance to gastric mucosal pH and abdominal compartment syndrome. J Trauma 44:1016–1021
27. Patel A, Lall CG, Jennings SG et al (2007) Abdominal compartment syndrome. AJR Am J Roentgenol 189:1037–1043
28. Maxwell RA, Fabian TC, Croce MA et al (1999) Secondary abdominal compartment syndrome: an underappreciated manifestation of severe hemorrhagic shock. J Trauma 47:995–999
29. Epelman M, Soudack M, Engel A et al (2002) Abdominal compartment syndrome in children: CT findings. Pediatr Radiol 32:319–322
30. Beasley CR, Ripley JM, Smith DA et al (1986) Pulmonary function in chronic renal failure patients managed by continuous ambulatory peritoneal dialysis. N Z Med J 99:313–315
31. Al-Bahrani AZ, Abid GH, Sahgal E et al (2007) A prospective evaluation of CT features predictive of intra-abdominal hypertension and abdominal compartment syndrome in critically ill surgical patients. Clin Radiol 62:676–682
32. Laffargue G, Taourel P, Saguintaah M et al (2002) CT diagnosis of abdominal compartment syndrome. AJR Am J Roentgenol 178:771–772

Index

MIX
Papier aus verantwortungsvollen Quellen
Paper from responsible sources
FSC® C105338

If you have any concerns about our products,
you can contact us on
ProductSafety@springernature.com

In case Publisher is established outside the EU,
the EU authorized representative is:
Springer Nature Customer Service Center GmbH
Europaplatz 3, 69115 Heidelberg, Germany

Printed by Libri Plureos GmbH
in Hamburg, Germany